ALSO BY DEAN ORNISH, M.D.

Stress, Diet & Your Heart

Dr. Dean Ornish's
Program for
REVERSING
HEART
DISEASE

Dr. Dean Ornish's

RANDOM HOUSE 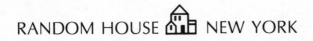 NEW YORK

Program for
REVERSING
HEART
DISEASE

The only system
scientifically proven
to reverse heart disease
without drugs or surgery

DEAN ORNISH, M.D.

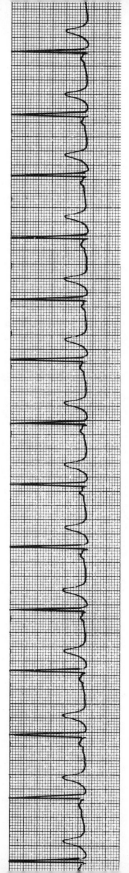

Owing to limitations of space, all acknowledgments
for permission to reprint previously published material
may be found on pages 603–604.

Library of Congress Cataloging-in-Publication Data

Ornish, Dean.
    Dr. Dean Ornish's program for reversing heart disease / Dean
    Ornish.
      p.   cm.
ISBN 0-394-57565-2
1. Coronary heart disease—Prevention. 2. Vegetarian cookery.
3. Relaxation. I. Title. II. Title: Doctor Dean Ornish's program
for reversing heart disease.
RC685.C6075 1990
616.1'2305—dc20   89-43544

Manufactured in the United States of America
    56789

Designed by Oksana Kushnir

For Gerald and Barbara Hines, who made the research possible;
for my parents, who made me possible;
for S.S. Satchidananda, who helped me to see what is possible;
and for Shirley, who makes all things possible

Commitment

Until one is committed there is hesitancy, the chance
to draw back, always ineffectiveness. Concerning all
acts of initiative (and creation), there is one elementary
truth, the ignorance of which kills countless ideas and
splendid plans: that the moment one definitely commits
oneself, then Providence moves too. All sorts of things
occur to help one that would never otherwise have
occurred. A whole stream of events issues from the
decision, raising in one's favor all manner of unforeseen
incidents and meetings and material assistance, which
no man could have dreamt would have come his way.

I have learned a deep respect for one of Goethe's
couplets: "Whatever you can do, or dream you can,
begin it. / Boldness has genius, power, and magic in
it."

—W. H. Murray,
The Scottish Himalayan Expedition

Acknowledgments

While I would like to take full credit for this book and for the success of the cardiovascular research on which it is based, it would be foolish of me to do so. Although this book is titled *Dr. Dean Ornish's Program for Reversing Heart Disease,* several people helped me develop this program, and many others provided the resources and support that enabled us to prove how powerful it can be. None of this work would have been possible without their dedication, generosity, and vision. (I wanted to call this book *Opening Your Heart,* since it describes the physical, emotional, and spiritual dimensions of opening the heart, but the publisher chose a more straightforward title.)

Each person named here made an important difference, without whom the research or this book would not have been possible. Although the list is somewhat long, it is incomplete. I've enjoyed writing this section because it's given me an opportunity to remember how meaningful each person's contribution has been and how grateful I am.

Whether research is considered "pioneering" or "fringe" is a matter of vision and faith. Several people provided encouragement and financial support at a time when this project was only a dream. Gerald and Barbara Hines not only provided major financial support but also encouraged many of their friends and business associates to do the same. In 1984, Mr. Hines and I founded the Preventive Medicine Research Institute, a nonprofit public research organization, to administer this research project, and he became chairman. (Tom Silk, Betsy Adler, and Barbara Ginsberg provided legal assistance.) Other board members included Martin Bucksbaum, Henry Groppe, Jenard Gross, Kenneth Lay, Frank Lorenzo, Stuart Moldaw, Ken Pelletier, Jay Pritzker, and Fenton Talbott. Mr. Lorenzo also provided air transportation on Continental Airlines for our research patients to fly to and from Houston for cardiac PET scans at the University of Texas Medical School.

Henry Groppe has been my friend, guardian angel, and confidante since 1979. In the academic world, Alexander Leaf, M.D., has been a mentor and role model. I feel very blessed to know both of them. Others whose advice was especially meaningful included Henry Blackburn, M.D., David Blankenborn, M.D., B. Greg Brown, M.D., William P. Castelli, M.D., Antonio M. Gotto, Jr., M.D., John Kane, M.D., Ph.D., Julius R. Krevans, M.D., Michael Lerner, Ph.D., Albert R. Martin, M.D., John O'Neil, William R. Owen, M.D., Doros Platika, M.D., John T. Potts, Jr., M.D., Rachel Naomi Remen, M.D., Jonas Salk, M.D., Steven A. Schroeder, M.D., John Stoeckle, M.D., as well as the scientific advisors, officers, and staff of the Institute for the Advancement of Health.

This study has allowed me to begin fulfilling another dream—to work with people who are both competent and compassionate. Foremost among these is Shirley Brown, M.D., with whom I have collaborated since our first cardiovascular research project in 1977. We've been collaborating and supporting each other ever since—in Houston, in Boston, and now in San Francisco. She was the co-director of the research that forms the basis of this book. Also, she is the person most responsible for Part 3 of this book. She organized, collected, and nutritionally analyzed each of the recipes, and along with Martha Rose Shulman, planned the 21-day menus.

Larry Scherwitz, Ph.D., is the other co-director of our research. We have been working together since 1980, when I was his student. Our skills and temperaments complement each other and made possible what neither of us could have accomplished alone. Richard J. Brand, Ph.D., is one of the country's preeminent theorists and biostatisticians, and he pioneered new methods of statistical analyses for our study. Richard, Larry, and I had endless discussions about the relative merits and disadvantages of different study designs and research protocols.

James Billings, Ph.D., M.P.H., brought a wealth of experience to our study, both as an accomplished researcher (including his position as co-principal investigator of the Multiple Risk Factor Intervention Trial) and a gifted therapist. Other counselors included Pamela Lea Byrne, R.N., M.S., M.F.C.C., Carol Naber, and Mary Dale Scheller, M.S.W., a social worker and gerontologist who also has been teaching the stress management classes since 1987. Sandra McLanahan, M.D., taught the stress management classes in the 1980 study and during the first two years of the current one. Chip Spann, PA-C, and Sarah Spann, L.V.N., taught the exercise classes at our retreats, and Terri Merritt, M.S., an exercise physiologist, has taught and supervised the exercise classes ever since. Terri also provided some background research for chapter 12. Pat McKenna, M.D., and Amy Gage donated their most precious resource to our study—their time.

One of the major challenges of our studies was to develop meals that are tasty and beautiful as well as healthful. We have worked with several gifted chefs, including Celeste Burwell, Mary Carroll, Alexsandra Chetrit, Carol Connell, Mark Hall, Christian Janselme, Donna Nicoletti, Sarah Reingold, and Jules Stenzel. These chefs also provided take-home meals for our study participants. (Although it's not on my résumé, we bought so much Tupperware that I became a certified Tupperware distributor in order to qualify for a discount.) Donna Nicoletti, Mark Hall, Jules Stenzel, and Pamela Morgan Maxwell tested all of the recipes in Part 3. Mark Hall created many of the recipes in Part 3. Most recently, Jean-Marc Fullsack has been our head chef.

I am grateful to renowned chefs Mollie Katzen (author of *Still Life with Menu,* the *Moosewood Cookbook,* and others), Deborah Madison (author of *The Greens Cookbook*), Wolfgang Puck (founder of Spago and author of *The Wolfgang Puck Cookbook*), Alice Waters (founder of Chez Panisse and author of *Chez Panisse Cooking*), and others who provided recipes for Part 3. Judy Gethers assisted Wolf-gang Puck.

The study would not have been possible without the break-throughs in medical technology pioneered by K. Lance Gould, M.D., including computer-assisted analyses of coronary arterio-grams and major advances in cardiac PET imaging. Besides his guidance and collaboration in every phase of the research, Dr. Gould and his colleagues (Richard L. Kirkeeide, Ph.D., Dale Jones, R.T., Mary Haynie, R.N., Richard Goldstein, M.D., Mary Tiberi, R.N., Yvonne Stuart, R.T.) performed cardiac PET imaging and quantita-tive analyses of coronary arteriograms on all of our study partici-pants. Ro Edens, his administrator, and Claire Finn and Kathy Rainbird, his assistants, were essential liaisons to our San Francisco research team. Ruth Ann Sparlin, Bonnie Lee, and Betty Hagen escorted our patients in Houston.

Myrna Melling (formerly Myrna Fast) is the person with whom I work most closely every day, and she is a blessing in my life. Myrna is the administrator of the Preventive Medicine Research Institute and the coordinator of all of our activities. Patricia Chung has been administrative assistant and research supervisor responsible for data collection. Recently, Barbara Musser joined our staff and will share Myrna's responsibilities.

I am especially indebted to the cardiologists, fellows, nurses, and technicians at Pacific Presbyterian Medical Center. William T. Armstrong, M.D., directed the cardiac catheterization laboratory and made our study possible. LaVeta Luce, R.N., and her colleagues obtained the quantitative angiography data. (LaVeta Luce and Myrna Fast considered the idea of starting a consulting firm, "Fast and Luce.") Arthur Selzer, M.D., Keith Cohn, M.D., Gabriel Gregorotos, M.D., and Bruce Brent, M.D., made important contri-butions to the study design. Washington Burns, M.D., directed the clinical laboratory.

Thomas A. Ports, M.D., directed the cardiac catheterization laboratory at the Cardiovascular Research Institute, School of Medi-cine, University of California, San Francisco, and made the study there possible. Georgie Hesse, R.N., and her colleagues obtained the quantitative angiography data. John Kane, M.D., Ph.D., and Steve Kunitake, Ph.D., performed the special lipoprotein and apolipo-protein assays. Richard J. Havel, M.D., Ph.D., directed the Cardio-vascular Research Institute. Steven A. Schroeder, M.D., and Albert

R. Martin, M.D., provided ongoing advice and support within the Division of General Internal Medicine, as did Richard Root, M.D., Floyd Rector, M.D., and George O'Keefe within the Department of Medicine.

Referring physicians and angiographers included: Damian Augustin, M.D., G. James Avery, M.D., Richard Axelrod, M.D., Wayne Bayless, M.D., Robert Blau, M.D., Craig Brandman, M.D., Bruce Brent, M.D., Roger Budge, M.D., Michael Bunim, M.D., Michael Chase, M.D., Ralph Clark, M.D., James A. Clever, M.D., Keith E. Cohn, M.D., James G. Cullen, M.D., Daniel Elliott, M.D., Richard Francoz, M.D., Gordon Fung, M.D., Kent Gershengorn, M.D., Gabriel Gregoratos, M.D., Lloyd W. Gross, M.D., Robert Hulworth, M.D., Timothy Hurley, M.D., Gerson Jacobs, M.D., Herbert N. Jacobs, M.D., Lester B. Jacobson, M.D., Thomas J. Kaiser, M.D., William Kapla, M.D., Hilliard J. Katz, M.D., John J. Kelly, Jr., M.D., Jonathan Keroes, M.D., Edward S. Kersh, M.D., Frederick London, M.D., Randall Low, M.D., Roy Meyer, M.D., Felix G. Millhouse, M.D., Frederick Mintz, M.D., Gene Nakamoto, M.D., Morris Noble, M.D., Philip O'Keefe, M.D., Paul Ogden, M.D., Thomas Olwin, M.D., James G. Reid, M.D., J. Patrick Robertson, M.D., John Sarconi, M.D., H.C. Segars, M.D., Arthur Selzer, M.D., Gene Shafton, M.D., Richard Strauss, M.D., Brian L. Strunk, M.D., Martin Terplan, M.D., William Thomas, M.D., Anne Thorson, M.D., Michael Volen, M.D., Mark P. Wexman, M.D. Radiologists included Robert Bernstein, M.D., Myron Marx, M.D., Gerald Needleman, M.D., and Jon Wack, M.D.

Alvin R. Tarlov, M.D., of The Henry J. Kaiser Family Foundation (Menlo Park) was the first major foundation to support our research. Other major foundation support came from J. Howard Creekmore of Houston Endowment, the National Heart, Lung, and Blood Institute of the National Institutes of Health (with special appreciation to Stephen Weiss, Ph.D., Fred Heydrick, Ph.D., Antonio M. Gotto, Jr., M.D., and Claude Lenfant, M.D.), the Department of Health Services of the State of California (with special appreciation to David Q. Bates, Assemblymen John Vasconcellos and Bill Filante, M.D., Senators Art Torres and Nicholas Petris, Kenneth Kizer, M.D., Neal Kohatsu, M.D., Theresa Parker, Lois Wallace, and Governor George Deukmejian), The John E. Fetzer Institute (with special appreciation to John Fetzer, Rob Lehman, Judith Skutch Whitson, Vic Eichler, and Bruce Fetzer), The Enron

Corporation Foundation (Kenneth Lay), Continental Airlines/ Texas Air Corporation (Frank Lorenzo), The First Boston Corporation (Fenton Talbott, William Mayer, John Harrison, Joseph Perella, and others), Texas Commerce Bank (Ben Love and Don Hawk), The Quaker Oats Company (Sandy Clingan Smith and others), The Emde Company, Corrine and David R. Gould, Dick and Kathy Dawson, General Growth Companies (Martin and Melva Bucksbaum), the Phyllis & Stuart Moldaw Philanthropic Fund, Gross Investments (Jenard and Gail Gross), Pritzker & Pritzker (Jay and Cindy Pritzker), Henry and Carol Groppe, Transco Energy Co. (W.J. Bowen), the Pacific Presbyterian Medical Center Foundation (Bruce Spivey, M.D., Aubrey Serfling, and Jerry Mapp), The Ziegler Corporation (Jack and Vyola Ziegler), Corporate Property Investors (Hans Mautner), The Ray C. Fish Foundation (Barbara F. Daniel, Christopher J. Daniel, James L. Daniel, Jr., Robert J. Cruikshank, CPA, and others), and the Nathan Cummings Foundation (Charles Halpern, Andrea Kydd, and others).

Additional support was provided by ConAgra, Inc. (Charles M. Harper, L. James Kennedy, Philip B. Fletcher, Scott W. Rahn, Stephen B. Hughes, Jim Seiple, Steve Van Tassel, John W. Bauer, and Blair Entenmann), the Physis Health Center (John Bagshaw, M.D.), The Jewish Community Endowment Fund, United Savings Association of Texas, Gross Investments (Jenard and Gail Gross), The Margoes Foundation (John Blum), Drexel Burnham Lambert (Michael Milken and Harry Horowitz), Hugh R. Goodrich, Edward O. Gaylord, Fayez Sarofim & Co., Eileen Rockefeller Growald, the Institute for the Advancement of Health, Lucy Rockefeller Waletzky, M.D., the Biopsychosocial Research Fund of the Medical Illness Counseling Center, United Energy Resources (J. Hugh Roff, Jr.), The Duncan Foundation (John Duncan), Mesa Petroleum (T. Boone Pickens), The Communities Foundation of Texas, Brown & Root, Inc. (T. Louis Austin, Jr.), The Sackman Foundation, Fenton and Judith Talbott, Leo Fields Family Philanthropic Fund, Richard and Rhoda Goldman, Burton I. Koffman, Charles & Louise Gartner Philanthropic Fund, Frank A. Liddell, Marianne Pallotti, Robert Finnell, T. B. Hudson, the Bob Hope International Heart Research Institute, Jeffrey Rhodes, Arnold and Carol Ablon, the Institute of Noetic Sciences (Brendan O'Regan), Werner and Eva Hebenstreit, Mel and Lenore Lefer, Thomas Russell Potts, Victor and Lydia Karpenko, Edwin and Natalie Ornish, Van Gordon Sauter, PPG

Industries, James and Margaret Keith, Howard B. Wolf & Co., Joseph Frelinghuysen, Edward F. Kunin, David Harrison, Kit Peterson, M.D., Joseph Forgione, and The William & Flora Hewlett Foundation.

Since 1984, Arthur Andersen & Co. has provided yearly financial audits and annual reports for the Preventive Medicine Research Institute on a pro bono basis. Paul Watson and Barbara Crist at Wells Fargo Bank provided us a line of credit to tide us over between grants.

Becky Ross, Christopher Hest, and the late Jim Graves of Fitzgerald, Graves and Company provided valuable advice, as did Bob Street, Ted Barash, and Ron Moskowitz. Henry Feldman of The Claremont Hotel and Resort gave us rooms at a discount, as did Manu Mobedshahi at The Sherman House, Ed Cohen at the Sherith Israel Kitchen, the Houston Marriott Hotel, and Marc Kaski at the Ft. Mason Center.

Henry Corra, Albert Maysles, and their colleagues at Maysles Films took an enormous gamble by deciding to film our patients from January 1986 when our study first began until the end of 1989 when I presented our final report at the American Heart Association's annual scientific meeting, even though they had no funds to make the film and we did not know if the study would be successful. The result was an extraordinary documentary in which the viewer can see the patients' struggles and transformations during the study, a much more powerful approach than simply having people talk about their experience in retrospect. The documentary will be shown on television later this year. I am grateful to them for their vision and for the enormous time and energy they invested. Many thanks to Peter Guber for his advice and support.

Betsy Rapoport has been the person most responsible for conceiving and editing this book (ably assisted by Peter Smith). We have worked closely together during the past year, and I have grown to have great respect for her intelligence, humor, and dedication, especially during the last nine months when she was developing a new project of her own, conceived with her husband, Ken Weiner. I thought I would deliver first, but I missed my deadline and she kept hers. (Her project is now known as Samuel Max Weiner.)

I am especially grateful to Peter Osnos and Robert Bernstein, who shared the vision of this book and made it possible. Their leadership and commitment to excellence are legendary, both in the publishing world and in the international human rights community.

For better or for worse, I wrote this book myself. My writing style is personal and somewhat idiosyncratic. Sometimes I use grammar that is not entirely proper in order to make the book more user-friendly, and occasionally I have chosen to be a little redundant in order to emphasize a point. Please do not hold the editors responsible for these lapses.

Esther Newberg and Michael Rudell are the best at what they do, combining integrity and intelligence, competence and compassion. Over the years I have learned to rely on their advice and perspective, and I have great love and respect for both of them.

Others at Random House who helped make this book possible include Bob Aulicino, Wanda Chappell, Dona Chernoff, Greg Euson, Joni Evans, Deborah Foley, Stacey Frankel, Ken Gellman, Debbie Glasserman, John Groton, Mary Beth Guimaraes, Nancy Inglis, Linda Kaye, Oksana Kushnir, Mary Beth Murphy, Elaine Panagides, Susan Reich, Amy Rhodes, Robert Singer, and Lisa Bankoff (ICM).

Alexander Laurant drew all of the illustrations, with the exception of the heart in chapter 2, drawn by Laurel Schaubert of Biomed Arts Associates.

I am especially grateful to my dear and generous friend, Ken Hubbard, and his new wife, Tori Dauphinot. They allowed me to stay in their beautiful home in New York for several months while writing the final draft of this book.

My parents, Edwin and Natalie Ornish, gave me the love, support, education, and skills that enabled me to do this work. My brother, Steven, is my closest friend and confidante. I am fortunate to have him, his wife Marty, and my sisters Kathy and Laurie, and Louvada Reeves in my family.

I learned the communication skills described in chapter 8 from Stephen J. Walsh, M.D., a psychiatrist in San Francisco.

Besides our research staff, participants, and my family, I am very appreciative to the following people who read the book manuscript and offered critical comments: Jan Abruzzo, M.S.W., Basil Anderman, Katharine Andres, Jim Autry, Herbert Benson, M.D., Joan Borysenko, Ph.D., Sybil Broyles, William Connor, M.D., Henry Corra, Norman Cousins, Robert E. Cunnion, M.D., Dick and Kathy Dawson, Michael DeBakey, M.D., Rachelle Doody, M.D.,

Larry Dossey, M.D., Vic Eichler, Ph.D., Robert Eliot, M.D., Melanie Elliott, R.N., Daniel Goleman, Ph.D., M.S., Antonio M. Gotto, Jr., M.D., Henry Groppe, T. George Harris, Carole and Bruce Hart, Margot Hennicke, Gerald and Barbara Hines, Stephen Hoffmann, M.D., Ken Hubbard, Dennis Jaffe, Ph.D., Yola Jurzykowski, Marla Kiess, M.D., Dinah Kilgore, Gini Kopecky, Ellen Langer, Ph.D., Alexander Leaf, M.D., George Leonard, Pamela Morgan Maxwell, Cindy Medich, R.N., Ron Moskowitz, Esther Newberg, Ken Pelletier, Ph.D., John and Julia Poppy, John and Lisa Pritzker, Rachel Naomi Remen, M.D., Rob Saper, M.D., Mary Dale Scheller, M.S.W., Stanley J. Schneller, M.D., Cynthia Scott, Ph.D., Bernie Siegel, M.D., Bob Tandler, Karen Thorsen, Anne Thorson, M.D., Art Ulene, M.D., Stephen J. Walsh, M.D., Andrew T. Weil, M.D., Stephen Weiss, Ph.D., Sharlene Weiss, Ph.D., and Margaret Williams, Ph.D.

As described in chapter 4, Swami Satchidananda began teaching me in 1972 the meditation and yoga techniques that evolved into the stress management program described in chapters 7–9. Since then, he has remained my teacher and close friend, for which I am deeply grateful.

Special thanks to Joyce Johnson of Wang Laboratories in San Francisco, who loaned me a laptop computer to use for making the final revisions in New York.

Most of all, I remain very grateful to the people who participated in both groups of our research project. They endured two coronary angiograms, two trips to Houston for PET scans, blood tests, thallium scans, questionnaires, electrocardiograms, interviews, and repeated blood tests in order to be in our study. Their primary motivation in volunteering was the possibility that it might make a difference in helping others to reverse or prevent their affliction. Their courage and commitment live on the pages of this book. Without them, there would have been no research and no book. As Swami Satchidananda once reminded me, "You are just the writing instrument." I hope that I have been a useful one.

Contents

AUTHOR'S NOTE

The Opening Your Heart program is an adjunct to, not a substitute for, conventional medical therapy. If you have coronary heart disease or other health problems, please consult your physician before beginning this program. Each person is different, and so this book is not suggesting that you do or do not have bypass surgery, angioplasty, other medical procedures, or take medications. These choices are personal decisions, ones that you should make only after talking with your physician. If you are taking cardiac medications, your physician may wish to decrease or discontinue some or all of these if your blood pressure, cholesterol level, or clinical status improve. Do *not* make any changes in your medication regimen without consulting your doctor; it can be very dangerous to suddenly stop taking some drugs.

In this book, the term "heart disease" is understood to mean "coronary heart disease" unless otherwise noted.

Except where indicated, the names of the patients who participated in our study have *not* been changed. All of these patients have given permission to publish their names as a way of sharing with you what they have learned and experienced.

No treatment program, including drugs, surgery, or lifestyle changes, is effective for everyone. The program described in this book may not cause reversal of coronary artery disease in everyone who follows it. Some people may become worse despite any treatments or lifestyle changes.

One of my goals in writing this book is to help increase your understanding of heart disease. Another goal is to strengthen the communication between you and your doctor. In this context, you may wish to share this book with him or her. Discuss it with your doctor so that the two of you can work together more effectively to help you achieve greater health and happiness.

"You can't expect insights, even the big ones, to suddenly make you understand everything. But I figure: Hey, it's a step if they leave you confused in a deeper way."

—Lily Tomlin, in Jane Wagner's
Broadway play,
The Search for Signs of Intelligent Life in the Universe

■

"I don't need faith. I have experience."

—Joseph Campbell, interviewed by
Bill Moyers

Introduction
Heart and Soul

This is a book about healing your heart: physically, emotionally, and spiritually. The Opening Your Heart program described in this book can help transform your life.

This program is based on cardiovascular research that I have directed during the past fourteen years, including a recent study my colleagues and I conducted that has proven—for the first time—that many people can begin to *reverse* their heart disease simply by changing their lifestyle. This is the only program scientifically verified to begin healing heart disease without using cholesterol-lowering drugs or surgical interventions. (At the time this is written, no other controlled studies in this country are even in progress to see if heart disease can be reversed without using drugs or surgery.)

Using medical technology never before

available, we found that the coronary arteries of many people with severe heart disease actually began to open when they followed our program. In other words, their arteries became less blocked and blood flow to the heart increased. And unlike with most surgical or medical therapies, the only known side effects from these lifestyle changes are desirable ones.

The participants in our program felt happier and more energetic; their chest pain decreased or went away completely; many were able to cut back on their medications or discontinue them altogether. Also, we measured greater reductions in their blood levels of cholesterol than have ever been reported without using drugs.

Although the incidence of heart attacks has been declining during the past decade, more people die from heart and blood vessel diseases each year than from all other causes of death *combined,* including cancer, AIDS, other infectious diseases, accidents, and homicides. (This is equally true for men and women.) Yet if heart disease can be reversed, then it may be preventable. We don't have to wait for a new drug, surgical procedure, or technological breakthrough.

Knowing what we now understand, heart disease may be preventable for the majority of people who are willing to follow the program described in this book. What our medical system can provide is much less important in determining our health than the lifestyle choices we make as individuals on a daily basis. This book can help you tailor a program that is right for you.

This program does not require deprivation, although the diet I describe may represent an entirely different way of eating for those raised on lots of red meat, cream sauces, and rich desserts. However, our program need not be all or nothing. If your doctor determines you have severe heart disease, you may be more interested in following each step of the program very strictly. However, we all have a spectrum of choices, and this book can help you to make intelligent ones. Somehow, many of us believe we must choose between leading an interesting, exciting, productive life that's filled with stress, great food, and dying young, or sitting under a tree, eating boring food, and watching our longer life go by—or maybe it just *seems* longer. Fortunately, that isn't really the choice. This program can help you to increase your productivity and happiness—*lasting* happiness—while decreasing your anxiety, stress, and the risk of illness. I'll explain how to make meaningful choices and how to tailor the program to best fit your needs.

While reversing coronary artery blockages is of great importance, I am even more interested in the power of this program to transform our lives in deeper ways. The goal of the program is not just to help you live longer—although you likely will do so. After all, none of us is going to live forever. And who wants to live longer if you're not enjoying life? My goal is not only to help you live longer but also to feel *better*. You can begin enjoying life more *now,* with less stress, more joy, and greater health.

On a deeper level, this book explores the psychological and spiritual dimensions of heart disease. Physical heart disease may be the final manifestation of years of abuse that first begins in the psyche and spirit. Susan Sontag notwithstanding, I am becoming increasingly convinced that heart disease is a metaphor as well as an anatomical illness. In poetry, art, and literature, the heart is often portrayed as the organ most affected by our emotions, and I think there is some truth in that.

Ultimately, the Opening Your Heart program is about learning how to feel freer and happier—a different type of "open-heart" procedure, one based on love, knowledge, and compassion rather than just drugs and surgery. We can learn how to open our hearts on emotional and spiritual levels as well as anatomical ones. While these changes are more difficult to measure scientifically than the improvements in coronary anatomy, I find them to be even more interesting and important for leading a happier, healthier life.

Physically, this program can help you begin to open your heart's arteries and to feel stronger and more energetic, freer of pain. Emotionally, it can help you open your heart to others and to experience greater happiness, intimacy, and love in your relationships. Spiritually, it can help you open your heart to a higher force (however you experience it) and to rediscover your inner sources of peace and joy.

In short, this is a program about how to enjoy living, not how to avoid dying. How to relax, not how to be lethargic (a difference well known to world-class athletes). How to manage stress, not how to avoid it. How to live in the world more fully, not how to withdraw from it. How to take care of yourself so that you can also give more fully to others.

The implications of this research go beyond treating and helping to prevent heart disease. Heart disease presents a rich model for examining the relationship between lifestyle and health. Lifestyle factors are important in most of the major killers, including the most common forms of cancer (breast, colon, lung, and prostate), arthritis, diabetes, and other degenerative diseases. However, the mechanisms by which lifestyle affects our health are better understood for heart disease than for other illnesses. Also, the diagnostic technology for examining the heart is highly advanced, so it is possible to actually measure if the disease improves, to what degree, and for whom. Finally, the heart is the place where the body, the psyche, and the spirit all converge.

This book is divided into three sections:

Part One begins with an overview of the relevant research and what this program can do for you. In it, I describe new concepts of heart disease and how lifestyle factors such as diet, emotional stress, and exercise affect your heart—for better and for worse. I also explain how substances such as nicotine, caffeine, cocaine, and alcohol can influence your heart's health. I hope that understanding how the lifestyle choices you make each day affect your heart will make it easier to understand the rationale for this program.

I'll also clarify some of the more common nutritional half-truths; for example, why olive oil and fish oil can actually *raise* cholesterol levels and may help *cause* problems, and why taking aspirin to prevent heart attacks may be ill-advised. I'll explain why cholesterol isn't the whole story behind heart disease, and why taking cholesterol-lowering drugs or niacin or eating oat bran isn't the best choice for most people. Most important, I'll examine the most common ways the medical community has chosen to treat heart disease, and why these interventions, while expensive and often dangerous, don't begin to address the root of the problem of why we feel stressed and get sick in the first place.

In later chapters I'll describe the psychological and spiritual aspects of illness and healing, using coronary heart disease as both example and metaphor. Unfortunately, this is an aspect of health that has until recently been largely ignored by the medical community. Yet through my research and through the studies of others, I am coming to believe that our emotional and spiritual health are exceptionally important to the health of our hearts. I'll share the latest scientific research in this exciting new field and explain how my own background helped to convince me of its value.

Part Two is a "how-to" section that describes the program in detail. (For an overview of the program, please turn to page 133.) For those interested in preventing heart disease, I'll present a spectrum of dietary choices, not a long list of "shoulds" and "thou shalt nots." For people who already have coronary heart disease, our all-you-can-eat Reversal Diet is much lower in fat and cholesterol, but it is not austere, with an emphasis on foods that are tasty, attractive, and familiar. Although you can eat virtually all you want on our program, you'll never have to count calories, and you'll probably find yourself losing excess pounds effortlessly. You'll also receive detailed instruction in how to exercise, how to quit smoking, and how to practice stress management techniques, including stretching, breathing, meditation, visualization, progressive relaxation, and skills to improve communication with your loved ones.

Part Three is a cookbook-within-a-book, with over 150 gourmet recipes by some of the country's most gifted chefs, including Wolfgang Puck, Deborah Madison, Alice Waters, Mollie Katzen, Mark Hall, and others, as well as some of the research participants who have been preparing and eating this food for years. They show how you can have food that is beautifully presented, delicious—*and* healthful. Each recipe has been nutritionally analyzed for fat, cholesterol, and protein content by Shirley Brown, M.D., to make it easier for you to customize a diet that works to meet your own individual needs. She and Martha Rose Shulman, author of *Mediterranean Light* and other best-selling cookbooks, have organized these recipes into twenty-one days of menus, as well as provided some helpful advice on making these meals.

References to all quoted studies are included for health professionals and the especially curious.

I write this book with passion and yet a certain amount of caution. As a physician, I want to share with you the joy that comes from seeing the amazing and powerful differences this program can make in people's lives. As a scientist, though, I want to take a more cautious position, making sure all of the uncertainties and "yes, but . . ." statements are included. In this book, I have tried to take a balanced position somewhere in between these points of view.

Also, I will be careful to distinguish what is scientifically proven from my speculations, personal experiences, and clinical observations. Please understand that my goal in writing this book is not to tell you that you have to change but rather to provide you with facts so that you can make informed choices. Whether or not you decide to change your lifestyle is up to you, but at least you will have accurate information upon which to base this decision.

Heart disease is not easy to reverse. Blockages in coronary arteries take decades to build up, and they do not simply melt away overnight. But they can improve, and more quickly than we had previously thought possible.

In short, this book provides a comprehensive personal system—the Opening Your Heart program—to help heal not only the heart, but also the soul. As Conrad Knudsen, one of our research participants, said, "Even if the tests showed my arteries hadn't opened up, I would still follow this program—because *I've* opened up."

But don't just take my word for it. Try it and see. In only seven days, see how much better you feel, whether or not you have a heart problem. In four weeks your cholesterol level will be significantly lower. After a few months, I hope you'll recognize even more profound and rewarding changes in how you look and feel. Experience the difference for yourself.

PART ONE

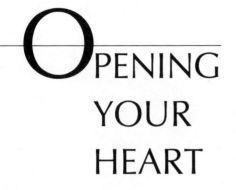

OPENING
YOUR
HEART

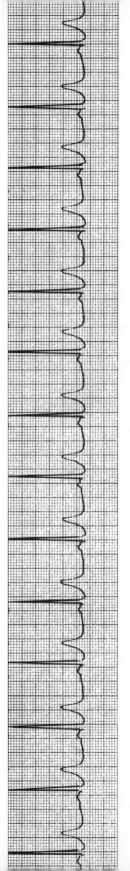

"Who are you gonna believe, me or your own eyes?"

—Groucho Marx, in *Duck Soup*

■

"Not everything that counts can be counted."

—Denis Burkitt, M.D., in
The Cancer Survivors

■

"Innovation is a very difficult thing in the real world."

—Richard P. Feynman, Ph.D., in
Surely You're Joking, Mr. Feynman!

■

"Keep an open mind, but not so open that your brains fall out."

—Unknown

1

"Why Don't You Do Something More Conventional?"

Forty million people in this country suffer from diagnosed cardiovascular disease, and an even larger number don't yet know that they have a heart problem. Sixty million people have high blood pressure. Eighty million people have elevated cholesterol levels. Over 1.5 million Americans have heart attacks every year. And for almost one third of them, having a heart attack was their first indication that they had a heart problem—clearly, not the best way to find out.

Although lifestyle factors play a major role in all of these, I was trained to treat hypertension, high levels of blood cholesterol, and coronary heart disease primarily by prescribing drugs. Yet increasing evidence indicates that medications to lower blood pressure and cholesterol prevent or reverse heart disease in only a small percentage of people. These drugs sometimes make people worse. And moderate dietary changes are not enough to reverse heart disease for most people.

Faced with this new information, many people are beginning to wonder, "Well, why bother? There's not much I can do to make a difference. Bring out the bacon and eggs!"

Fortunately, my colleagues and I are finding that the comprehensive lifestyle program described in this book can lower cholesterol and blood pressure more than has ever been reported without drugs and can even begin to reverse severe coronary heart disease in many people without using cholesterol-lowering drugs or surgery. Of course, none of us is going to live forever, but we don't have to suffer the *premature* death, disability, and cost that come from heart disease.

I first became interested in conducting research on heart disease in 1975 when I was a medical student at the Baylor College of Medicine in Houston. In 1977, I had the privilege of studying with Dr. Michael DeBakey, assisting in the operating room when he performed coronary bypass surgery. His surgical skill was amazing, the technology was impressive, and the circumstances were dramatic. After a while, though, I became a little disheartened as I saw the limitations of technological approaches that literally and figuratively *bypassed* the underlying causes of the problem. It was the difference between temporizing and healing.

Bypass surgery became, for me, a metaphor for the inadequacy of treating a problem without also addressing the underlying causes. We would operate on patients, their chest pain would usually go away, and they were told that they were cured. Most would go home and continue to do the same things that led to the problem in the first place. They would smoke, eat a high-fat, high-cholesterol diet, manage stress poorly, and lead sedentary lives.

At that time, even the hospital had several cigarette machines in the lobby, and just about the only foods available in the hospital cafeteria were cheeseburgers, fried fish, and french fries. In many hospitals, it's still that way. Some even have McDonald's or Burger King franchises right in the hospital. (Now, though, Baylor has a lowfat gourmet restaurant.) Several years ago, Dr. Robert Wissler, an eminent pathologist at the University of Chicago, fed his patients' regular hospital diet to baboons. The baboons developed arterial blockages.

I began to wonder: What would happen if, instead of bypassing the problem, patients began to change what seemed to be the under-lying *causes* of their heart disease?

I went to the medical library and began reading extensively. There were many research studies proving that diets high in fat and cholesterol cause blood cholesterol levels and blood pressure to go up, whereas low-fat, low-cholesterol diets cause blood cholesterol levels and blood pressure to go down. Epidemiological studies showed that high blood cholesterol levels increase the risk of heart disease in virtually all countries throughout the world.

Other studies indicated that emotional stress increases blood pressure and blood levels of cholesterol independent of diet—the type of stress is not that important. Indianapolis 500 race car drivers have higher cholesterol levels after the race than before. Tax accoun-tants have increased cholesterol levels around April 15 when com-pared with the rest of the year. Medical students have higher cholesterol levels during exams. Likewise, other research studies demonstrated that stress management techniques can lower choles-terol levels and blood pressure independent of diet. Furthermore, evidence showed that smoking increased the risk of heart disease, and regular exercise helped to decrease the risk.

Each investigator worked in his or her own area—for example, Dr. Herbert Benson studied meditation, Dr. Ralph Paffenbarger studied exercise, Dr. Frank Sacks studied diet, and so on. Surpris-ingly, no one at that time had studied a comprehensive lifestyle program that used *all* of these lifestyle interventions, and no one had examined the effects of these lifestyle changes not only on risk factors such as cholesterol and blood pressure but also, more importantly, the effects of a comprehensive lifestyle program on the underlying heart disease process.

It seemed like an exciting opportunity, so in 1977 I decided to take a year off between my second and third years of medical school in order to conduct a small pilot study of ten patients using this combined lifestyle program. The Chief of Medicine, Dr. Antonio Gotto, was very supportive and provided most of the testing facili-ties, and the Franzheim Synergy Trust provided a grant to help support the study. The Plaza Hotel in Houston donated ten rooms to us for one month.

One of the advantages of being a second-year medical student was that I hadn't had enough clinical experience to be jaded, to know that it was "impossible" to reverse heart disease, so I told the patients that this program might help them get better. Since most of them had heard from their physicians that their heart disease was only likely to stabilize or worsen over time—the so-called natural history of the disease process—I was unwittingly giving many of them hope for the first time since their illness had been diagnosed.

It was hard to find eligible patients. We were looking for people who had documented coronary heart disease and chest pain but who were not going to have bypass surgery. More bypass surgery is performed in Houston than anywhere in the world, so if a patient had anigiographically documented heart disease and chest pain, then most of the time he or she underwent bypass surgery. As a result, we had to look through over ten thousand patients' charts to find even one hundred patients who were eligible for the study.

Eventually, ten people volunteered. They all experienced remarkable improvements after one month on our program. People who had had incapacitating chest pain with even minimal exertion— showering, shaving, gentle sexual activity, walking short distances— became essentially pain-free and were able to do all of these activities without difficulty. In most cases, these improvements began to occur after only a few days. Many of those who had been out of work for years now were able to return to work full-time. Everyone reported feeling more energy, less depression, and a greater sense of well-being.

The participants' cholesterol levels dropped significantly. Their blood pressures decreased so much that we often had to reduce or even discontinue the anti-hypertensive medications that many of them had been taking for many years (and had been told they would need to take for the rest of their lives). Exercise capability improved in everyone.

Most participants not only felt better, they *were* better. We used what was at that time a new test called an exercise thallium scan, a type of nuclear medicine study now in use in most hospitals. This test noninvasively measured how much blood flow the heart received. Using this test, we found that most patients showed significant improvements in coronary blood flow—after only thirty days!

This was thought by most doctors to have been impossible— "There must be some mistake," many of them told us at the time. "The tests must be wrong." Nuclear medicine tests such as the thallium scan were sometimes called "unclear medicine" by doctors because the images were not always 100 percent reliable—although they were accurate enough to serve as the basis for clinical decisions every day. Since the pilot study hadn't included a randomized control group for comparison, some critics asked, "How do you know that patients wouldn't have gotten better anyway?" even though it would have been highly unusual for anyone's thallium scan to improve without drugs or surgery. Nevertheless, we published a summary of our results in the journal *Clinical Research.* A few years later, similar improvements in blood flow and function were found in studies by Dr. Gerhard Schuler in West Germany, by Dr. William Haskell at Stanford, and by Dr. Victor Froelicher in San Diego.

I then learned that a few physicians (including Dr. Lester Morrison, Dr. William Castelli, Dr. Walter Kempner, and others) and some laypeople such as Nathan Pritikin speculated that coronary artery blockages could be reversed in humans by a low-fat diet and exercise, whereas most cardiologists dismissed this idea as a lot of nonsense. Unfortunately, there was little scientific evidence to prove or refute these claims, so the public became confused and the medical community became polarized. Other physicians such as Dr. Robert Eliot, Dr. Carl Simonton, and Dr. Bernie Siegel and people such as Jeanne Achterberg, Joan Borysenko, and Norman Cousins discussed in their books and lectures the importance of managing emotional stress and interventions such as visualization in treating chronic diseases. Again, due to the lack of scientific proof, there were more debates, misunderstandings, and disagreements.

I went back to medical school and graduated in 1980. Before beginning my medical internship and residency at Massachusetts General Hospital and Harvard Medical School, I decided to take another year off to conduct a larger study designed to address some of the limitations of the first one. This new study would have a usual-care control group for comparison.

In this second study, my colleagues and I (including Dr. Shirley Brown, Dr. Sandra McLanahan, and Dr. Larry Scherwitz) enrolled forty-eight patients and randomly divided them into two groups: one group lived together in a condominium and followed our lifestyle program for twenty-four days, whereas the other group followed the advice of their physicians. (We scientifically chose this time interval because the owner donated the use of his facilities to us for twenty-four days . . . .) We tested both groups at the beginning and end of the study and compared the results.

Once again, we measured significant improvements in the participants who followed our program: an *average* 91 percent reduction in the amount of chest pain (angina), a 55 percent improvement in exercise capability, a 21 percent reduction in cholesterol levels, and significant reductions in blood pressure at rest and during emotional stress. The participants reported improved well-being, and greatly reduced anxiety, fear, worry, and depression. Using a different nuclear medicine test called a gated blood pool scan, we measured overall improvements both in the ability of the heart to pump blood and in how uniformly it was contracting, two indirect indications that the heart disease was improving after only twenty-four days. All of these improvements were statistically significant when compared with the usual care group, whose heart disease either stayed the same or became slightly worse during the same time interval. We published the results of this second study in the *Journal of the American Medical Association.* These two studies formed the basis for my earlier book, *Stress, Diet & Your Heart.*

While these studies were encouraging and intriguing, they did not provide definitive evidence that heart disease could be reversed. Also, it's not very difficult to motivate people to change their lifestyle when they are "captive" in a hotel or condominium—but could we motivate patients to make comprehensive changes in their lifestyles while living in the real world? And, what would happen to risk factors such as cholesterol levels and blood pressure in participants who'd been in the program over a period of years rather than weeks? Finally, and most important, could we measure reversal in their coronary artery blockages?

From 1981 to 1984, I completed my internship and medical residency in Boston. In July 1984, I moved to San Francisco to begin planning this study at Pacific Presbyterian Medical Center and the UCSF School of Medicine.

Although several experiments during the past decades had established that coronary heart disease could be reversed in *animals*—including dogs, cats, rats, rabbits, pigs, and monkeys—this had never been proven in *humans.* In part, this was because conventional recommendations for lifestyle changes did not go far enough to reverse heart disease, and also because the technology for measuring heart disease had not been accurate enough.

Recent breakthroughs in medical technology—including computer-assisted quantitative coronary arteriography and cardiac PET (*P*ositron *E*mission *T*omography) scans—finally made it possible to measure precisely even small changes in coronary artery blockages and blood flow, thereby giving my colleagues and me the tools to measure the extent and severity of heart disease with confidence. From July 1984 until December 1985, we designed a new study that used these state-of-the-art, high-tech, expensive diagnostic tools to measure the power of lifestyle changes that were ancient, low-tech, and freely available. These tests were developed and performed by K. Lance Gould, M.D., of the University of Texas Medical School at Houston, whose $25 million PET scanner is the best available.

When we first began, Dr. Gould believed that lifestyle changes were unlikely to reverse heart disease, so we made a good team. We reasoned that whatever happened, the results of our research would be very interesting. If we found that heart disease could be reversed, then, of course, that would be important news. If we found that people could not be motivated to make comprehensive lifestyle changes or that these modifications had no effect on heart disease, then that also would be interesting; in that case, drugs and surgery might be the only effective answers to treating and trying to prevent heart disease.

At first, we found it very difficult to obtain funding for this new study. It was discouraging. We applied to the American Heart Association, to the National Institutes of Health, and to the major foundations, but these grant requests were rejected. The reviewers wrote: "It's impossible to reverse heart disease, and even if it could be done, one year is not long enough to prove it. Lifestyle changes may reduce the risk of getting heart disease but not reverse it—and people won't change their lifestyles to that degree anyway. You have to use cholesterol-lowering drugs to show reversal. No one would volunteer to have repeat coronary angiography, since that test is dangerous." And so on.

Some of the criticisms of our approach indicated how powerful and yet topsy-turvy cardiology had become in its approach to treating heart disease—what seemed like common sense to me was often viewed as radical heresy, and what seemed to me like terribly invasive approaches were viewed as simply routine. A well-known cardiologist at one of the major foundations to which we applied for funding asked me, "Why are you doing this radical intervention? Why don't you do something more conventional to treat heart disease?"

"Well, like what?"

"Like plasmapheresis [a technique in which a patient's entire blood volume is filtered *every week* through a dialysis-like machine to remove cholesterol], or partial ileal bypass surgery [in which one end of the intestine is spliced onto the other, bypassing most of the intestinal tract so that the body doesn't absorb as much cholesterol], or high doses of cholesterol-lowering drugs, instead of your approach of changing diet, exercise, stopping smoking, and stress management training!"

Yet our research team believed in our vision. I flew to Houston and met with Gerald D. Hines, the renowned real estate developer. He made a major contribution in support of our research and agreed to help us raise the rest of the funds needed to conduct the study. We received additional pledges from a number of Houston-based individuals, corporations, and small foundations, including Continental Airlines, the Enron Corporation, Texas Commerce Bank, the Emde Company, Gross Investments, the Ray C. Fish Foundation, Transco Energy Company, Arthur Andersen & Co., and others.

With those assurances, my colleagues and I began our study. Unfortunately, six months later, oil prices plummeted and the Houston economy collapsed. As a result, the support we expected did not always materialize and fund-raising became much more difficult.

For the next three years, we continued the research, not knowing from one month to the next where the funds would come from to pay our expenses. Somehow we managed to raise enough each month to get by. After we began demonstrating that we were accomplishing our objectives, some of the larger foundations and corporations provided support for our work, including Houston Endowment, The Henry J. Kaiser Family Foundation, The Fetzer Institute, the State of California, The First Boston Corporation, Quaker Oats, and several others (please see the acknowledgments section).

In our current study, patients with severe coronary heart disease were randomly divided into two groups. Patients in one group were asked to follow the program described in this book. Patients in the usual care comparison group were asked to follow their doctors' advice: to make moderate dietary changes (eat less red meat, more fish and chicken, margarine instead of butter, and no more than three eggs per week), to exercise moderately, and to quit smoking. We tested both groups of patients at the beginning of the study and one year later and compared them. The angiograms were made in San

Francisco, and these films were sent to Dr. Gould and Dr. Richard Kirkeeide in Houston for quantitative analyses. These data were then sent directly to Dr. Richard Brand in Berkeley for statistical analysis.

After only one year, the majority (82 percent) of the patients who made the comprehensive lifestyle changes described in this book demonstrated some measurable average *reversal* of their coronary artery blockages. (Not every blockage in each artery was reversed, but the majority were.) Overall, the average blockage reversed from 61.1 to 55.8 percent; more severely blocked arteries showed even greater improvement. These blockages took decades to build up in the arteries, so they don't just melt away completely in only a year. But even a small amount of reversal after one year in a severely blocked artery causes a great improvement in blood flow to the heart (as measured by a cardiac PET scan). As a result, these participants began to feel better very quickly, as you will read in chapters 2 and 6. Also, four arteries that had been completely blocked began to open, even those that had been totally occluded for years. The average amount of reversal would have been even greater if we had included these changes in our analysis.

All five of the women in our study showed some overall reversal of their arterial blockages, even those who made only moderate lifestyle changes. These findings suggest that women may show reversal easier than men.

In contrast, the majority of the heart patients in our comparison group who were following their doctors' advice became measurably *worse* during the same interval. Thus, for people who have heart disease, conventional recommendations for changing lifestyle may not go far enough.

Our research findings were published in *The Lancet* (the most well-respected international medical journal) in summer 1990, as well as in other medical journals and at scientific meetings. Recently, the National Heart, Lung, and Blood Institute of the National Institutes of Health and the Fetzer Institute awarded us a major grant that allows us to extend our research for four more years to determine if the participants' coronary arteries become even less blocked as they continue in the program over a longer period of time.

Apparently, it's never too late to begin making these changes. In our research, the amount a participant improved was primarily related to how well he kept to the lifestyle program, not to his age or the severity of his disease. We measured the greatest improvement in the oldest patient in our study (Werner Hebenstreit, age seventy-four) and in the patient with the most severe coronary artery blockages (Bob Finnell, age fifty-two, whose three major coronary arteries were blocked 100, 100, and 79 percent). This was different from what I'd expected—I had predicted that the younger patients with earlier, less advanced disease would show the most improvement, but (fortunately) I was wrong. In fact, the most severely blocked arteries are the ones that showed the greatest amount of reversal. While some aspects of the program that we used in our third study are similar or identical to those we used in our first two studies, there are many important differences. For example, the role of communication skills and the importance of establishing intimacy were a major focus of our third study, and as you'll read in chapter 4, I've personally come to believe that these may be critically important to healing our hearts on several levels. The program also expands the use of visualization as part of the healing process. Also, my understanding of how these techniques are best used has evolved considerably.

We don't know the relative contribution of each component of the program. That is, we can't say how much of the improvement was due to the changes in diet, how much was from the stress management techniques, how much was due to the group support, and so on. Our data indicate that each part of the program is important, but some parts may be more important than others for different people. In our study, adherence to each component of the program was directly correlated with the degree of reversal in coronary artery blockages.

For example, dietary changes may be more important for a person who has been eating a high-fat, high-cholesterol diet but who is not under much stress, doesn't smoke, exercises, and has a lot of emotional support. Likewise, the stress management techniques may be more important for someone who is in a high-stress job but whose blood cholesterol level is only 150. The point is that while there may be some individual differences, it is the program as a whole that has been demonstrated to begin reversing coronary heart disease in most of our study participants.

During the past few years, the public and medical community have become more aware of the importance of cholesterol in heart disease. The medical community has gone from one extreme—saying that cholesterol has little to do with heart disease—to the other, portraying cholesterol as the primary cause of heart problems.

While cholesterol *is* very important, it is not the whole story. Neither is high blood pressure, or smoking, or lack of exercise. All of the known risk factors explain only about one half of the heart disease that we see. Clearly, something else is going on.

When I first began planning this third study in 1984, I thought that participants' cholesterol levels would need to decrease to below 150, or at least below 180, in order to show reversal of their coronary artery blockages. Again, I was wrong, and this is one of our most interesting findings.

Let me illustrate with an example. Robert Royall is a fifty-three-year-old priest with severe coronary heart disease. His cholesterol levels are elevated primarily because of a genetic condition known as familial combined hypercholesterolemia.

In November 1986, he had a coronary angiogram (cardiac catheterization) that revealed a 37 percent blockage in one of the main coronary arteries (known as the left anterior descending artery) that supplies the front of the heart with blood (see figure 1.1). At that time, I invited him to enroll in our research project.

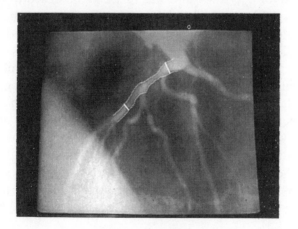

Figure 1.1

He had a prior commitment to move to North Carolina and lead a church congregation there, so he declined. He followed his doctor's advice and began to reduce the amount of fat and cholesterol in his diet from 40 to 30 percent (less red meat, chicken with the skin removed, fewer eggs) and began exercising more. He did not smoke. His cholesterol decreased from 390 to 360.

After a while, though, the frequency of his chest pains began to increase. In November 1987, he returned for another angiogram. The test revealed that the 37 percent blockage had dramatically worsened to 77 percent (see figure 1.2).

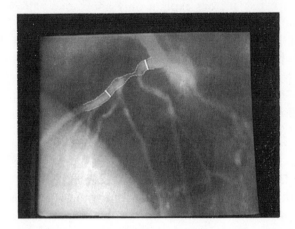

Figure 1.2

Because of this evidence that his disease was worsening, he volunteered for our study and was randomly assigned to the group making comprehensive lifestyle changes. He followed the program described in this book, and his cholesterol level decreased from 360 to about 250—a large reduction, but his blood level was still much too high, I thought. I was tempted to prescribe cholesterol-lowering drugs for him, but we decided to wait until his next angiogram since he seemed to be improving in so many other ways: he had lost fifty-five pounds, he had only rare chest pain, and he'd opened up emotionally to the other group members in ways that were sometimes startling.

After one year in our program, we repeated his angiogram again. This time, the 77 percent blockage had reversed to only 59 percent, and blood flow through that artery increased by 270 percent (see figure 1.3).

In summary, then, conventional lifestyle recommendations had caused his coronary artery blockage to worsen dramatically after one year, whereas our program caused the same blockage to improve one year later. It is possible that some people with genetically high cholesterol levels may benefit from a combination of the Opening Your Heart program plus cholesterol-lowering drugs, but drugs alone are not optimal and may not even be necessary.

Hank Ginsberg is a sixty-three-year-old investment banker who had tried everything to control his heart disease. He first tried car-

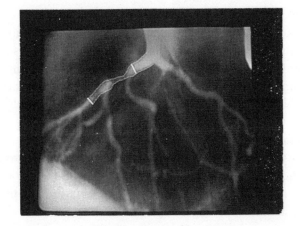

Figure 1.3

diac medications, but his chest pain kept getting worse. Then he underwent bypass surgery in 1983, but a few years later the bypassed arteries clogged up again. He had an angioplasty four years later, but the arteries closed up within a few months.

He then entered our program. Although he followed it closely, his cholesterol level decreased from 271 to 192—still too high, I thought. Yet his angiogram one year later showed significant reversal in his coronary artery blockages.

In contrast, one of the patients in the comparison (control) group of our study took lovastatin (Mevacor), a powerful cholesterol-lowering drug, for one year, and he stopped smoking. His cholesterol level decreased from 248 to 172 during the year, yet his coronary artery blockages worsened substantially and he had a heart attack at the end of the year.

Only two other controlled studies besides ours have demonstrated that reversal of coronary artery blockages can occur in humans. The first was published in June 1987 by a pioneering researcher, David Blankenhorn, M.D., at the University of Southern California School of Medicine. (Dr. Blankenhorn's earlier studies demonstrating that blockages in the arteries to the legs can begin to reverse helped inspire me to do my research.)

In the 1987 study, Dr. Blankenhorn and his colleagues randomly divided patients into two groups. One group received very high doses of two cholesterol-lowering drugs in combination—30 grams per day of colestipol (Colestid) plus 8 to 12 grams per day of niacin—and the other group did not. Both groups were placed on a 30 percent fat "low-fat" diet along the guidelines of the American

Heart Association (a diet much higher in fat than the one outlined in this book). A 30 percent fat diet includes lean red meats, chicken with the skin removed, fish, and no more than three eggs per week. Only patients whose blood cholesterol levels were substantially lowered by drugs were included in this study. The patients who received cholesterol-lowering drugs reduced their cholesterol levels to below 180.

Coronary angiograms were performed at the beginning of the study and two years later. Only 16 percent of the participants who took the cholesterol-lowering drugs showed some measurable reversal of their coronary artery blockages; 44 percent of the people had no change in their blockages and almost 40 percent of the people actually got worse despite intensive drug treatment. Also, the participants reported no overall reduction in the frequency of their chest pain.

The second important investigation was conducted by B. Greg Brown, M.D., and his colleagues at the University of Washington Medical School in 1990. (Dr. Brown, along with K. Lance Gould, M.D., developed the technique of quantitative coronary angiography, which was the major test used in our research.) In Dr. Brown's important study, men with heart disease and elevated cholesterol levels were divided into three groups. Group A was given high doses of niacin (4 grams per day) plus colestipol (30 grams per day); Group B was given high doses of lovastatin (40 milligrams per day) plus colestipol (30 grams per day); Group C was given a 30 percent fat "low-fat" diet. After two and one-half years, patients in Group A showed a slight amount of overall reversal (0.9 percent) of their coronary blockages and patients in Group B showed even less reversal (0.3 percent). The majority of patients in both groups became worse, that is, their coronary arteries became more blocked despite drug treatment. Group C patients also became worse, showing a 1.7 percent worsening of their coronary artery blockages.

If lowering cholesterol were the primary factor in causing reversal of heart disease, then the blockages of most of the patients in the studies by Dr. Blankenhorn and Dr. Brown who were taking cholesterol-lowering drugs should have shown reversal, since almost all of these patients had substantial decreases in blood cholesterol levels due to these drugs. Yet only the minority showed reversal. In fact, the majority of these patients stayed the same or worsened despite treatment with cholesterol-lowering drugs.

Overall, in both Dr. Blankenhorn's and Dr. Brown's studies, patients who took the cholesterol-lowering drugs did somewhat better than those who did not take drugs and who made only moderate changes in diet. In contrast, the majority of patients in our study showed a greater degree of reversal in coronary artery blockages over a shorter period of time—without using cholesterol-lowering drugs.

Thus, taking cholesterol-lowering drugs has value, and it is better to take these drugs than to do nothing. Even better, though, may be to make comprehensive lifestyle changes described in this book, certainly at least as a first step.

Both Dr. Blankenhorn and Dr. Brown found that the coronary artery blockages worsened in patients who ate a 30 percent fat diet and did not take cholesterol-lowering drugs. My colleagues and I found similar results in the comparison group patients in our study who ate a 30 percent fat diet. Thus, the conventional dietary recommendations may not go far enough for people who have a heart problem. Dr. Blankenhorn's research also indicated that a 30 percent fat diet helps to prevent *new* arterial blockages from forming, but it is not usually enough to *reverse* existing blockages. In other words, more moderate changes may help *prevent* heart disease, whereas more comprehensive changes are needed to *reverse* it. This is the rationale for the Prevention Diet and the Reversal Diet described in chapter 10. An ounce of prevention is indeed worth a pound of cure.

In our research, we found that there was a "dose-response" effect to our program. That is, the more closely people followed our program, the better they felt and the less obstruction they had in their coronary arteries. So even a 30 percent fat diet is more beneficial than a 40 percent fat diet. The coronary artery blockages may worsen on a 30 percent fat diet, but more slowly than on a 40 percent fat diet. But *reversing* the coronary artery blockages usually requires a diet even lower in fat as well as other lifestyle changes described in this book.

While there was a direct correlation between adherence to each part of our program (diet, stress management, exercise, and stopping smoking) and the degree of improvement, there was very little correlation between blood cholesterol levels and degree of change in their arteries. (In particular, reversal did not correlate with blood levels of total cholesterol, HDL, LDL, total cholesterol/HDL, LDL/

HDL, or changes in any of these. These terms are defined in chapter 10.) Dr. Blankenhorn's study also found that there was little correlation between changes in any of these blood cholesterol levels and arterial blockages.

Why? Although difficult to prove scientifically, I believe that heart disease needs to be examined and treated at a deeper level. The use of cholesterol-lowering drugs is based on the presumption that cholesterol is the primary determinant of atherosclerosis, whereas I am becoming increasingly convinced that other factors, including emotional stress, perceived isolation, lack of social support, hostility, cynicism, and low self-esteem, also play important roles, so examining these issues is an important part of the Opening Your Heart program. Working with a relatively small group of patients on an intensive basis over a long period of time has given my colleagues and me special opportunities to gain insight into some of these factors and to begin working to address them more directly and effectively.

This program is based on the premise that there are different levels of healing. That is, *the farther back in the causal chain of events we can address a problem, the more powerful the healing can be.* The physical manifestations of an illness—the symptoms—need to be addressed. But if we treat the problem *only* at a physical level, then the patient's improvement is less than it could be and the illness is more likely to recur, either in the same form or in a different one.

For example, we know that the arteries that supply the heart with blood can become progressively clogged over time with cholesterol and other deposits. When these blockages become severe, the heart does not receive enough blood and it becomes starved for the oxygen carried in the blood. If this deprivation is brief, the result is chest pain (angina); if prolonged, the part of the heart not receiving enough blood actually dies and turns into scar tissue. This is called a heart attack. If the scar tissue is small, then the person may live. If a large part of the heart dies, or if the heart attack occurs in an important part of the heart (such as the pacemaker area, for example), then the person may not survive. (Similarly, blockages in an artery that leads to the brain can cause a stroke, in which part of the brain dies from lack of blood flow.)

On one level, therefore, blockages in the coronary arteries lead to chest pain and heart attacks, and blockages in the brain's arteries leads to strokes. To address this level of disease, doctors began performing coronary artery bypass surgery over twenty-five years ago as a way of bringing more blood around the blocked arteries. In this procedure, a vein is taken from the patient's leg and spliced around the obstructed artery, thereby increasing blood flow to the heart.

A more recent approach to treating closed arteries is called coronary angioplasty, in which a small balloon is inflated inside a blocked coronary artery, thereby "squishing" the blockage and widening the vessel, allowing more room for blood to flow to the heart.

Bypass surgery, angioplasty, and cholesterol-lowering drugs do not address the deeper questions of why the blockages in the coronary arteries occur in the first place. You might ask, "Well, so what? I mean, who needs philosophy when you have drugs and surgery? They work, don't they?"

Yes and no. Temporarily, these approaches can be lifesaving for many people. I use them sometimes. When a patient comes into the emergency room with severe chest pain, saying, "Doc, please get this elephant off my chest," I don't just feed him broccoli and ask him to start meditating—I use whatever cardiac drugs, electrical shocks, and surgical procedures are necessary to treat the acute, life-threatening condition. Even if a person decides to follow the Opening Your Heart program, I will usually prescribe cardiac medications (such as calcium channel blockers or nitrates) and gradually reduce the dosage over time as the person's symptoms, blood pressure, and cholesterol improve.

Once the person is stabilized and is recovering, then we can begin discussing why heart disease occurred and what he or she can do to avoid a return trip to the emergency room. There is a real window of opportunity when a person first learns that he has heart disease: the doctor has his or her full attention. At that time, the illness and suffering can be powerful catalysts for changing not only behaviors such as diet and exercise, but more important, for helping to transform more fundamental determinants of health, including the patient's values, relationships, self-perceptions, and self-esteem.

Coronary heart disease—the blockages in the coronary arteries and reduced blood flow to the heart—is the end product of a chain of events that occur over a lifetime. A fundamental and recurring theme of this book is that *treating only the physical manifestations of heart disease without addressing the more fundamental causes will provide only temporary relief, and the disease is likely to recur. At best, we will trade one set of problems or illnesses for another.* This is true for all conventional treatments of heart disease, including drugs, surgery, and angioplasty. These themes are more fully explored in chapter 2.

It has been difficult to measure the role of emotional stress on the heart, so its importance is often not recognized. Modern medicine is based on science, and scientists tend to believe only what can be measured and observed, even though what can be quantified may not be what is most important. Like the man who looks under the street lamp for his wallet "because the light is better there" even though he lost it over in the dark alley, we may be looking in the wrong place if we study only what can be measured.

Cholesterol and blood pressure can be measured easily, and powerful drugs are available that can lower both of these. This makes both doctors and drug companies very happy: doctors can simply write a prescription instead of spending much time teaching patients about lifestyle changes, and drug companies reap the profits.

Also, the third-party reimbursement system (health insurance, Medicare, etc.) encourages the use of drugs and surgery rather than health education. In America, more money is spent on treating heart disease than any other illness—*$78 billion* annually. Last year, over $7 billion was spent on bypass surgery in this country. If I perform bypass surgery on a patient, the insurance company will pay at least $30,000. If I perform a balloon angioplasty on a patient, the insurance company will pay at least $7,500. If I spend the same amount of time teaching a heart patient about nutrition and stress management techniques, the insurance company will pay no more than $150. If I spend that time teaching a well person how to *stay* healthy, the insurance company will not pay at all.

It's not surprising that doctors tend to spend time on what is reimbursed, especially since we do not learn much in medical school about nutrition or how to motivate patients to change their lifestyles. We are not taught skills for coping with stress in our own lives or for teaching these skills to our patients. So we doctors practice medicine in ways that we are trained to do and in ways that we are paid to do.

I remember making rounds on my first day of internship in Boston in 1981. I was a little intimidated by how smart everyone seemed to be. We rolled the chart rack down the hall and stood outside the first patient's room.

The resident turned to me and said, "Dean, this is a fifty-three-year-old man who had a heart attack three days ago. He's depressed and he wants to talk to someone, but we don't have time—we have to round on forty-five patients plus six more in the coronary care unit during the next two hours. Just go in his room, listen to his heart and lungs, and get out!"

The following year, while making rounds (this time, *I* was the resident), a prominent cardiologist, looking very frustrated, walked over to me on the wards. He said, "You're taking care of my patient, Mr. Smith. He's scheduled for bypass surgery later today and he's so worried he's bouncing off the walls. I send patients for bypass surgery every day, so I don't understand why he's so worried—it's no big deal to *me.*"

We doctors don't set the best examples. Besides learning not to value or hear the emotional needs of our patients, we often learn to deny and split off our own feelings as part of our medical training. As a profession, we have among the highest rates of drug addiction and divorce of any identifiable group, and the average physician dies ten years prematurely. Each year, enough physicians commit suicide to equal a large medical school's entire graduating class. And that's just the known suicides. So it is not very surprising that many doctors do not believe that emotional distress or spiritual isolation can contribute to heart disease. It's easier not to.

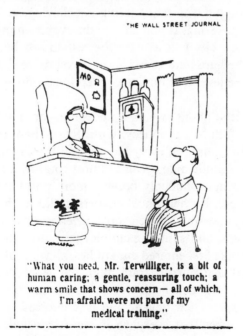

THE WALL STREET JOURNAL

"What you need, Mr. Terwilliger, is a bit of human caring; a gentle, reassuring touch; a warm smile that shows concern — all of which, I'm afraid, were not part of my medical training."

From the *Wall Street Journal*—permission, Cartoon Features Syndicate.

Part of the value of this comprehensive lifestyle intervention research is that it can build bridges to both the medical community and to the general public. When I speak to doctors at hospital conferences and medical meetings, I begin by describing the scientific evidence from our research—the data, the PET scans, the angiograms, and so on. Then, when they ask, "What did these patients do to get these results?" I reply, "We began them on an exercise program." "Yes, of course, what else?" "We gave them a different diet and helped them to stop smoking." "Yes, of course, what else?" "Well, while I think diet, exercise, and stopping smoking are important, I also believe that working at a deeper level is also very important: teaching people how to quiet down the mind and to gain more control over it; how to listen to others' feelings and to their own; how to feel more connected to others and to themselves; how to give and to receive love more fully."

And the scientific data often open the door—and the heart—for doctors to begin hearing these ideas, which are new to many of them. I have never been to a cardiology scientific meeting where anyone has studied or discussed the importance and the power of love—ironic, as the heart is the symbol of love.

Research also has another important value: redefining what is possible. While it's true that "seeing is believing," it's equally true that believing is seeing. If you believe that you're hungry, when you drive into a new city you will see the restaurants but you may not be aware of the hardware stores, even if you drive right by one. We see what we believe, and our preconceptions influence our perceptions.

Our beliefs about what is possible—or impossible—often become a self-fulfilling prophecy. Until Roger Bannister ran a mile in less than four minutes, everyone thought it was impossible. Soon after, the four-minute mile became almost routine. I don't think this was because people suddenly became more physically fit (steroids notwithstanding). Rather, once one person did it, the belief shifted about what was possible. Once people *believed* it was possible, it *was* possible. We can find similar examples in many other arenas.

When people first entered our studies, all we could tell them was that we hoped that our program might be beneficial. Now we are demonstrating how beneficial this program can be. Suddenly, we have new evidence, new beliefs, and new choices.

I don't expect that everyone in the world will suddenly say,

"Hey, this is something I want to do 100 percent." But many people will. At least you will know what your choices are, and you can choose intelligently. And you have a spectrum of choices. The more you do, the more benefits you will receive. It's not all or nothing.

No matter how much we learn, though, there is always an element of mystery, genetics, perhaps even destiny in explaining why some people improve while others do not. We may not always be cured (that is, our arterial blockages may not become unclogged), but we can learn to be healed—for the real issue is not just how to delay death but also how to be more fully alive, freer from our self-imposed limitations. Now, using this program, we can often have both.

"Judge not, that ye be not judged."

—Matthew 7:1

■

"My strength is as the strength of ten,
Because my heart is pure."

—Tennyson,
Sir Galahad (1842)

■

"Only the brave know how to forgive."

—Laurence Sterne,
Sermons

■

"I was angry with my friend:
I told my wrath, my wrath did end.
I was angry with my foe:
I told it not, my wrath did grow."

—William Blake,
A Poison Tree

■

"Blessed are the pure in heart: for they shall see God."

—Matthew 5:8

2

"I Mean, What Could Be Wimpier Than *That?*"

One of the participants in our research is Dwayne Butler, a man with severe coronary heart disease. I found him to be a particularly inspiring example of how illness can be a catalyst for transforming and improving the quality of a person's life, not simply his behavior. This chapter is a transcript of an interview with him recorded on July 27, 1989, seven months after he entered our study. His angiogram one year after he started revealed some overall reversal in his coronary artery blockages. The scientific basis for the Opening Your Heart program is described in the next chapter.

My name is Dwayne Butler. I'm fifty-three years old and I'm a general manager for Haula-way Container Corporation.

I was born in New Mexico. I'm just, I

guess, a bull-headed type of person who felt he'd been an all-American boy, proud of strength and honor and glory and all of that other stuff. Some people called me a redneck. Any wimps or weaklings or anybody else were not tolerated.

And that's not right. I know that's not right. And even when I feel that way, I know it's not right. It's just an outward appearance, it's just a facade that I put up there to look mean and tough and ornery and all of that. And we like to do that. We being, as I grew up, the kids I messed around with and the people I hung out with. The way I was raised did not tolerate anything or anyone different, and all that goes with it. And that's wrong, I know that's wrong.

But throughout my time in the service, it was the same way. When I played sports, it was the same way. Back then, we weren't called jocks, but we were supposed to be tough so we didn't put up with any nonsense. And when we went into the service I can remember they asked whether you were a homosexual or not or even had those tendencies—and you had better say no. Or they wouldn't take you. No way.

You know, that was a thing that was drilled into you that it was wrong, absolutely wrong. And I'm not saying it's right. But you are supposed to love your fellow man and your neighbor as yourself and all of this, but you don't. You just don't.

Because you judge people. You feel you are better than they are, but you're not. And after years of that type of training, so to speak, it's hard to get rid of, until you finally face life full and then face reality and ask, "Who am I?" I'm not trying to quote the Bible, but "Judge not, lest you be judged." You are not supposed to judge people. Yet that's what we do every day.

Back then, though, in the crowd I was running around with, if you didn't measure up in the manly category, they would reject you. You would be out. You would lose face, you would lose friends. Because you would be isolated, you wouldn't have *any* friends. And when I was young, I didn't have a whole lot of friends. When I got up to junior high I had to fight my way through school. I mean physically. Fist fights. Because, for some reason, I didn't make friends too easily.

It was a small town and I came from a very strict Christian family. There were many times that we went to church three times on Sunday and once on Wednesday and some other times as well.

Younger kids are very tough on different types of people, and we were the minority.

I can remember that there was a group of boys that didn't really like me. After school, they would have one of their buddies at each door and I would have to pick the easiest door to head out. I would head out and I would get caught and we would go out and have a fist fight.

In junior high, I was fearful most of the time. We even made appointments to fight: "Be on the library lawn at nine o'clock Saturday morning—and you better be there!" And if you weren't there, you were a wimp. Then you got met at the door. So I learned to take it. I grew up with that kind of philosophy, and it was the survival of the fittest.

When I got to high school, I went out for sports and got onto the football team. They were the toughies, they were the ones with the cheerleader girlfriends. They didn't do so good in school, but they seemed to be on the right track at the time.

So when I went through high school I seemed to do very well because I was good in sports and I had all of this, you know, I was the king of the mountain. I said to myself, "This must be the way to go." And you are supposed to hate certain kinds of people and give them trouble—people of different colors, different religions, different educations, wimps, etc.—and to love other kinds of people. But that is just absolutely wrong.

We saw ourselves like pro wrestlers, big and tough. I can remember going down Main Street, and we would challenge anybody. We would stop a car full of kids from school and we would challenge them to fight. Other guys. There would be four or five guys in the car and one or two of us, and we'd pull them over and challenge them right there. They would normally have one or two girls and we would show those girls that our group was tougher than theirs. It was just a show.

Inside, we were hoping they were going to back down, but sometimes they didn't. And so we would go outside the town, and two or three of us would take on five or six of them and we would have a knock-down drag-out. It wasn't over drugs or booze or women. It was over machismo, you know, toughness. Proving yourself.

I went to college for a while on an athletic scholarship, but I finally decided to give that up and went into the service. In the service I had the same situation. You had the wimps and you had the other guys. So, I can remember many, many fights in the service.

And I drank heavily in the service. I also drank in high school. 'Cause that was part of the tough show.

Then the gay lifestyle became more popular, and that was one thing my friends and I really hated. We always joked about it during high school.

I'm just going to unburden my soul here. You get to a place where you think there is something wrong with these people and the world would be better off without them. I never went out gay bashing. That wasn't really the thing in the 1950s. The first time I really heard it was here in San Francisco, much later. But if it had been, if my friends were doing it, then I would have been there, too. No doubt. Because that was my mental makeup.

I finally got out of the service and started back to school. And I caused trouble, occasionally got drunk, and got put on probation. I was doing everything against the school rules because it was such a mousy place, I thought. All of them were such weaklings, such a bunch of wimps in there.

I got into some fights. Thought I was quite the fellow. There were two or three of us there who thought we were, and we used to cause a lot of trouble. You know how that goes. So they put me on probation for the rest of the year and wouldn't let me come back the next year.

That really irritated me, so I just went back and started working on an oil rig. I figured that's all I'd do. So my life went on for a couple of years there, and I said to myself that there had to be a better way to make a living than that, throwing that iron around and always being covered with dirt. I was strong, but I was working seven days a week and almost twelve hours a day. I was getting tired of that lifestyle.

While I was there, I met Kathy through a friend. She came up from Phoenix, and three months later, we got married. She settled me down. We moved to Farmington and I went to work for Frontier Airlines.

Not long after, I got into another fight. This supervisor got me upset, so I pushed him. He said, "Don't you ever push me again." So I just popped him, I busted his nose. I was a very violent person and I wore a chip on my shoulder all the time. Just don't pop off around me.

Later, we moved to Seattle. But I still got in some fights. Once, a guy gave me lip and I just almost killed him. He popped off at me and I said, "Don't you *ever* talk to me like that again." I hit him. And he staggered back and tried to hit me, and I hit him again. And I said to myself, "Man this is *fun.*" It brought back twenty years of life in me. I hit him again, picked him up, and threw him on the floor. I could have killed him. They had to take him to the hospital. I saw how easy it was to kill a man.

Another time I was in Missoula hanging out with a bunch of guys. And we said, "You see this guy coming?" "Yeah." So we just pushed another guy back into him and that started it. We just wanted a fight. So we had a rip-roaring one. I thought this one guy was going to kill this other guy. It was snowing, but we finally got out of there.

When I first met Dr. Ornish, I was very bitter. I guess I was bitter over a number of things. I weighed too much and I couldn't cope with it. I'd lose weight and then I'd gain it back and couldn't lose it again. I had a heart problem. And it really disgusted me when I found out because I thought I was strong. I said, "I don't really have a heart problem, I can overcome this if I just act ornery, work hard, and keep doing what I'm doing and go back on a diet." Just stop eating breakfast and lunch. Almost just a starvation diet. But I found out when I did that, I'd lose twenty or thirty pounds until I went off it and I ate twice as much and I gained back twenty or thirty pounds plus even more. That was really getting to me.

And then my age was getting to me. I couldn't handle being fifty years old. I'd look around and I could see my life just passing me by. And all I could say was "What a waste." And I only get one chance at life. I felt like I'd blown fifty years. My wife said, "You haven't. Look at the three beautiful girls we've raised." I said, "Yeah, but I treated them all badly because I was a very selfish person."

Every time I did something, I didn't consult my wife, I didn't consult my girls, I didn't care. If I got a promotion, I would say, "Hey, we are moving tonight or tomorrow. We are selling the house." I didn't come home and talk to my wife about it first.

I was fat, I had a heart problem, and there had to be something better in life than that. Then Dr. Ornish called me up and asked, "What's more important, your job or your family?" And I immediately replied, "My job." And that really blew my mind. I asked myself, "What did I say that for?" And I realized that my job really was more important to me than my family at that time.

So, I really got to thinking. I said to myself, "If this guy's got a program that can help me with my weight and my heart, then maybe it will help me in other ways." So I signed up.

Although he described the program to me, it didn't really sink in. If I had understood that I was going to have to do meditation and I was going to have to get in a group and talk about my life, I wouldn't have enrolled, because I thought it showed weakness. Talking about myself and telling you that I've got a problem. Telling you that I have done some things to my wife and others and that I feel like I need to ask them for forgiveness. Telling you that I feel like I've been a no-good-bum husband and a bad father. I wouldn't have come. Because that wasn't my lifestyle. I am telling you like it is.

I had been telling myself, "I can handle these problems myself. I don't need your help. If I need your help, you can operate on me and fix my heart physically, but don't touch me mentally or emotionally because I have it all together." That's the type of person I was.

When I went to the research retreat and some of these things were thrown at me, I said to myself, "You know, I think I'll try this. I'm going to try it on for size. If it helps me a little, then I'm going to take another step." Even though I thought at the time that just about everything that we were doing was about as wimpy as you could imagine—eating vegetarian food, meditating, talking about our feelings. I mean, what could be wimpier than *that?*

To me, physicians are heroes. They've got all this education, and they really do something. And don't get me wrong, but psychologists, yeah, I thought they were all wimps. But when the psychologist in the study, Dr. Jim Billings, first met me, he said, "Now I'm your shrink and you had better watch what you say around me," immediately I liked the guy. I said, "Hey, this guy isn't a wimp, he's a pretty nice guy. He talks my language." We got along.

The food was a big change for me. When I came to the retreat and started to eat the food, I said, "What in the world did I get myself into? Where's my meat and my cheese?"

I don't know why I stayed. When Dr. Ornish first called me, it surprised me. Because no one outside my family had ever taken a concern for my well-being. And all of a sudden, here I have a doctor and some other people that said, "Hey, Dwayne, you've got a problem. We've got a program. We think it may help you, and we'd like for you to join us and find out."

At the retreat, I first said, "Well, I don't really think I have a problem with my life, I only have a heart problem. It's the only problem I've got." And then when I got in there and heard the other people talking, and when I met the other staff people, I said, "Wow, these are neat people. Not just a bunch of wimps, they're neat people. I'll give this another week or two." And I started to feel better. So I said to myself, "Okay, I'll give it six months."

Although I minimized my heart problem, I was under a lot of emotional stress at the time. I was charged, unfairly, with a crime I didn't commit (and for which I was later found to be not guilty). So I had to go to court. And that just about destroyed me.

I'm married with three grown girls, with two grandkids. I was afraid some people might think I was guilty. I was afraid to tell my wife, Kathy. So I was really feeling *bad.* I had gone through a lot of thoughts, including what would happen if I committed suicide? And if I did, what would be the easiest way to do it? Because I don't like pain. I don't want to think about it. Close my eyes and never wake up again. Enter eternity without God. I had even gone to *that.* And suicide had *never* entered my mind before. I was at the bottom.

I was very short-tempered. Moody. I was going through hearings and attorneys hours upon end. Had a huge attorney bill. Trying to keep that undercover. Kathy knew something was up.

Finally, she said, "There's something wrong. I haven't been living with you for twenty-five years and not know that something's wrong." I said, "There's nothing wrong. It's just my job. Don't worry about it." But every night I'd come home and I'd see her. And it really got to me.

So my whole relationship with her was slowly deteriorating. Not on her part but on mine. Because I couldn't face ever telling her. And I couldn't face ever telling my girls. It was just all inside, right here, and it couldn't come out. Attorneys knew it. People I was involved with knew. But none of my friends, not my family—nobody. "I'll handle this myself." But it was destroying my relationships.

I was hard on Kathy. I was hurtful. I would say things that would hurt her just to make her hush up. And our love relationship was just nothing—I just went through the motions. Because I had such guilt. And with that, you know, you have no feelings. It's just dead.

Because it was too painful to feel. It was too painful to realize that someone that loved me was being hurt. It was so painful that it was easier just to block out my feelings altogether. I'd block them out totally. I just wanted to block out the pain, but after a while, I was just numb. I couldn't feel pain or pleasure.

One night I told my pastor, and he said, "Dwayne, you've got to tell Kathy. You've got to do it one of these days." Well, that was on a Monday morning. I had been having too many bad thoughts. I said to myself, "What if I run away? Just vanish into the sunset. Hop on a train and nobody'll ever see me again." I was afraid to tell her, because I thought she'd leave me. She'd be hurt, and she wouldn't want to have anything to do with me. And take the kids with her.

On Tuesday night, I told her because I just couldn't hold it in any longer. And I didn't know if she would understand. I was afraid I'd be rejected. So I had to act tough and fight and pretend I wasn't afraid. I was so angry and hostile—physically and emotionally—because I was so afraid of being rejected and left all alone.

And I always thought that I could handle loneliness and aloneness, being by myself. That's what I always thought I wanted to be. I didn't want to make friends. I didn't want to get close to people. If I didn't get close to them, they couldn't hurt me.

To this day, I don't like to be rejected for anything. I don't like it. Yet I do that to other people, so why is it so hard for me to have people do that to me? I don't know. I have a double standard, I guess. Maybe it's like football—my coach used to tell me that the best defense is a good offense. I try not to do that to people anymore. But I was. I was doing it to gays.

I'm not now. There are certain people I don't like to associate with. But it's not just because they're gay, or whatever; it's on an individual basis.

If I had known there were going to be a few gay people in the study, I wouldn't have volunteered. Before I went to the retreat, I used to think I could spot them. But most of them look just like me and you.

When I met the people on the first day of the study, I said, "Hey, these guys look pretty good." But I found out that Oscar [not his real name], one of the men in the study, was gay. He was somebody who had treated my wife Kathy and me with exceptional grace and was just very pleasant, so I had to stop and think. She liked him immediately, and we would go to the room and say, well, he really *is* a nice guy. And then when he talked about or mentioned that he was gay,

I said, "Why do I feel that way towards gays?" I started to question myself and my motives and my attitude. And how I was really taught to love people but I wasn't doing it. I really took a second look at myself.

Kathy has been such a helpmate. We don't agree on everything, and we are very different from each other. Opposites attract, I guess. She has been my steady rock for thirty years. She comes up with some pretty neat things. And she loves people that I don't love. And she sees the good side of people when I don't see it.

She said something very positive about Oscar, so one day in our group discussion at the retreat I just decided, hey, maybe someday I need to talk to him, and this might be a good time to do it. We have two physicians and we have a psychologist here. Maybe they can spot me and figure out what's wrong with me.

During one of the group discussions at the end of my first week in this program, I told Oscar how I used to feel about gay people, how wrong that was, and how much I loved him. Afterwards, I walked over and gave him a hug.

I thought that I would be totally embarrassed. I really hadn't planned to do it. Kathy was totally taken aback—she didn't realize I had it in me to do that. I wanted to get something out of my system that had been there for years and years.

And it felt good. I felt a release of tension. I can remember it just like it was last night. I just felt a release. I felt, "Hey—this is what life is all about. It's made me feel better. Now I think I'll face some other things in this group. This group is going to help me." And I later shared with the group how I was falsely accused. And when *I* opened up, *they* opened up. Instead of rejecting me, we all felt a lot closer.

You know, we all have our lifestyles. I am a Christian, and it's really, really hard for me to profess because I don't want people to reject me. And people get nervous around people like that for some reason. I guess that's the way gays feel sometimes. You know, they hide in the closet and they don't like people to know they are gay because they don't want the rejection or whatever. So we have something in common—we don't like to be rejected.

I used to notice how different I was from other people—"You're a wimp, you're a different religion, you're a different race, you're from a different part of the country." You're this and I'm not. Like that.

Now, I'm beginning to find ways that we're similar as opposed to finding ways that we're different. And you know what's happening? We're smiling and looking at each other instead of grimacing and wanting to fight. And it feels great. I want to tell other people how great that feels.

Before, I was all in a knot inside. I was tight all the time. My muscles were tight. I even learned that my blood vessels were tight and restricted. When you walk around that way for years and years and you're uptight all the time, then it takes its toll on your body.

And that's not only with other people. That's true even in the family. If you're not getting along with your spouse or you're trying to keep things from her and you've got secrets that you should've told her, then you're like this all the time. You're always on edge. You're sitting there watching TV, you're afraid you're going to say something wrong. Or you're going to slip and say something, and she's going to say, "What did you mean by that?" And it's out of the bag. It's just like teenagers hiding smoking, they don't want their folks to know it. Or somebody taking drugs and they don't want their friends to find out.

And that fear of being found out creates a feeling of tightness and stress. Because if you're found out, you fear you'll be rejected and left all alone.

But I wasn't rejected. I confided to Kathy, my wife, about these things and found out she still loved me. Our relationship grew even stronger. Now, I'm not saying that would happen in every case, but in this case it did. And that *release* was there. She accepted me. And she still loves me. She knows all about my past. And now she loves me even more.

And then talking to Oscar and talking to Ralph [not his real name]—two gays in the study with me. "Say hey, guys, I have these hard, bad thoughts about your lifestyles. But I'm trying to change them. And I'm sorry. And, you know, I love you." And, *wham!* It just feels clean. You feel clean. Inside, the pressure leaves you. The chest pain and chest tightness leave you.

Sometimes, after I'm on my way home, I can't believe what I've said in the group. "What did I say that for?" But I feel so much better, I'm glad I did. Because I feel released. It feels like a burden has been lifted off of me when I've told somebody how I really feel about him.

And even though I showed who I really am, I wasn't rejected.

I was accepted. And you know what? The group opened up to me, showing me who they really are. There was a fellowship with some people who I'd been rejecting all along because I thought they didn't measure up to my standards. And what standards do I have to hold up, you know? I'm no better and no worse than they are.

And when I told the truth to Kathy, and when I found out that she didn't reject me, I felt loved for who I really am for the first time. I could stop pretending and hiding parts of myself. I could take off the masks I'd been wearing.

You can't put it in words, really. You can say all these words that you feel great. You feel released and you feel like you are sitting on top of the world, but there's no way to describe it.

You look at the world from a different perspective. You lose a lot of hate. You lose a lot of fear. You start loving more. It affects your love toward your family and others more than you realize—you thought you loved them but you didn't *really* love them. I took Kathy for granted a lot of the time. Now, all of a sudden, she's proven to me, "Hey, Dwayne, I really love you. Now trust me, tell me when it hurts. Tell me about your problems. And let me tell you about mine." We're able to share our secrets more.

And you really need somebody to share your secrets with. Because you just kind of go crazy inside if you don't. Your self-worth goes to pot, and you've always got a facade up there. You know you're trying to be somebody that you're really not.

Before the trial, I went there and did my breathing exercises and positive meditation and visualized what would happen in the courtroom. That, hey, I'm innocent and I'm going to tell it like it is. And I did. During the trial, the meditation and stress management techniques helped me through it. I felt very comfortable about it and I told the truth.

And it came out all right. Last week, the judge ruled in my favor. I'm not guilty. Of course, it's a big relief. But telling Kathy about being charged with a crime I didn't commit, and having her love and accept me before the judge ruled—that was a much bigger relief.

And I'm not saying that I'm perfect. I've got a long way to go. I've got a lot of things to ease up on, to become more comfortable with. But I've come a long way.

This program has helped in a lot of other ways, too. I've lost eighty-five pounds. When I started the program seven months ago I weighed 280 pounds. Now I'm right at 195.

Before, I was nothing but a meat-and-potatoes man. That's all I ate—I loved cheese and I loved meat. We used to like to go out and barbecue when we had the family and kids over—all big meals.

But if I could change, anybody can change. I'm serious about that. It was a struggle at first, but not after a few weeks. Once in a while, I miss a little cheese, but I don't miss eating meat.

And I don't go around feeling deprived or hungry. That's another thing about this program. If I get hungry, I know that I can eat whenever I want as long as it's the food on this program.

I've been on a lot of diets, and I went around hungry most of the time, starving. Lettuce didn't go very far. On every other diet I've been on, I had to count calories. I had to be careful not to eat too much. Now, I eat until I'm full. Before, I'd lose weight and gain it back like a yo-yo, but now I keep it off. It's just like regular eating habits. You eat three good meals a day, plus snacks. I feel great.

It's not a daily battle. I take a lot of customers to lunch—a lot of business lunches. And they order their fish or steak or whatever. And I'll order a salad and a fruit or some spaghetti with nothing on it and fruit. I eat until I'm full, and I'm satisfied.

My cholesterol has dropped from 310 down to 149, 161 points! And I'm not taking niacin or any other cholesterol-lowering drugs.

Before I started on this program, my blood pressure was high, around 150/90 even when I was taking blood pressure medicine [Corgard, a beta blocker]. My doctor told me I'd have to take it the rest of my life even though it made me tired and depressed. After a few months on the program, my doctor took me off it—said I didn't need it any more. Now it's 124/72 without medication. And it stays there. It's not a fluke. It's that low every time they test it.

Also, I was taking medication for my gout [Zyloprim]. And I stopped taking those pills, too, and I haven't needed them. Before, I'd have flare-ups of my gout every three or four months even when I was taking the medication.

And I don't snore any more. Now, that might not seem very important to some people, but it was a big problem for me. The snoring was so bad, my daughters could hear me all the way downstairs. My wife started wearing some earplugs but that didn't help, so she had to sleep downstairs. She never slept with me.

Now Kathy sleeps with me every night, all night long and I

don't snore at all. The snoring ceased when I lost about forty pounds. And I've never had that since.

Also, I have a lot more energy. I never have chest pain. I walk five miles a day now, almost every day. Before, my wife couldn't get me out of the house. I mean, I'd groan, moan, and complain. *I* drag *her* out of the house now. We really laugh about that now, and we enjoy walking together, but I used to really be ornery. I'm still a little ornery, but I used to be really *mean.* She'd ask, "Can we walk just a little further?" So I'd just head out and I'd leave her behind. And I'd walk as fast as I could. I knew it was hurting me, it was making me feel bad, and I wished I hadn't even done it, but I would keep going until I knew she was really upset and I'd put her in her place. But I wouldn't dream of doing that now.

I feel so much better about myself now that I've made all of these changes. I just changed jobs. I've been in the leasing business—a high-pressure business—for twenty-four years. Three months ago, I decided to get out of it and do something I liked better. I don't believe I'd have really been able to handle the stress of losing a job and the stress of trying to find another one if I hadn't been in this program. I would go out for interviews, and I felt comfortable, confident, assured. I knew I looked halfway decent, I didn't look like a Porky Pig. I didn't sweat, and I could cross my legs, and I felt good about myself.

I mean, it's totally different. I go down the road, I can drive without yelling at people. I look at people differently. I look at myself in the mirror and I'm beginning to like what I see. I don't say bad things when I walk past the mirror anymore. I have more respect for myself. I just feel like a new human being.

I love my wife. I told the group tonight that we've fallen in love again. It's a whole new life. I just wish everybody could have this.

And I love the meditation and stress management. When I come home from work, I have a light snack. Then Kathy and I go for a walk for an hour and fifteen minutes. When we get back, we eat, play with the dogs a little bit—then she says, "Let's go do our stress management." She loves doing it. If I say, "Let's skip tonight," then she says, "Nooooo, c'mon, let's do it." So we go upstairs and we do it for a whole hour.

I tell you, if I can do it, anybody can do it. And not only just the diet and exercise, but also the psychological part—getting rid of some of your animosities, hates, bigotry, all of that stuff that goes along with feeling bad about yourself. It's very helpful to have support of some kind. If you don't have it at home, then get some kind of group support like this.

And so, I guess, confessing your faults and sharing your feelings and your secrets with one another helps. My religion tells me to do that. But I never practiced it. And to love your brother as yourself—I never practiced that, either.

When you ask for forgiveness, when you ask for understanding, when you ask for love, then you're able to give these, too. That must be what the human body needs and what being human is all about. You know, it must be. Because it works.

"We all agree that your theory is crazy, but is it crazy enough?"

—Niels Bohr (Nobel Laureate/physics)

■

"All great truths begin as blasphemies."

—George Bernard Shaw,
Annajanska

■

"Whenever a new discovery is reported to the scientific world, they say first, 'It is probably not true.' Thereafter, when the truth of the new proposition has been demonstrated beyond question, they say, 'Yes, it may be true, but it is not important.' Finally, when sufficient time has elapsed to fully evidence its importance, they say, 'Yes, surely it is important, but it is no longer new.' "

—Michel de Montaigne (1533–1592)

■

"Be patient towards all that is unsolved in your heart and try to love the questions themselves."

—Rainer Maria Rilke,
Letters to a Young Poet

3

"Yes, That's True, But What Is the *Cause?*"

When I was a student, one of my teachers, a very wise man, had a habit of asking the same question over and over: "Yes, but what is the *cause*? And what is the cause of *that*? And what underlies *that* cause?" And so on.

His questions were a simple yet powerful means of getting to, well, the heart of what is really important. Once the underlying causes are identified, then a problem can be addressed at more fundamental levels. As introduced in chapter 1, a primary theme of this book is that *the farther back in the causal chain of events we can begin treating the problem, the more powerful can be the healing.*

Ideally, a problem can be addressed at many levels simultaneously. The opposite is also true: if we treat only the apparent problem without also dealing with the underlying causes, then (1) new problems may occur, (2) the old problem may recur or persist, and (3) treatments tend to be more difficult, expensive, and invasive, with greater side effects than if the underlying causes were also addressed.

Let's examine heart disease in this context.

What is coronary heart disease? What is a heart attack? What causes these to occur?

The bottom line is simply this: the heart becomes starved for the oxygen carried in the blood. As described in chapter 1, if the oxygen deprivation is brief, then chest pain (angina) occurs; if prolonged for more than a few minutes, the result is a heart attack.

What causes the heart to become starved for oxygen and blood?

CORONARY ARTERY BLOCKAGES

The heart pumps blood to feed itself through what are called coronary arteries. Oxygen is food for the heart, and it is carried in the blood.

Three major coronary arteries feed the heart. The right coronary artery feeds the right side of the heart. Two other coronary arteries feed the left side of the heart: the left anterior descending artery (which feeds the front of the heart) and the circumflex coronary artery (which curves around to feed the back of the heart). These major coronary arteries branch into smaller ones farther downstream (see figure 3.1).

Until relatively recently, most of what we knew about heart disease was learned at the autopsy table, since tools were not available to observe and study the living heart. When someone who died from a heart attack was autopsied, in most cases *blockages* were found in one or more of the coronary arteries, so these obstructions (also called *plaque, atherosclerosis,* or *arteriosclerosis*) were thought to be the main cause of chest pain and heart attacks. On further analysis, these blockages were found to be comprised of cholesterol and other deposits. This was one of the first clues that dietary cholesterol played a role in causing the blockages to form.

Over time, plaque can build up inside the lining of the coronary arteries, somewhat like rust accumulating inside a pipe. Studies of soldiers who were killed in World War II, Korea, and Vietnam indicated that most of these young men already had some mild

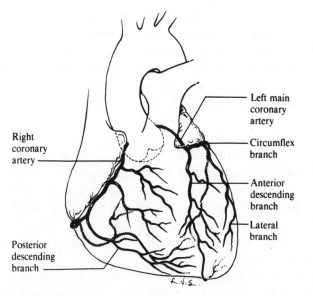

Figure 3.1. Heart and Arteries

blockages forming in their coronary arteries. More recent studies of children who died accidentally in the town of Bogalusa, Louisiana, revealed that many of them already had some blockages forming in their coronary arteries, especially if their cholesterol levels were elevated. In most people, the blockages form slowly and chronically over a period of decades.

The first step back in this causal chain was the realization that coronary artery blockages led to reduced blood flow to the heart and thus to chest pain and heart attacks. So in the 1950s, surgeons invented new ways of trying to increase blood flow to the heart. This was an appealing idea, but limited, since it only went back one step in the chain: The surgery tried to improve blood flow around the blockages without dealing with the more fundamental question of what causes the blockages.

The first surgical approach was called the Vineberg procedure, named after the surgeon who devised it in 1946. In this operation, the internal mammary artery that supplies blood to part of the chest wall was redirected and spliced into the coronary artery downstream from the coronary artery blockages in an attempt to increase the blood flow to the heart. The procedure sounded good in theory, and many thousands were performed.

After a few years, through, controlled scientific studies determined that the operation was worthless. While the chest pain was reduced in many people who had this operation, studies found that performing *sham* operations caused patients' chest pain to be equally relieved. In these procedures (unethical by today's standards), patients would undergo anesthesia, have their chests cut open and then sewn up without anything else having been done.

In 1961, the first coronary artery bypass operation was performed. In that procedure, a vein was removed from the patient's leg and spliced around the coronary artery blockages.

During the 1960s and 1970s, cardiac surgeons became the most powerful doctors in many medical centers, while the status of cardiologists declined somewhat. When I was an intern, the demand for bypass surgery was so great that patients would sometimes wait in the hospital for weeks—we called it "orbiting"—before a surgical date was available.

Surgeons became so enthusiastic about this operation that for many years they refused to participate in randomized, controlled clinical trials to determine whether or not the operation was beneficial in prolonging life. (In one hospital, the chief of cardiology prudently moved to Florida soon after he wrote an article questioning the value of bypass surgery.) Two decades later, in the early 1980s, three major randomized, controlled clinical studies finally were published demonstrating that bypass surgery provided only marginal benefit for most patients with moderate to severe heart disease when compared with conventional medical therapy (that is, drugs). In other words, many of the patients who underwent bypass surgery didn't really need it. By 1987, however, over 200,000 patients were undergoing the operation each year at an average cost of over $30,-000 each. A report from Harvard's Dr. Thomas Graboys and Dr. Bernard Lown, published in the *Journal of the American Medical Association* in 1987, stated that at least one fourth of bypass operations were unnecessary.

Bypass surgery did prolong life somewhat in patients with extremely severe disease. But compared to what? All of these studies compared patients undergoing bypass surgery only with those who were taking cardiac medications (but not cholesterol-lowering drugs), not with patients who were making comprehensive lifestyle changes.

So bypass surgery is another example of what happens when we do not go back very far in the chain of causation. New problems occur (heart attacks, strokes, infection, or death can occur during bypass surgery, and up to one third of patients who undergo bypass surgery suffer some transient or permanent neurological damage or decrease in IQ), the old problem may recur or persist (50 percent of bypassed arteries clog up again within five years, and 80 percent become blocked after seven years). Similarly, a recent study found that the incidence of strokes was *higher* in people who underwent cerebral bypass surgery. Both operations are very expensive and extremely invasive. Coronary bypass surgery consumes more health dollars than any other procedure.

So many bypass operations are performed each year that it almost seems routine. Most people do not fully appreciate how invasive and traumatic a bypass operation can be.

In 1977, Dr. Andreas Gruentzig invented balloon angioplasty, a somewhat less invasive approach than coronary bypass surgery. In this procedure, a small balloon is passed through a tube inside a blocked coronary artery. The balloon is inflated, squishing the blockage and making more room for blood to flow.

Because it was less traumatic for patients, angioplasty had important advantages over bypass surgery. Angioplasty also gave cardiologists a tool to regain from cardiac surgeons much of their lost status and income. Within a few years, many cardiologists all over the world began performing angioplasty—first only on single arterial blockages, then on multiple blockages. Many of the cardiologists who had criticized heart surgeons for not performing controlled clinical trials of bypass surgery when it was first introduced began performing angioplasty on a regular basis before knowing its long-term effectiveness. In only five years, the number of angioplasties skyrocketed from about 32,000 in 1983 to about 200,000 in 1988, with proportionate increases in costs.

Again, we can see the same pattern emerging from not going back very far in the chain of causation. New problems occurred (sometimes coronary arteries dissect or rupture when the balloon is inflated, requiring a quick trip to the operating room for emergency bypass surgery), and the old problem often recurred or persisted. *One third* of arteries dilated by angioplasty will clog up again *within four to six months,* and this approach is expensive and invasive, although less so than bypass surgery. (Our program does not seem to affect whether or not these dilated arteries stay open, although it often benefits the nondilated arteries. The damage that the angioplasty balloon causes to the lining of the coronary artery appears to override the effects of lifestyle factors.) Although designed to prevent heart attacks, however, angioplasty sometimes causes it. In the first 3,000 cases, about 4.5 percent of the patients had a heart attack during angioplasty, and 8.8 percent required emergency bypass surgery. (With practice, those figures are now better.)

Heart transplants and the artificial heart are perhaps the epitome of this approach in treating coronary heart disease, of what happens when we fail to go back very far in the chain of causation.

Dr. Christian Barnard captured the imagination of the world when he performed the first heart transplant in 1967. This was the zenith of heart surgery's golden era, and it seemed then as though anything would be possible.

Unfortunately, the same pattern again emerged. New problems occurred (rejection of transplanted hearts), the old problem recurred (even hearts with normal coronary arteries at the time of transplant often became clogged within a few years, since patients hadn't changed their lifestyles), and the approach was extremely expensive (at least $100,000 per operation) and invasive. In general, heart transplants are now performed primarily to treat cardiomyopathy in younger people, a degenerative disease of the heart muscle that is usually unrelated to coronary heart disease and for which this operation can be better justified.

Twenty years later, Dr. William DeVries implanted the first artificial heart in Barney Clark. Again, however, the technology did not fulfill the initial expectations. New problems occurred (infections, psychosis, limited mobility), the old problem recurred (blood clots formed in the artificial heart and lodged in the arteries of Mr. Clark's brain, causing strokes), and the approach was even more expensive and invasive than heart transplants. Even after surgery, the patient remained tethered to a large external pump. These problems were so severe that the National Institutes of Health voted to discontinue spending millions of dollars on the artificial heart program.

All of these technologies have their place, and sometimes, when appropriate, I recommend most of them, especially during a life-threatening crisis or if a patient does not wish to make lifestyle changes. I have great respect and admiration for the skill, training, and dedication of cardiologists and cardiac surgeons, and they are doing what they sincerely believe is best for their patients.

The point is simply this: none of these approaches—drugs, bypass surgery, angioplasty, heart transplants, or an artificial heart—addresses the more fundamental causes of heart disease, so *all trade one set of problems for another.* Instead of trying to find more effective ways of undoing the damage, why don't we concentrate on finding out what causes heart disease in the first place?

WHAT CAUSES CORONARY BLOCKAGES TO FORM?

Let's go back another step in the causal chain. What causes coronary artery blockages to form? If we can address this at a more fundamental level, then we can design treatments that are more effective and less expensive and that produce fewer new problems and side effects.

Blockages form when the lining of a coronary artery is damaged. The body attempts to repair this insult by putting the physiological equivalent of a Band-Aid over the damaged area. This band-aid is made of cholesterol, collagen, and other materials.

If the injury to the lining is chronic, then the band-aids begin to pile up, one on top of another. Over time—decades—these begin to build up and form coronary artery blockages. Like the fight-or-flight mechanism discussed later in this chapter, the body's attempt to heal itself becomes destructive and even deadly when the injury is chronic and repetitive.

What injures the lining of the coronary arteries?

- high blood cholesterol levels
- excessive dietary cholesterol and saturated fat (independent of blood cholesterol levels)
- high blood pressure
- nicotine

Let's examine each of these.

High Blood Levels of Cholesterol and Excessive Intake of Saturated Fat and Cholesterol
Besides providing the building blocks for the blockages, high blood levels of cholesterol can actually injure the lining of the arteries. This double-whammy is one reason why cholesterol plays such an important role in causing the formation of coronary artery blockages.

A recent report in the *Journal of the American Medical Association* stated that *one half of all adult Americans have cholesterol levels high enough to require treatment.* But what kind of treatment?

Most people—and even drug companies—agree that the first step is diet. The American Heart Association and the National Cholesterol Education Program guidelines advise patients with elevated cholesterol levels to reduce their daily fat intake from 40 percent to 30 percent of total calories (since your body converts saturated fat to cholesterol), and to reduce cholesterol consumption from 500 milligrams to 300 milligrams per day. This is a good first step.

Unfortunately, this type of diet will cause only small reductions in blood cholesterol levels in most people and their cholesterol levels will still be too high. A study published in the *New England Journal of Medicine* reported that even a diet with only 20 percent fat did not reduce cholesterol levels significantly more than a diet containing 30 percent fat.

So, both patients and their doctors get very frustrated. "I'm eating a low-fat, low-cholesterol diet, but my cholesterol level won't come down very much. What can I do?" Many doctors will reply, "Well, I guess you'll have to start taking cholesterol-lowering drugs for the rest of your life."

All of the physicians I know are motivated primarily by the desire to be useful, not just to make money. But the influence of drug companies is so pervasive that, from the first day of medical school, it affects and in many ways determines how medicine is practiced and how disease is viewed.

Drug companies spend millions of dollars educating physicians. Drug companies are the major advertisers in all medical journals. They fund clinical trials to determine the effectiveness of their drugs and they pay these researchers to speak at hospitals and medical schools. And if a drug company that makes a cholesterol-lowering drug provides most of the funds to conduct research on the effectiveness of that drug, then there is a potential for bias, even if unwittingly, despite independent monitoring committees that sometimes oversee these studies. Drug companies provide sandwiches and doughnuts at hospital conferences and for the doctors' lounges. They provide free samples of their products. Drug companies also sponsor scientific meetings on the importance of lowering cholesterol, often emphasizing the importance of cholesterol-lowering drugs. These meetings are sometimes held in resorts, and doctors who attend may even be given free transportation and expenses in addition to their food and entertainment.

There is nothing inherently wrong with any of this, and it is all very comfortable and familiar. But in subtle and sometimes overt ways, the message to doctors gets through: "Drug companies are your friends. Patients are not really willing to change their diet and lifestyles very much, so why waste your time? Why bother? It's so much quicker and easier to prescribe our drugs, and they work."

The problem with cholesterol-lowering drugs is that they are expensive and they have side effects, both known and unknown. The newer cholesterol-lowering drugs, such as lovastatin (Mevacor), are *very* expensive, costing up to $2,000–3,000 per person per year. Since there are 100 million Americans with elevated blood cholesterol levels, treating everyone with these drugs would cost *$200–300 billion* per year, which is clearly not feasible.

Besides the expense, these drugs have side effects. Short-term side effects of lovastatin may include liver damage and possibly cataracts. Side effects of other cholesterol-lowering drugs include intestinal problems, nausea, bloating, and abdominal pain. No one even knows the long-term effects of putting millions of Americans on the newer cholesterol-lowering drugs for the rest of their lives.

High doses of niacin are sometimes used to lower cholesterol. Although niacin is a vitamin and is available without prescription, the amount of niacin required to lower cholesterol is so high that it becomes a drug when taken in large doses. Side effects of niacin include liver damage (usually reversible when the niacin is discontinued), glucose intolerance, gout, headaches, itching, and skin flushing.

As described in chapter 1, only two studies to date have demonstrated that cholesterol-lowering drugs may reverse heart disease, and reversal occurred in only the minority of patients. Other investigations, including the $170 million dollar National Heart, Lung, and Blood Institute "Type II" study, found that cholesterol-lowering drugs did not reverse coronary heart disease. In contrast, most of the people in the lifestyle-change group of our study showed some overall reversal of their heart disease.

Currently, there are several other ongoing investigations to determine if cholesterol-lowering drugs can reverse heart disease. Eventually, some studies may find that they do. Even if this were so, though, I don't believe that using drugs to lower cholesterol would be the best approach.

I prescribe cholesterol-lowering drugs only for people who do not wish to change their lifestyle according to our guidelines—i.e., as an adjunct or as a last resort, not as a first choice. Following the Opening Your Heart program is a better first choice, since it may be more effective than cholestrol-lowering drugs, the only side effects of this program are good ones (as described in chapters 2 and 6), it is inexpensive, and it addresses the emotional and spiritual dimensions of heart disease as well.

I prefer to educate, not to dictate. If a person has heart disease, then I might say, "Mr. Jones [or Ms. Smith], you have severe heart disease, and you may want to do something about it. If you are willing to make comprehensive lifestyle changes, we now have evidence indicating that your heart disease may be stopped and often even reversed. I may ask you to take some cardiac drugs for a while until the lifestyle changes begin to take effect. If, for whatever reason, you think this approach is not right for you and you do not wish to make these lifestyle changes, then you may need to take cholesterol-lowering drugs and other medications for the rest of your life and you may need angioplasty or bypass surgery."

The Opening Your Heart program described in this book may cause reductions in blood cholesterol comparable to the decreases caused by cholesterol-lowering drugs. Instead of categorizing some people as diet-responsive and others as unresponsive to diet, we are finding that *the vast majority of people are diet-responsive if the diet is sufficiently low in cholesterol and saturated fat.*

The two studies most frequently cited that examined the value of cholesterol-lowering drugs on reducing heart attacks are the Lipid Research Clinics trial and the Helsinki Heart Study. A recent article in the *New England Journal of Medicine* by Dr. Allan Brett of the Harvard Medical School raised important questions about how these two investigations have been interpreted.

These two studies produced similar results. Both enrolled asymptomatic middle-aged men with high blood cholesterol levels (averaging about 290). In each study, patients in one group were given a cholesterol-lowering drug—cholestyramine (Questran) or gemfibrozil (Lopid)—whereas patients in the other group were given a placebo, a pill with no drug effects.

After seven years of follow-up in the Lipid Research Clinics study, 155 of 1906 men who were given a cholesterol-lowering drug had heart attacks as compared with 187 of 1900 patients who were given a placebo (8.1 percent versus 9.8 percent). After five years in the Helsinki study, 56 of the 2051 men who were given a cholesterol-lowering drug had heart attacks as compared with 84 of 2030 patients who were given a placebo (2.7 percent versus 4.1 percent). In interpreting these data, Dr. Brett made the following points:

- Most of the people who were treated with a cholesterol-lowering drug did not benefit from drug treatment. "Treatment improves one's chances of not having a cardiac event form about 96 percent to a bit more than 97 percent over five years."
- "Many people must be treated [with drugs] to benefit relatively few. When an intervention is not burdensome and is free of risk [like the Opening Your Heart program described in this book], this issue becomes less important. But when a large population undergoes a [drug] treatment alleged to benefit only 1 or 2 percent of its members, the balance of burdens and benefits requires close scrutiny."
- "Neither the Lipid Research Clinics nor the Helsinki Heart Study demonstrated a reduction in overall mortality." In other words, taking cholesterol-lowering drugs didn't help most participants to live longer.
- There was an excess of violent and accidental deaths among the patients who took cholesterol-lowering drugs in the Lipid Research Clinics study. A similar trend occurred in the Helsinki study. It's unclear whether this is an unanticipated side effect of these drugs.
- "Some physicians may find it easier to focus on the serum cholesterol level than on a careful assessment of a patient's lifestyle and values. . . . Patients need to be reassured that the cholesterol level is only one variable in the highly complex equation that determines how long and how well we live."

In the same issue of the *New England Journal of Medicine,* Dr. Alexander Leaf, Chairman of the Department of Preventive Medicine, at Harvard Medical School, made the following observations:

- "In societies in which the mean cholesterol levels are 150 or lower without the use of drugs, coronary heart disease is essentially unknown as a public health problem."

- "Life expectancy is not unlimited. . . . Adding days of vigorous well-being or reduced morbidity would seem more rational goals for a health care system, although they are more difficult to quantify, than the extension of life expectancy."
- "Elevated cholesterol levels are very important in the genesis of atherosclerosis, but they are not synonymous with the disease. Many genetic factors and environmental risk factors can increase or decrease the tolerance to elevated cholesterol levels."

There *is* a genetic variability in how efficiently (or inefficiently) a person metabolizes dietary saturated fat and cholesterol. Some people can eat almost anything yet their blood cholesterol levels do not increase very much. (These are the people who sometimes live to be one hundred, and when interviewed attribute their longevity to the twelve eggs and sausage they have been eating for breakfast every morning.) Others find that even a small amount of dietary fat or cholesterol makes their blood cholesterol levels increase. Most people are somewhere in between on this spectrum.

Why? Drs. Michael Brown and Joseph Goldstein won the Nobel Prize in Medicine in 1985 for their discovery of *LDL-cholesterol receptors.* These receptors are located primarily in liver cells, and they bind and remove cholesterol from the bloodstream.

The more cholesterol receptors you have, the more efficiently you can metabolize and remove cholesterol from your blood. The fewer cholesterol receptors you have, the more your blood cholesterol level will increase when you eat saturated fat and cholesterol.

The number of cholesterol receptors is, in part, genetically determined. However, if the amount of saturated fat and cholesterol in your diet is low enough, then your blood cholesterol level will be low even if you don't have very many cholesterol receptors. In other words, even if you are not very efficient at removing fat and cholesterol from your blood, it doesn't matter if you don't eat very much of it.

The amount of fat and cholesterol in the diet described in this book is so low that these genetic differences become much less important. As a result, almost everyone in our program showed significant reductions in their cholesterol levels. On the other hand, for many people—and for most people who have heart disease—even a 20 percent fat diet has too much saturated fat and cholesterol in it.

Only about 5 percent of people have genetically high cholesterol levels that remain elevated regardless of lifestyle. Even in some of these cases, our lifestyle program may help, as in the case of Robert Royall described in chapter 1. That is, when people followed our program 100 percent, their arteries begin to open even when their blood cholesterol levels did not fall below 200.

Lifestyle factors also influence the number of cholesterol receptors. A diet high in saturated fat and cholesterol produces what Drs. Brown and Goldstein termed "double trouble." The dietary fat and cholesterol not only saturate the receptors, they also decrease the number of receptors—a bad combination. Fortunately, the Reversal Diet (described in chapter 10) gives a double benefit: it increases the number of cholesterol receptors and it does not saturate these receptors.

Your body makes all the cholesterol it needs, even if you don't eat any cholesterol in your diet and even if you reduce your saturated fat intake. In fact, three fourths of the cholesterol in your blood is made by your body. It's the *excessive* amounts of cholesterol and saturated fat in our diet that lead to coronary heart disease.

Besides drugs, there are a variety of other substances that will lower blood cholesterol levels to some degree. Eating alfalfa will help. So will psyllium husks. Eating garlic will lower cholesterol levels somewhat (it will also help reduce your stress by keeping people away from you). Ingesting the insecticide DDT will raise your HDL or "good" cholesterol (which I'll discuss in chapter 10), but that's not an advisable way to do it. Eating oat bran or rice bran is another popular way of trying to lower cholesterol.

Like drugs, though, these substances do not go far enough back in the causal chain. Instead of limiting the amount of saturated fat and cholesterol in their diet, many people believe that eating oat bran or other soluble fibers will somehow magically protect them and lower their blood cholesterol levels. (Some oat bran muffins contain more fat than a chocolate cream donut.) They use it almost like an amulet to protect them from heart disease instead of changing their lifestyle. Thirteen years ago, in the first study I conducted, one of the patients came up to me and said, "Dean, I had a cheeseburger today—but I had it on a whole wheat bun." Another patient said, "I've stopped eating red meat—now I order it well-done."

High Blood Pressure

Hypertension, or high blood pressure, also injures the coronary artery lining and leads to the formation of coronary blockages. When blood pressure is elevated, the blood hits the side of the arterial wall with increased force, thereby causing some injury or damage to the lining of the artery. In response to this injury, blockages begin to form as described earlier.

This creates a vicious cycle: as the artery becomes increasingly blocked, the blood pressure increases—like a garden hose whose nozzle becomes smaller and smaller. As the pressure increases, more injury to the lining occurs, causing more blockages, increasing the pressure, and so on.

Many studies clearly indicate that high blood pressure—systolic or diastolic—increases the risk of coronary heart disease. Most physicians treat high blood pressure by prescribing anti-hypertensive drugs. These drugs are effective in lowering blood pressure in most people. Like the cholesterol-lowering drugs, however, the problem with anti-hypertensive drugs is that they are costly and have side effects, both known and unknown.

The side effects of anti-hypertensive drugs can be considerable, including impotence, fatigue, depression, and blood cell disorders. So it is not surprising that up to 90 percent of patients who are prescribed these drugs do not take them as directed.

Sometimes these side effects are deadly. Although most physicians strongly believe that treating high blood pressure with drugs is a good thing to do, new data raise some important questions about this. A recent report from the National Heart, Lung, and Blood Institute published in an American Heart Association journal, *Hypertension,* reviewed the designs and major results of the seventeen large-scale, controlled, clinical trials that reported the effects of drug treatment of hypertension on cardiovascular disease. Of these seventeen studies, nine analyzed populations with less severe hypertension (diastolic blood pressure less than 105). This analysis, called a "meta-analysis," reached a very surprising conclusion.

In these 43,000 patients with moderate hypertension who were followed for an average of 5.6 years, *decreasing blood pressure with drugs did not significantly reduce coronary heart disease mortality.* In approximately one half of the studies, the nonintervention control group had fewer nonfatal heart attacks and fewer fatal heart attacks than the group treated with drugs!

Why? For many years, diuretics (such as Dyazide) have been prescribed as the first-line drug to treat high blood pressure. Unfortunately, diuretics *increase* blood sugar and blood cholesterol levels (especially the LDL, or "bad" cholesterol). Also, they *decrease* blood levels of potassium and magnesium, which increases the risk of sudden cardiac death.

A beneficial effect of anti-hypertensive drugs was clearer in patients who had severe hypertension. But most people who have hypertension have only mildly elevated blood pressure, and it is for this group that our lifestyle program can be most beneficial.

At least 60 million Americans are considered to be hypertensive (that is, they have blood pressures greater than 140/90). In a recent article, Dr. Norman Kaplan, a renowned hypertension expert, pointed out that "readings in as many as 80 percent of patients are lower when taken out of the office. . . . This study and many more document the inescapable fact that, for some patients, the doctor's office may be the only place where the blood pressure is high." Dr. Kaplan terms this phenomenon "white coat hypertension" and estimates that at least 20 percent of people with diagnosed high blood pressure may not really need treatment.

In our research, we originally intended to keep everyone with high blood pressure on the same medications to avoid confounding the interpretation of our results. What we found in all three of our studies was that *most of the patients who followed our lifestyle program had to decrease or discontinue their blood pressure medications.* Their blood pressures were getting so low that many were becoming lightheaded or even faint.

Other researchers have confirmed that comprehensive lifestyle changes reduce blood pressure. A recent study by Dr. Herbert Benson at Harvard Medical School found that patients' blood pressure remained significantly reduced three to five years after making lifestyle changes that included meditation, group support, diet, and exercise.

All of which illustrates another major theme of this book: if you go far enough back in the causal chain—that is, if you treat the cause of the problem—then the patient won't need to take so many—or any—drugs. If drugs are used to control a patient's symptoms without also treating the underlying causes of the illness, then that patient will probably have to take these drugs for the rest of his or her life, often in ever-increasing dosages and with unpleasant and sometimes dangerous side effects.

Many studies have examined the effects of anti-hypertensive drug treatment on severe illness and death. Despite increasing evidence that diet, weight loss, stress management, stopping smoking, and exercise can help reduce blood pressure, there has never been a single long-term, randomized, controlled study to determine the effects of nondrug treatments of high blood pressure on severe illness or death. The same is true for high cholesterol levels. Treating high blood pressure does significantly reduce the incidence of stroke (although strokes are much less common than heart disease), but we do not know if nondrug approaches are equally effective since all of these studies use drugs.

Mild hypertension is very common. Some studies have found that up to 40 percent of people over age fifty have mild hypertension, comparable to the percentage of people with elevated cholesterol levels. Are we going to treat that many people with drugs? Wouldn't it be better to try other approaches that are less expensive, safer, and with healthful rather than harmful side effects? Is this really such a radical idea?

As Dr. H. L. Langford wrote recently, "We can theoretically prevent hypertension if we can change the environmental factors that interact with the genetic components to raise blood pressure."

A large-scale study in Helsinki compared 612 people who were intensively treated with anti-hypertensive and cholesterol-lowering drugs to a control group of 610 people who received usual medical care with fewer drugs. Although these drugs produced a 35 percent overall reduction in risk factors (primarily blood pressure and cholesterol levels) in the drug-treated group, *the participants developed twice as much heart disease* after five years when compared with the control group of patients that took fewer anti-hypertensive and cholesterol-lowering drugs!

In the U.S., blood pressure levels tend to rise as people age. Likewise, blood cholesterol levels tend to rise as people get older. In other countries though (including most of Asia and Africa) where peoples' lifestyles are similar to the Opening Your Heart program, neither blood pressure nor blood cholesterol rise with age, and the incidence of heart disease is also very low.

As with cholesterol-lowering drugs, I sometimes prescribe anti-hypertensive drugs, but usually not as the primary treatment. In patients with severe hypertension (usually if greater than 160/100), and in those who already have evidence of end-organ damage (for example, those with an enlarged heart, kidney disease, or eye disease), then I will begin treating elevated blood pressure with medication while simultaneously recommending the lifestyle program outlined in this book. Patients who follow this program will often show significant reductions in blood pressure, and I will taper or discontinue blood pressure medications slowly as this process occurs. If, for whatever reason, patients with high blood pressure or high cholesterol levels do not wish to change their lifestyle or if their blood pressure remains high despite lifestyle changes, then I recommend that they continue taking medication to lower their blood pressure or cholesterol indefinitely (or until they decide to change their lifestyle).

One of the nice side effects for many patients who are following the Opening Your Heart program is renewed sexual vigor, since patients are often able to reduce or discontinue the anti-hypertensive and cardiac drugs that can cause impotence, as discussed earlier in this chapter. Also, when someone has blockages in his coronary arteries, he likely has some blockages in *all* of his arteries, including the vessels that supply blood to the penis. Erection problems sometimes appear before obvious heart disease is diagnosed. So if improving your coronary arteries is not sufficient motivation to begin changing your lifestyle, perhaps improving your sexual function will be.

Nicotine

Most people know that cigarettes are the major cause of lung cancer. Less well known is that smoking causes many more deaths from heart disease than from lung cancer, in both men and women.

It's easier to see why smoking leads to lung cancer, since the smoke is inhaled into the lungs. Why does smoking help cause heart attacks?

The nicotine and other toxic substances in tobacco are absorbed into the blood and injure the lining of the coronary arteries. As I will describe later in this chapter, nicotine also causes the coronary arteries to constrict and blood clots to form and lodge in the coronary arteries.

What is the current first-line treatment that most doctors give their patients who want to stop smoking? Another drug—in this case, nicotine gum. Since nicotine can injure the lining of the coronary arteries, this is not much better than smoking as far as your heart is concerned (although your lungs will be pleased).

Of course, quitting smoking is not easy (see chapter 11 for help).

Paradoxically, though, most people I work with find it easier to quit smoking if they also change their lifestyle in comprehensive ways. At first, though they may ask, "How do you expect me to change my diet, begin to exercise, and learn stress management techniques when it's hard enough to just quit smoking?" Since many people smoke when they feel stressed, then it's easier to quit when they have alternative ways of managing stress that aren't centered around smoking. Also, when a person makes comprehensive lifestyle changes, they begin feeling so much better that the harmful effects of smoking become more apparent. So the craving and daily battle of not smoking become much easier.

CORONARY ARTERY SPASM, PLAQUE HEMORRHAGE, AND BLOOD CLOTS

Besides coronary artery blockages, what else causes the heart to become starved for blood? Let's go another step back in the causal chain.

In the late 1970s, studies in Italy by Dr. Attilio Maseri and others demonstrated that the cause of heart disease was more dynamic and complex than had previously been thought, and that other mechanisms besides blockages played important roles in reducing blood flow to the heart. He demonstrated that the coronary arteries are not rigid, like lead pipes; the arteries are flexible and are lined with smooth muscle that can constrict, thus reducing coronary blood flow. This constriction of the artery is known as *coronary artery spasm,* or just spasm.

When a coronary artery goes into spasm, it can injure the lining of the artery, leading to cholesterol deposition and plaque buildup as described earlier. Also, another mechanism known as *plaque hemorrhage* can result: the spasm can injure the lining of the coronary artery so badly that bleeding occurs into the wall of the vessel, causing the wall of the artery to bulge into the artery, thus obstructing blood flow through the artery.

Another important mechanism that can reduce blood flow to the heart is a *thrombus,* or *blood clot.* Small blood clots can form and lodge inside a coronary artery, thereby obstructing blood flow to the heart.

In most people, these mechanisms work in combination. That is, if a coronary artery is already 70 percent clogged with plaque, then even a small blood clot can lodge in the artery and reduce blood flow to the heart (causing chest pain) or block it completely (leading to a heart attack). Likewise, the more blocked with plaque an artery is, the less coronary artery spasm is required to reduce or shut down blood flow to the heart (see figure 3.2).

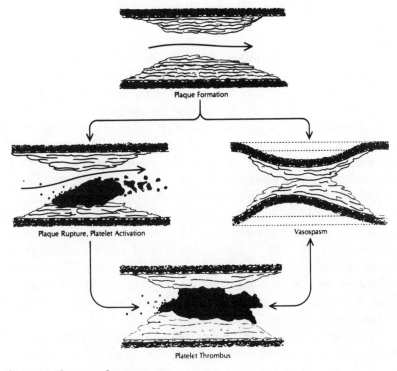

Figure 3.2. Coronary Spasm
BY ALAN ISELIN

All of these mechanisms interact and interrelate. As these became better understood and accepted by the medical community, doctors began to look for ways to keep these mechanisms from being activated. For example, it has been known for a long time that aspirin interferes with blood clot formation (this is the reason surgeons often instruct patients not to take aspirin before an operation, which would increase the risk of bleeding). For many years, this was viewed simply as a troubling side effect of aspirin when it was given to reduce pain. (Americans consume over thirty million *pounds* of aspirin every year!) Doctors then began to wonder if aspirin could reduce the incidence of heart attacks by helping prevent blood clots from forming inside the heart.

A large clinical trial was established to see if aspirin prevented heart attacks. The Physicians' Health Study, as it was called, randomly divided over 22,000 doctors into two groups: one group took an aspirin every other day, the other group took a placebo. Until the study was completed, only an independent data monitoring board knew who took which. (Bristol-Myers, maker of Bufferin aspirin, helped to fund this study.) Neither group was asked to make lifestyle changes.

After five years of follow-up, the group that took aspirin had 44 percent fewer nonfatal heart attacks than the placebo group. For ethical reasons, the study was stopped early, news was made, and it seemed that everyone should start taking aspirin.

A closer look at the results of that study revealed that while aspirin did reduce the incidence of heart attacks, it increased the risk of hemorrhagic strokes: bleeding into the brain. The group that took aspirin had over twice the incidence of moderate to severe hemorrhagic strokes when compared with the placebo group. Also, the incidence of sudden cardiac death was almost twice as high in the aspirin group, and the incidence of gastric and duodenal ulcers was almost twice as high in the aspirin-treated group. Although the group taking aspirin had fewer heart attacks, *overall, there was no difference between the two groups in number of deaths resulting from heart disease or from all causes of death.* Similar results were found in the British Doctors' Trial.

This is not surprising. Heart attacks usually occur when a small blood clot lodges in an artery that is already significantly blocked with cholesterol and other deposits—so the blood clot is the final blow in a person who already has significant coronary atherosclerosis. Since aspirin interferes with blood clot formation, the incidence of heart attacks decreases. For the same reasons, though, the risk of bleeding in your stomach or brain or heart *increases.*

So, using the same model that we have been discussing throughout this chapter, taking aspirin is only one step farther back in the causal chain than bypass surgery, and we see a similar pattern. New problems occur (hemorrhagic strokes, gastrointestinal bleeding, sudden cardiac death, etc.) and the old problem recurs (aspirin does not affect coronary atherosclerosis, so the blockages continue to build up over time). Since we are a step farther back in the causal chain, however, aspirin is much less expensive and invasive than bypass surgery. Other drugs, like dipyridamole (Persantine), heparin, and warfarin (Coumadin) are sometimes prescribed to help prevent blood clots and heart attacks, with similar side effects. (Some patients, especially those who have had massive heart attacks or who have what are called ventricular aneurysms, bulging areas of the heart damaged by a heart attack, are at much higher risk for blood clot formation. For them, the benefits of aspirin or Coumadin may outweigh the risks.)

Fish oil capsules also interfere with blood clotting. It has long been known that Greenland Eskimos have relatively low rates of coronary heart disease even though their diet is high in fat. Scientists learned that the fatty fish they consume is rich in omega-3 fatty acids, also called EPAs (for eicosopentanoic acid). Television and magazine advertisements began to appear, showing Eskimos sitting around a fire, eating blubber, while the announcer promoted fish oil capsules. What these advertisements failed to mention is that Eskimos have among the highest rates of hemorrhagic stroke in the world. Also, fish oil capsules tend to *raise* cholesterol levels. EPAs may have some beneficial effects, and these can be obtained from *The Reversal Diet* discussed in chapter 10 without consuming fish oils.

A new category of drugs, known as calcium-channel blockers, was developed to help prevent the occurance of coronary artery spasm. Like other cardiac medications, these drugs (Calan, Cardizem, and Procardia) also can be useful but are expensive and have side effects, and none address the underlying cause of the problem.

WHAT ACTIVATES THE MECHANISMS THAT CAUSE CORONARY BLOCKAGES, BLOOD CLOTS, AND SPASM?

Let's go another step back in the causal chain. Instead of asking, "How can we prevent the blood from clotting and the coronary arteries from constricting?" the more interesting and fundamental questions to me are, "Why does the blood clot where it's not supposed to in the first place?" and "Why do the arteries go into spasm?" and "What activates the mechanisms that causes coronary artery blockages to form?"

What I find tremendously interesting is that *lifestyle factors can activate all mechanisms known to cause coronary heart disease and heart attacks.* In other words, lifestyle choices we make each day— what we eat, how we respond to stress, how much we exercise, and whether or not we abuse tobacco, alcohol, and other drugs—can lead to heart disease.

Here are some examples of how lifestyle choices affect coronary artery spasm and blood clot formation:

Diet

As described earlier, a diet high in saturated fat and cholesterol provides the building blocks for coronary atherosclerosis. The role of diet in heart disease has been studied for years. What's new is that we now know diet affects the heart very quickly, not just over a period of years. Even a single meal high in fat and cholesterol may cause the body to release a hormone, *thromboxane,* which causes the arteries to constrict and the blood to clot faster—one reason why heart patients often get chest pain after eating a fatty meal, and why so many of them end up in the emergency room after a rich Thanksgiving or other holiday feast.

The good news is that improvements also can occur very quickly when people follow the program in this book. We can make different lifestyle choices to begin healing ourselves. In our research, we found that blood flow to the heart could begin to improve in just a few weeks. Our diet allowed participants' arteries to dilate and blood to flow more freely because the fat and cholesterol content was so low.

Nicotine

In addition to injuring the lining of your coronary arteries, nicotine in cigarettes causes your blood to clot faster, and causes your arteries to constrict, leading to the buildup of blockages.

Recent studies by Dr. Judith Ockene and others have demonstrated that quitting smoking rapidly decreases the risk of a heart attack. Within three years after stopping, the risk of heart disease was decreased by 64 percent. Why? Because the primary reason that smoking leads to heart attacks is the effect of nicotine on blood clot formation and coronary spasm, not just blockage formation. When a person stops smoking, nicotine is eliminated from his or her body fairly quickly and the risk of blood clots or coronary artery spasm falls rapidly. A recent study by Dr. Lynn Rosenberg found even better news: when women stop smoking, their risk of heart attack becomes nearly identical to nonsmokers after quitting for at least three years.

Stimulants

Cocaine (especially "crack") and amphetamines are perhaps the most potent stimulants of arterial constriction, blood clot formation, and plaque hemorrhage. The deaths of world-class athletes such as Don Rogers, Len Bias, and others who were young and very fit were tragic examples of how their alleged cocaine use caused intense constriction of their coronary arteries, resulting in fatal heart attacks even though they had no significant arterial blockages. (You can be fit—that is, well conditioned, well muscled, and athletically gifted—yet not be very healthy if your coronary arteries are blocked.) Other stimulants, such as caffeine, may do this but to a much lesser degree.

Exercise

In people with coronary artery blockages, exercise actually *increases* the tendency of blood to clot and arteries to constrict during the time of activity—one reason why even athletic people sometimes die while jogging (like Jim Fixx) or playing basketball (like Pete Maravich). When people exercise regularly, however, these mechanisms are less likely to be activated during the rest of the time when they are not exercising.

Vigorous exercise may actually increase the risk of sudden cardiac death in people who eat a high-fat diet, who smoke, who manage stress poorly, and who use stimulants, whereas moderate exercise can be very beneficial when combined with other lifestyle changes. The risk of exercise is in direct proportion to its intensity, so moderate exercise conveys most of the benefits while decreasing the risk. In chapter 12 I describe how to exercise safely.

Emotional Stress

How does emotional stress lead to coronary heart disease? Most physicians and scientists accept the roles of diet, lack of exercise, and smoking in causing heart disease, but the importance of emotional stress as a cause of heart disease is only now achieving widespread acceptance. As described in chapter 1, the reasons for this are varied.

Until recently, it was rare to see a research study on stress and heart disease, but during the past few years there has been a surge of interest in this area. Even now, though, most cardiac rehabilitation programs do not teach stress management skills and most physicians don't advise their patients to learn them.

Emotional stress comes in two basic categories: acute and

chronic. We are designed to cope with acute stress much better than with chronic stress.

The body responds to stress—whether emotional stress (perceived danger) or physical stress (extreme temperature changes or exertion)—by activating a series of mechanisms collectively known as the fight-or-flight response, which prepares us either to fight or to run.

The body does this in two ways. First, there are direct connections between your brain and your heart. These nerves, called the sympathetic nervous system, stimulate receptors in the heart that make it beat faster and harder and can cause the coronary arteries to constrict. Second, the brain causes other organs, such as your adrenal glands, to secrete stress hormones such as *adrenaline* and steroids such as *cortisol,* which circulate in the blood until they reach the heart. Acute stress tends to cause rises in production of adrenaline and its relative, *noradrenaline,* whereas chronic stress causes increases in cortisol production.

As a result of signals from these hormones, a series of physiological reactions occur:

- Our muscles begin to contract, thereby fortifying our "body armor." We are more protected from bodily injury.
- Our metabolism speeds up, providing more strength and energy with which to fight or run. Both our heart rate and the amount of blood pumped with each beat increase.
- Our rate of breathing begins to increase, providing more oxygen to do battle or to run from danger.
- Our digestive system begins to shut down, diverting more blood and energy to the large muscles needed to fight or run.
- The pupils of our eyes begin to dilate, aiding vision. Other senses such as hearing also become heightened.
- We feel an urge to urinate and move the bowels, to reduce the danger of infection if abdominal injury should occur.
- Arteries in our arms and legs begin to constrict, so that less blood will be lost if we become wounded or injured. (You may notice that your hands get cold during times of stress, which is the principle behind the "stress cards" in which the color of the card you hold begins to change as you become more relaxed.)
- Our blood clots more quickly, so we'll lose less blood if we become wounded or injured.

These mechanisms have evolved over the centuries to help us survive danger. They work best when the danger is clear, well defined, and short-term. An example of an acute stress graph is shown in figure 3.3. It illustrates the following situation. You are crossing a street on your way home (point 1), when suddenly, out of the corner of your eye, you notice a car coming at you at high speed. Your muscles tense, you feel a surge of energy, and you lunge backward, smashing into a newspaper vending machine and cutting an artery in your hand, which quickly stops bleeding (point 2). These fight-or-flight mechanisms help to save your life. After the danger has passed, you may experience a compensatory parasympathetic response (point 3): your knees feel shaky, you feel weak, your muscles relax, and your arteries dilate. After a few minutes, you return to baseline (point 4). (This syndrome is described by Kenneth Pelletier, Ph.D., in his book, *Mind as Healer, Mind as Slayer.*)

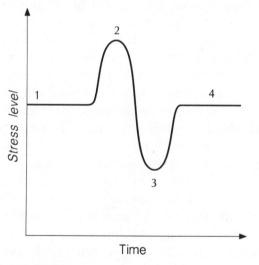

Figure 3.3. Acute Stress Graph

Unfortunately, emotional stress in modern times tends to be chronic rather than acute. The pace of life in the past ten years seems to be increasingly faster—the so-called acceleration syndrome. Like Alice in Wonderland, we go faster and faster while remaining in the same place. Federal Express overnight service is no longer quick enough—that letter needs to be sent by fax immediately. Even the traditional places of refuge in the twentieth century—the car and the home—are transformed, with fax machines and computers at home, telephones in the car, even fax machines for the car. With portable telephones and laptop computers, anywhere can be an office.

Of course, the technology is not to blame. These same devices can be used to decrease stress by allowing people more flexibility in choosing their work environments. (I have a fax machine, portable phone, and laptop computer, and these allow me to work out of my home.) It's what we do with technology that determines its effects on our lives.

Likewise, our "inner technology" is correct—we're built right—but we are designed to cope with acute stress, not the chronic stress of modern life. We often don't have time to recover from one stressful situation before we get hit with another. An example of a chronic stress graph is shown in figure 3.4. It illustrates the case of a mythical Mr. Jones:

Mr. Jones is already having a tough day. The alarm clock jars him out of bed, but he's already late for an important morning meeting at work—daylight savings time began last night and he forgot to set the clock ahead. He turns on the radio while shaving and hears that another airplane began losing important pieces of its fuselage while in flight, and he's scheduled to fly across the country the next day. Ouch—suddenly there's blood all over the towel. Damn razor! While reading the newspaper over breakfast, he learns that his stocks are down; now he's not sure how he's going to make the mortgage payment and send his son to college. No time to talk with his family over breakfast—he's late! He gulps down two cups of coffee, bacon, eggs, and toast and rushes out the door. Trouble ahead: An eighteen-wheeler jackknifed, and traffic is backed up for miles—not today! He arrives at work over an hour late, just as the important meeting is ending. Both his boss and his main competitor smile at him as they walk by. He goes into his office as his secretary tells him that the IRS called to schedule an audit of his tax returns for the last five years. And his day is just beginning!

When our stress mechanisms are *chronically* activated, the same responses that are designed to protect us can become harmful—even lethal. Arteries constrict not just in our arms and legs but also inside our hearts. Blood clots are more likely to form inside our coronary arteries.

Thus, most of our muscles constrict during times of chronic, intense emotional stress, ranging from the large muscles (causing tension and pain in the neck, back, shoulders, etc.) to the smooth

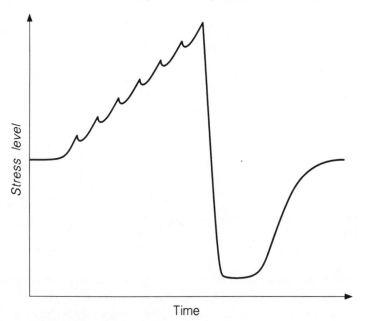

Figure 3.4. Chronic Stress Graph

muscle that lines the coronary arteries (leading to spasm) to the fibers of the heart muscle itself (leading to contraction band necrosis, described later in this chapter.).

Dr. Andrew Selwyn at Harvard Medical School and Dr. John Dearfield at the Hammersmith Hospital in London used cardiac PET scans to measure blood flow to the heart in patients with heart disease. While patients were being scanned, he asked them to begin doing simple arithmetic problems. Just the emotional stress of doing mental arithmetic caused a measurably reduced blood flow to the heart. Similarly, Dr. Alan Rozanski at the University of California, Los Angeles, School of Medicine found that mental stress caused the heart to beat less effectively in people who had coronary heart disease.

As I briefly mentioned in the last chapter, there are a lot of misconceptions about stress and the heart. *The ability to respond to stress and the ability to relax are equally important in being able to function effectively while remaining healthy.* I'm not saying we should all be laid-back, avoid stress, and never get mentally or physically aroused. Both arousal and relaxation are healthy responses.

The ideal response is to respond to challenges or difficult situations fast and efficiently and then to relax. Many people are better

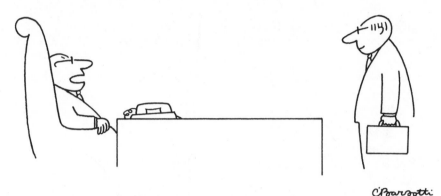

"YOU STOPPED TO SMELL THE FLOWERS? WHAT THE
HELL KIND OF EXCUSE IS THAT?"

at getting pumped up than at relaxing afterwards. During acute stress, the hormones adrenaline and noradrenaline give us more energy and help us to think more clearly to deal with the challenge. It is when we lose the ability to return to baseline—to relax—that the stress response becomes chronic. When this happens, the noradrenaline and adrenaline levels remain high, causing anxiety and insomnia, coronary artery spasm, and increased blood clotting. Also, excessive cortisol and other steroids are produced, causing blockages to build up more rapidly in the arteries as well as, emotional depression, impotence, acne, and immune system impairment. These effects are independent of diet and other factors. (Athletes who have been taking steroids to build up muscles are beginning to find that they can also build up coronary artery blockages.)

Recent research shows that the lining of normal coronary arteries produces a substance called endothelium-derived relaxation factor, or EDRF, that dilates the coronary arteries, allowing more blood to flow to the heart. When the lining of the coronary arteries is damaged by atherosclerosis, much less EDRF is produced, so the arteries tend to constrict and reduce coronary blood flow. As a result, atherosclerotic coronary arteries tend to be hyperresponsive to stress. In other words, the same amount of stress hormones cause partially blocked coronary arteries to constrict even more than normal ones. The more blocked with plaque an artery is, the less EDRF is produced, so the more likely the artery will go into spasm at the site of the coronary artery blockage.

Normally, exercise causes the arteries to secrete more EDRF, causing the coronary arteries to dilate despite the increase in sympathetic nervous system stimulation. In people who have coronary artery blockages, however, the coronary arteries constrict during exercise, making an already bad situation even worse. This occurs because less EDRF is produced in coronary arteries that are partially blocked with atherosclerosis. Smoking also decreases the production of EDRF from your cells.

Dr. David Harrison and his colleagues fed monkeys a high-cholesterol diet and found that they developed coronary artery blockages and their production of EDRF decreased. Here's some good news: He then fed these monkeys a very low-fat, low-cholesterol diet similar to our Reversal Diet and found that the monkeys' EDRF levels returned to normal even though the coronary artery blockages only partially reversed.

"You know, it's a real jungle out there. I mean, sometimes my office is a zoo. Just when I think I've finally got it made and get some respect, along comes someone else to challenge my authority. I feel stressed all the time, trying to keep my position and worrying about others trying to get what *I've* got." A typical day in the business world? Yes, but it's monkey business.

Studies by Dr. Jay Kaplan, Dr. Thomas Clarkson, and their colleagues at the Bowman Gray School of Medicine have given the best scientific evidence to date of the role of emotional stress in causing coronary artery blockages. Dr. Kaplan and his colleagues studied cynomolgus monkeys, which are very similar to people in how they develop coronary artery blockages. These monkeys, like humans, have a complex social organization; like many people, these monkeys are very aware of their social ranking and social status.

The investigators determined social rankings among these monkeys on the basis of fight outcomes or competitions among individual monkeys. Winners of fights or competitions were judged dominant to losers.

In their first experiment, thirty monkeys were divided into two groups. Half were placed in a chronically stressful, socially unstable environment, and the other half were maintained in a nonstressful, socially stable environment. Both groups were fed a high-fat, high-cholesterol, typical American diet.

After twenty-two months, the dominant, highly aggressive, and competitive monkeys in the chronically stressed, socially disrupted, unstable groups had developed coronary artery blockages *over twice as severe* as the dominant monkeys in the unstressed group. These dominant, stressed monkeys also had twice as much blockage as monkeys in the subordinate groups (who did not fight to achieve or maintain social status). *These differences in coronary artery blockages occurred even though blood pressure and cholesterol levels were comparable in all groups.*

The investigators then repeated this study, but this time the monkeys were fed a diet that was somewhat lower in fat (the "prudent diet" of the American Heart Association). As expected, the monkeys developed less extensive blockages than in the first study, but the dominant, chronically stressed monkeys had significantly more blockages than the other groups of monkeys. Again, both the stressed and unstressed monkeys had comparable blood pressure and cholesterol levels, so the effects of stress on the heart must have been caused by other mechanisms.

The authors wrote, "We concluded from this study that psychosocial influences on coronary artery atherosclerosis were not dependent on the presence of large amounts of fat and cholesterol in the diet." In other words, stress caused formation of coronary artery blockages even when monkeys were fed a diet lower in fat and cholesterol. When the diet was higher in fat and cholesterol, the influence of stress on causing arterial blockages was magnified thirty times! Therefore, in monkeys, both emotional stress and diet are powerful influences on the development of coronary artery blockages.

In other experiments, Dr. Kaplan found that chronic stress increased the permeability of the monkeys' arterial walls to cholesterol—in other words, stress makes the coronary arteries absorb more cholesterol. Also, stress decreases levels of HDL ("good") cholesterol.

The investigators also found that monkeys whose heart rates and blood pressures showed the largest increases when the monkeys were stressed also had the greatest severity of coronary artery blockages. The dominant, chronically stressed monkeys showed the widest swings in heart rate and blood pressure when they went from a relaxed to a stressed state. Even the presence of the investigators was enough to cause a marked rise in the heart rate of dominant monkeys. (Dr. Robert Eliot has termed people who react to stress in this way "hot reactors," and his research and the work of others indicate that hot reactors are at higher risk of dying from heart disease.)

The dominant monkeys were chronically stressed by trying to maintain control in a constantly changing social environment. That is, each dominant monkey had to keep fighting to maintain his high-status position when new monkeys were continually introduced to his group—similar to what is often seen in organizations and corporations.

In monkeys and in humans, chronic stress causes overproduction of the stress hormone cortisol which, in turn, increases the formation of coronary artery blockages. Chronic stress also decreases estrogen production—one reason that stressed women sometimes have irregular menstrual cycles. This disruption of estrogen production by the ovaries can contribute to coronary heart disease in women.

Dr. Kaplan's experiments also demonstrated that *subordinate* female monkeys developed almost as much coronary atherosclerosis as the *dominant* male monkeys. (In monkeys, at least, perhaps males need to learn to be less dominant and females to be less subordinate.) Almost half of the subordinate female monkeys developed menstrual abnormalities, and most had low estrogen levels, another side effect of chronic stress.

Dominant male monkeys tended to spend significantly more time alone than the other monkeys. In contrast, monkeys who engaged in friendly, positive behaviors such as grooming or passive body contact had lower heart rates (indicating relaxation) than the same monkeys when they were alone. Female monkeys who were isolated in individual cages had twice the atherosclerosis as those who were allowed to live together with other monkeys.

A brutal study from Dr. Boris Lapin and Dr. Genja Cherkovich, published in a Soviet scientific journal, also demonstrated that emotional stress can cause coronary artery blockages to form. In a series of experiments conducted several years ago, a male baboon was taken from his female mate and placed in a separate cage. Then the male was forced to watch his mate copulate with a rival monkey. After four or five months of this, the isolated male monkeys had significant increases in coronary artery blockages, blood pressure, and heart attacks.

Even in monkeys and baboons, social isolation is a major cause of emotional stress. I think the same is true for humans as well: when we go far enough back in the causal chain, we find that feeling isolated leads to emotional stress and, in turn, to heart disease. I will explore these ideas in greater depth in the next chapter.

Chronic emotional stress may cause coronary artery blockages to form in humans as well as in monkeys. A recent study by Dr. Abla Sibai found that people exposed to the stress of fourteen years of war in Beirut had significantly more coronary artery blockages at angiography than visitors who were not under this chronic stress, independent of other risk factors such as blood pressure and cholesterol.

A recent study by Dr. Peter Schnall at Cornell found that workers who faced high psychological demands without having much control over day-to-day decisions had three times the risk of having high blood pressure. *All* of these chronically stressed workers had thickened or enlarged hearts.

SUDDEN CARDIAC DEATH

It's as bad as it sounds. Approximately 40 percent of people who die from heart disease didn't even know they had a heart problem until they died from it—clearly not the best way to find out. So no matter how good we get at treating heart disease, the major focus needs to be on prevention.

Sudden death due to heart disease occurs in two ways:

· Blood flow to the heart is reduced, causing a heart attack;
· The heart begins to beat erratically.

So far, we have been discussing what causes heart attacks. Not surprisingly, the same lifestyle factors that can lead to heart attacks also can lead to an irregular or erratic heart rhythm, known as an arrhythmia.

Irregular heart beats are of two types: life-threatening and harmless. Almost everyone has an occasional "skipped beat," which is harmless. (Actually, "skipped beats" are usually extra or premature beats.) An electrocardiogram helps a doctor figure out if a person is having irregular heartbeats that may be dangerous. The most dangerous type is called *ventricular fibrillation.*

Ventricular fibrillation is caused when blood flow to the heart is suddenly reduced by any of the mechanisms already discussed (including coronary artery blockages, blood clots, spasm, and so on), even if a heart attack does not occur. Ventricular fibrillation can also occur when the electrical conduction system of the heart is disrupted, usually by emotional stress or stimulants.

Studies by Dr. Bernard Lown at Harvard Medical School and by others have shown that emotional stress—even just the sight of the experimenters—can cause ventricular fibrillation to occur in dogs. Similar work by Drs. Mark Entman and James Skinner at Baylor College of Medicine showed that emotional stress caused ventricular fibrillation to occur in pigs when coronary blood flow was reduced, whereas putting pigs in a familiar and relaxed environment helped to prevent sudden cardiac death even when coronary blood flow was reduced.

A study by Dr. Michael Brodsky, reported in the *Journal of the American Medical Association,* examined six patients who had life-threatening irregular heartbeats and who had no coronary artery blockages. Five of these six patients reported marked psychological stress. For example, one patient was a Cambodian refugee who had been separated from her husband and six children for years during the Khmer Rouge takeover. She later found her children in a refugee camp, where she began having fainting spells and palpitations. Closer to home, Dr. Thomas Graboys of Harvard Medical School reported that one of his patients began to have life-threatening irregular heartbeats while watching the closing minutes of a close Boston Celtics basketball game. And the Japanese government recently began funding a $2 million study of karōshi, or "sudden cardiac death from overwork."

In humans, unfortunately, all of the drugs used to *treat* irregular heartbeats can *cause* irregular heartbeats and sudden cardiac death in some people. And there is no way to predict whether or not these drugs will make a patient better or worse. Recently, a large-scale clinical trial of two new anti-arrhythmia drugs sponsored by the National Institutes of Health was discontinued when the researchers realized that sudden cardiac deaths were much *higher* in the patients who were receiving these drugs.

CONTRACTION BAND NECROSIS

Recently, another mechanism was discovered that can cause damage to the heart muscle independent of coronary blood flow. It, too, is dependent on lifestyle. Stress hormones such as adrenaline and steroids open calcium channels at the cellular level in the heart, causing the coronary arteries to constrict (spasm). (This is why calcium-channel blocking drugs like Cardizem and Procardia are often prescribed.) Under conditions of intense chronic stress, even the muscle fibers inside the heart itself can begin to contract so vigorously that the normal architecture of these fibers is disrupted, damaging the heart muscle. This mechanism is known as "contraction band necrosis," "myofibrillar degeneration," or "coagulative myocytolysis," and it can lead to a condition called cardiomyopathy in which the heart doesn't pump blood very well. This, in turn, can cause heart failure.

Although obscured by these medical terms, what we are really seeing is, to me, an amazing metaphor: the inability of the heart to relax causes the heart's muscle fibers to constrict to the point that it damages itself—like clenching your fist so hard and for so long that the bones and knuckles in your hand begin to break. This inability to relax and the resulting chronic constriction manifest themselves throughout the body, from the large muscles in the back down to the smallest fibers in the heart. I think this metaphor even extends to a constricted and limited sense of self, described in chapter 9.

In summary, when we go far enough back in the causal chain, we can see that heart disease is usually due to excess: too much fat and cholesterol, too much stress, too many cigarettes, and so on. What this means is that we have the power to change our lifestyles to begin healing ourselves.

The body has a great capacity to heal itself when given a chance to—unfortunately, most people eat more fat and cholesterol than the body can metabolize, so it builds up in the arteries. People often feel chronically stressed, so the body never has a chance to recover from one stress before getting hit with another one. And many people compound the problem by smoking a pack or two of cigarettes every day and leading sedentary lives. When we identify and remove the excess, then the heart can begin to heal itself. Best of all, this healing process can begin to take effect sooner than we had thought possible. Chapter 4 takes us another step back in the causal chain.

"You don't understand! I could've had class! I could've been a contender! I could've been *somebody*. Instead of a bum, which is what I am, let's face it."

—Marlon Brando, in
On the Waterfront

■

"We are what we pretend to be."

—Kurt Vonnegut, Jr.,
Mother Night

■

"In this world there are only two tragedies. One is not getting what one wants, and the other is getting it."

—Oscar Wilde,
Lady Windermere's Fan

■

"In all abundance there is lack."

—Hippocrates (460–400 B.C.),
Precepts

■

"Need and struggle are what excite and inspire us; our hour of triumph is what brings the void."

—William James,
Is Life Worth Living?

■

"I do mean it when I say I need you—'cause I'm lonely. You think I'm lying, don't you?"
    "Nobody ever lies about being lonely."

—Donna Reed and Montgomery Clift, in
From Here to Eternity

4

Lifestyle Changes of the Rich and Famous

In the previous chapter, I discussed the causal chain of coronary heart disease and the idea that the farther back in that chain we can begin treating the problem, the more powerful the healing can be. So far, I've focused on conventional treatments of heart disease—drugs and surgery—and the roles of lifestyle factors such as diet, emotional stress, exercise, smoking, and stimulants in causing heart disease.

However, we know that the traditional risk factors—cholesterol, blood pressure, age, gender, genetics, smoking, diabetes, obesity, sedentary life—explain only about 50 percent of heart disease. At least half of the reasons why people get heart disease are unknown. So why is it that some people get heart disease while others don't? Clearly, all of these risk factors are important, but I don't think that any of them go to the core of why people develop heart disease. I'm not entirely sure what does, but I'm becoming more certain than I have been in the past.

Let's go another step back in this causal chain. Are there common psychological—and perhaps even spiritual—factors that lead to coronary heart disease?

In the 1950s, Drs. Meyer Friedman and Ray Rosenman described a syndrome they termed Type A behavior that they believed caused heart disease. The Type A syndrome describes someone who is hostile, self-involved, impatient, and always in a hurry. Type As make obsessive attempts to achieve poorly defined goals and have a strong need for recognition and advancement. They have a tendency to do two or three things at the same time, such as talking and moving quickly, and so on. At first, studies indicated that Type A behavior was linked with heart disease; later, more conclusive studies failed to substantiate this connection.

More recent evidence has helped to explain this discrepancy. Research by Dr. Larry Scherwitz at the University of California, San Francisco, Dr. Redford Williams at Duke University, and others indicates that certain elements of Type A behavior are linked with heart disease whereas other components are not. (In his book, *The Trusting Heart*, Dr. Williams describes how this research evolved.) In particular, the factors most toxic to the heart are self-involvement, hostility, and cynicism.

Dr. Scherwitz, Dr. Lynda Powell, and others found that the frequency with which a person refers to him- or herself—that is, how frequently he or she used the words "I," "me," "my," and "mine" in an ordinary conversation—actually predicted the recurrence of a heart attack. The more frequently a person used those words, the greater the likelihood he or she would die from a heart attack.

In another study, Dr. Scherwitz analyzed tape-recorded interviews from a nine-year research study involving almost 13,000 men. This study, called the Multiple Risk Factor Intervention Trial (MRFIT), was designed to determine if moderate lifestyle changes could help prevent heart disease. Dr. Scherwitz found that people who used frequent self-references later developed heart disease more often than people who didn't. Most striking was the even greater degree of self-involvement in those who ultimately died from heart attacks.

Well, why should that be true? Certainly, saying the words, "I," "me," "my," and "mine" isn't harmful per se. Instead, our speech reflects how we view the world we live in. When we feel isolated from others, we focus more on ourselves—"*I* need this, *I* want that."

These research studies have taken us a major step in the right direction, but they raise even more basic questions. I wonder: *Why* are we self-involved? *Why* are we cynical? *Why* are we hostile? Is there a more fundamental cause for these emotions that can lead to coronary heart disease and other illnesses?

I believe that there is. Living with patients for a month at a time in our two earlier studies and meeting with them frequently and intensively during the past four years of our third study has provided me with some special opportunities. The majority of doctors see a lot of different patients but are not able to spend very much time with most of them, whereas this research allows me to work with the same relatively small group of people for several years. In the current study, we live together for a week in a retreat, where participants learn the fundamentals of our program. We then meet two evenings every week for four hours each session, including one hour each meeting of what we call group support led by clinical psychologist Jim Billings, Ph.D., Shirley Brown, M.D., Mary Dale Scheller, M.S.W., and me.

So we get to know each other very well, and I am learning all the time. At first I viewed our support groups simply as a way to motivate patients to stay on the other aspects of the program that I considered most important: the diet, exercise, stress management training, stopping smoking, and so on. Over time, I began to realize that the group support itself was one of the most powerful interventions, as it addressed what I am beginning to believe is a more fundamental cause of why we feel stressed and, in turn, why we get illnesses like heart disease: the perception of isolation.

In short, *anything that promotes a sense of isolation leads to chronic stress and, often, to illnesses like heart disease.* Conversely, *anything that leads to real intimacy and feelings of connection can be healing* in the real sense of the word: to bring together, to make whole. The ability to be intimate has long been seen as a key to emotional health; I believe it is essential to the health of our hearts as well.

There are two general strategies for achieving intimacy: *horizontal intimacy*—developing the connections and relationships between ourselves and others—or *vertical intimacy*—developing the connections between us and the higher parts of ourselves.

Horizontal intimacy can be increased through participation in support groups, development of communication skills, learning forgiveness, developing feelings of trust, practicing altruism, and so on. Prayer and meditation are two ways of realizing vertical intimacy. These are described more fully in chapters 7, 8, and 9.

Therefore, even though we now have evidence that our lifestyle choices can cause heart disease, it's not enough just to change our behaviors; we have to go a step farther back in the causal chain of why people get sick. Ultimately, the stress management techniques described in this book are not designed simply to "manage" stress, to "cope" with stress, or to "deal" with stress; they can be used to help us transcend our sense of isolation so that real healing can begin—that is, so our psychological and spiritual hearts can begin to open, not just our arteries.

In this context, *heart disease can be a catalyst for changing not only our behaviors but also for transforming ourselves in more fundamental ways.* The stress management techniques described in chapter 7 are not simply another type of tranquilizer. These techniques do not *bring* relaxation or peace from outside oneself. Instead, they help us to quiet down the mind and body sufficiently to experience an inner sense of peace, self-esteem, and happiness, one that came not from getting but rather from being, not from doing but from undoing.

Someone once asked Swami Satchidananda, a spiritual teacher, "What are you, a Hindu?" "No," he replied, "I'm an Undo. I'm trying to teach people how they can undo the patterns that cause damage to their minds and bodies so they can begin to heal." It's a simple statement, but one that reflects a different conception of health and healing.

I wrote *Stress, Diet, and Your Heart* in 1982. When I conducted the two earlier studies that formed the basis of that book, I was only beginning to explore these ideas. There was not much scientific literature at that time to support my clinical observations. Since then, though, increasing scientific evidence is demonstrating that isolation and suppression of feelings often leads to illness, whereas intimacy and social support can be healing. Let's examine a few of these studies:

· In the Alameda County Study (6,928 men and women living near San Francisco) and in the North Karelia Study (13,301 men and women living in Eastern Finland) participants were studied for five to nine years. Those who were socially isolated had a two- to three-fold increased risk of death from both heart disease and from all other causes when compared to those who felt most connected to others. *These results were independent of other cardiac risk factors* such as cholesterol level, blood pressure, genetics, and so on. Similar results were found in 2,059 subjects from Evans County, Georgia, where the greatest mortality was found in older people with few social ties.

Even being a member of a club, church, or synagogue significantly decreased the risk of premature death and significantly protected people from heart disease even when they had high blood pressure. In a subsequent nine-year period, those whose social connections decreased experienced a greater risk of death from heart disease.

· In the previous chapter, I discussed Dr. Jay Kaplan's research with monkeys in which he found that disrupting the social networks of monkeys caused them to develop coronary artery blockages twice as severe as unstressed ones, *even when their cholesterol levels and blood pressures were comparable.*

· At the University of Houston, Dr. Robert Nerem unwittingly studied what happens when rabbits are given social support. Genetically similar rabbits were placed on a high-cholesterol diet designed to cause atherosclerosis so the investigators could study their blockages. The researchers expected all of the rabbits to develop atherosclerosis. Instead, they found that rabbits (who were stacked in cages up to the ceiling) in the higher cages developed more atherosclerosis than ones in the lower cages. This made no sense to the investigators.

After further investigation, they found that the lab technician, who was short, would play with rabbits who were in the lower cages when she came in at night to feed them because she could reach them. The rabbits in the higher cages were isolated and ignored. The scientists repeated the study, and they found that rabbits who were individually petted, held, talked to, and played with on a regular basis (and then killed to study their arteries . . .) showed more than a *60 percent* reduction in the percentage of atherosclerosis they developed when compared to genetically similar rabbits that were given the same diet and only routine laboratory animal care. *This was true even though blood cholesterol levels, heart rate, and blood pressure were comparable in both groups of rabbits.*

· Studies by other investigators have shown that people who live alone have more heart disease than those who live with someone or even something—a plant or a pet, even a goldfish. So being the petter or the pettee has many health benefits, probably because it decreases isolation.

· The quality of the social support is more important than the number of people involved who provide support. At Yale University School of Medicine, scientists studied 119 men and 40 women who were undergoing coronary angiography. They found that the more people felt loved and supported, the less coronary atherosclerosis they had at angiography, *independent of other risk factors* such as age, sex, income, hypertension, serum cholesterol, smoking, diabetes, genetics, and hostility.

· In one study reported by Dr. Ruberman in *The New England Journal of Medicine,* interviews with 2,320 male survivors of heart attacks revealed that patients who were classified as being socially isolated and having a high degree of life stress had more than four times the risk of death from heart disease and from all other causes when compared with men who had low levels of both stress and isolation.

· A study of 4,251 men of Japanese ancestry living in Hawaii found that social networks protected them against heart attacks, chest pain, and coronary heart disease during a seven-year period, *independent of known health hazards* such as cigarette smoking and high blood pressure.

· At the Duke University Medical Center, Dr. D. G. Blazer studied 331 people in Durham County, age 65 or older. Risk of mortality was almost four times greater in people who did not have much social support, even when taking into account other factors such as gender, race, economic status, physical health status, depression, stressful life events, and smoking.

· At Southern Methodist University in Dallas, Dr. James Pennebaker conducted a series of studies concluding that sharing feelings is good for the soul, or at least for the immune system. Researchers asked a group of students to spend twenty minutes each day over a four-day period writing about a traumatic event in their lives. A second group was asked to write about trivial events. Blood samples were taken from both groups before and after this four-day period.

Results showed an increase in immune activity in the group that was self-disclosing, whereas the other group showed no change. The researchers wrote, "Failure to confide traumatic events is stressful and associated with long-term health problems. Inhibition of thoughts, feelings, or behaviors was associated with physiological work, resulting in increased autonomic nervous system activity." In other words, holding feelings in puts a chronic stress on the heart and on the immune system.

- At Ohio State University College of Medicine, scientists found that patients who scored above the average in loneliness had significantly poorer immune functioning.
- In Sweden, a ten-year study of 150 middle-aged men found that social isolation was one of the best predictors of mortality, both from all causes and from coronary heart disease.
- At the Medical College of Wisconsin, Dr. James Goodwin and colleagues found that unmarried persons with cancer had decreased overall survival, even after adjustment for disease severity and type of treatment. In another study, he found that among 256 healthy elderly adults, individuals with good social support systems tended to have lower blood cholesterol levels and higher indices of immune function. These findings were independent of age, smoking, alcohol intake, and degree of emotional stress.
- At Stanford University School of Medicine, Dr. David Spiegel, conducted research in which patients with metastatic breast cancer were randomly divided into two groups. One group received the usual medical care, while the other received the usual medical care plus weekly ninety-minute group support meetings for one year. Although he planned the study expecting that there would be no difference in life span between the groups, five years later he found that the patients who attended the weekly group support meetings had *twice* the survival rate of the control group.

· A report published in the journal *Science* reviewed the mounting evidence that social isolation heightens people's susceptibility to illness. According to Dr. James House, one of the authors of this article, "It's the 10 to 20 percent of people who say they have nobody with whom they can share their private feelings, or who have close contact with others less than once a week, who are at most risk."

The report said that "social isolation is as significant to mortality rates as smoking, high blood pressure, high cholesterol, obesity, and lack of physical exercise. In fact, when age is adjusted for, social isolation is as great or greater a mortality risk than smoking. After controlling for the effects of physical health, socioeconomic status, smoking, alcohol, exercise, obesity, race, life satisfaction and health care, the studies found that those with few or weak social ties were twice as likely to die as those with strong ties." The authors concluded by stating, "Thus, just as we discover the importance of social relationships for health, and see an increasing need for them, their prevalence and availability seem to be declining."

All of these studies indicate that isolation from others can lead to illness, whereas feeling more connected and intimate with others can enhance health, well-being, and even survival. This seems to be true both for animals and for people. Unfortunately, we often go about trying to feel connected with others in ways that can be self-defeating. These studies indicating that social support and intimacy may even prolong life are in sharp contrast to the investigations of cholesterol-lowering drugs, aspirin, and other interventions that do not seem to prolong life and often trade one set of health problems for another.

What I'd like to do now is to shift from what is scientifically proven and to share with you some clinical observations and personal experiences of how I got interested in this area of research and what I'm learning.

Our research patients are a very diverse group of people in age, gender, race, religion, ethnic background, sexual preference, socioeconomic status, and educational level—in all the different ways that we ordinarily categorize and define people, emphasizing our differences instead of our similarities, a process that ultimately leaves us feeling more isolated and lonely. (Or as Swami Satchidananda once said, "We're born fine until we de-fine ourselves, and then we use these definitions to see how we are different rather than how we are alike. So now we must re-fine ourselves.") Our participants were people who would not have had a lot to do with each other except for the fact that they had all volunteered for an unusual research project. At first it seemed like the only thing they had in common was that they all had heart disease.

Over time, we began to learn that they had something much more profound in common: how they tended to view themselves and their relationship to the world. Underneath the various definitions and seeming differences, most of them shared a view of the world that was remarkably similar: "I really feel isolated and alone, and I don't want to feel that way. I want to feel connected, close, and intimate. I must be lacking something or I wouldn't feel so isolated. I have to become special in order to be loved."

Most of us know—if only as a dim memory—how good it feels to be emotionally intimate with other people and to be reconnected with our thoughts and feelings. In trying to regain a lost sense of intimacy and connection with other people, we tend to get into patterns of behavior that are stressful and ultimately self-defeating or self-destructive. Over time, these patterns can lead to vicious cycles, as I will describe later. With a sense of isolation comes a perception of *lacking*—either not *having* enough or not *being* good enough.

cathy®   **by Cathy Guisewite**

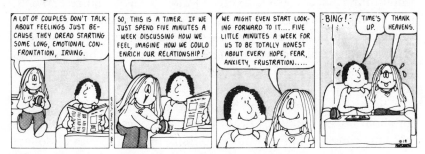

What generally follows from this is the belief that: "*If only* I had more money, *if only* I had more power, *if only* I had sex more often or with more people, *if only* I had more accomplishments, *then* I'd be happy and everything would be fine and I'd be okay, and people would love me and I'd feel connected with them and I'd be happy." Or: "*If only* I were smarter, or thinner, or heavier, or more beautiful, or more muscular, *then* I'd be happy and everything would be fine and I'd be okay, and people would love me and I'd feel connected with them and I'd be happy."

Of course this way of viewing the world is not unique to heart patients, but I think it helps to explain why unhappiness, chronic stress, and heart disease are so prevalent in our society, even where there is material abundance. We desire what we think will allow us to feel loved and respected, and thus to feel reconnected, to transcend our feelings of being isolated and alone. Most advertising is designed to increase these desires—the modern American mantra of want, need, and buy.

Unfortunately, no matter how it turns out, "it" doesn't really bring us the lasting happiness we wanted and then we are left feeling more isolated and disappointed. *Until we get it,* we feel anxious and worried. *If we don't get it,* then we feel stressed. *If somebody else gets it,* it's even worse, and it reinforces this dog-eat-dog, zero-sum view of the world: the more you get, the less there is for me, and you only go around once so you've got to grab all the gusto you can, because life is passing you by, so hurry up and do more, and more, and still more . . .

But *even if we get it,* whatever *it* is, it doesn't really bring us the lasting contentment and meaning in our lives that we thought it would. First, success tends to breed jealousy, envy, and resentment, all of which further isolate us. We may suddenly have more "friends," but not necessarily ones who really care for us, causing a wariness and suspicion that interferes with intimacy. The people who really love us do so despite our external trappings, not because of them.

Second, it's almost never enough. As one patient said, "It's good for about fifteen minutes," or, as Peggy Lee sings, "Is that all there is?" One patient told me, "I used to think that ten thousand dollars would make me happy, and then I made ten thousand. Then I'd think if only I made a hundred thousand, certainly that would be enough and I could relax and be happy, but it wasn't."

In the movie *Wall Street,* one of the characters asked Gordon Gekko (a character loosely based on the financier Ivan Boesky), "How many yachts can you water-ski behind?" It's a cliché to say that money doesn't buy happiness, but for people who define themselves by what they do or by how much money they make, then it's a cliché based in truth. Ivan Boesky already had more money than he could ever spend before he began selling insider information in hopes of making even more money. For some people, money is the only way of keeping score. For others, the currency of self-esteem is job title, academic rank, or athletic statistics. The arena may differ for each of us, but the pattern is similar. (I will discuss my own arenas in the next chapter.) Sometimes it's worse to get what we think will make us happy when we find out it doesn't; before, at least, we had our illusions to keep us going.

Marilyn Chambers starred in a different type of movie: hardcore pornography. In a recent interview, she described Chuck Traynor, who "discovered" her and Linda Lovelace, star of *Deep Throat:* "He's lived out most of his fantasies, but he still doesn't know what'll make him happy."

We've all seen kings, presidents, and other political figures who did not seem very happy, despite their powerful positions. This research has provided me the opportunity to spend some time with some very wealthy and (by conventional standards) powerful people, some of whom contributed to our study and helped make it possible. The company chairmen and presidents that I've spent time with who are happy usually feel that way *despite* their money and success, not because of it. Many others feel isolated and unhappy notwithstanding great wealth and accomplishment.

One need only to pick up a magazine or newspaper to read the same themes:

"I've always been an outsider," said Boris Becker. "The only way to be together with other boys, to be accepted by them, was through sports. I wanted to find love and friendship through sports. That's where I found my self-approval.

"After tough tournaments I frequently go through phases of deep depression. I walk up and down in my apartment and see no reason why I should go on. These are nightmares. And I say to myself a thousand times, 'Man, what are you doing?'

"I very frequently think about the meaning of life because I live through so many extreme moments. I am one of very few people who reach the limit, where I feel that I cannot go any further. I cannot do more than win Wimbledon, Davis Cup and Flushing Meadows. I cannot really go any further than becoming No. 1. I therefore reach a level that most people never reach in their lives.

"I thought more than once that it wouldn't be so bad if I died at that moment." [*World Tennis,* 4/90, p. 38]

Failure seems an especially painful prospect for Michael Jackson, for whom satisfaction apparently comes not from within but from outside things like sales and awards, which can be fickle. . . . After his new record won "only" one Grammy, Michael told another reporter, "It bothered me. I cried a lot. My family thought I was going crazy because I was weeping so much about it." The down side of his astronomical success is that Michael is no longer competing with anyone but himself: he has been catapulted forever into his own lonely stratosphere. [*Rolling Stone,* 9/24/87, p. 57]

"I have problems like anybody else," says Eddie Murphy, who is soft-spoken and easygoing at close range. "In fact, I have more because I have this strange existence. It's funny. When I sit back with people like Stallone, we can trade stories. It's like the same identical things happen: the way power isolates you, and everybody tries to get close to you. It's just a bunch of stuff." [*People,* 8/8/88, p. 78]

"I guess I used to think that rock could save you," Bruce Springsteen says later. "I don't believe it can anymore. . . . As you get older, you realize that it is not enough. Music alone—you can take some shelter there, and you can find some comfort and happiness, you can dance, you can slow-dance with your girl, but you can't hide in it. And it is *so* seductive that you want to hide in it. And then if you get in the position of somebody like me, where you *can* if you want to, you really can."

He stops himself. "Well, you *think* you can, anyway. In the end you really can't because no matter who you are, whether it's me or Elvis or Michael Jackson, in the end you really can't. You can use all your powers to isolate yourself, to surround yourself with luxury, to intoxicate yourself in any particular fashion that you so desire. But it just starts eating you away inside, because there is something you get from engagement with people, from a connection with a *person,* that you just cannot get anyplace else." [*Rolling Stone,* 5/5/88, p. 40]

Happiness often eludes us, just beyond our grasp, like a carrot on a stick dangling in front of a donkey. And like the fabled musk deer that wanders the forest, searching for the source of the beautiful odor and not realizing the scent comes from itself, we often seem to be looking in the wrong place for our happiness and sense of self-worth.

The self-involvement, hostility, and cynicism that predispose us to heart disease are really effects of a more fundamental cause: the perception of isolation. When someone feels isolated and alone, then his focus is on himself: *"I* feel alone, *I* am lacking, if only *I* had _____, *then* I'd be happy." The perception of isolation leads to self-involvement. Likewise, the chronic frustration and recurrent disappointments and disillusionments of not getting what we think will make us happy—or getting it and finding that the happiness doesn't last—can lead to chronic hostility and cynicism.

So, a real paradox is that we try to set ourselves apart from other people as a way of trying to become more intimate with them: "Look at me—I'm special! I'm worthy of your attention and respect! Love me!"

And yet, what does it mean to be special? To be special means to be different, to be set apart from other people—so *the irony is that we set ourselves apart and further isolate ourselves in a futile attempt to feel reconnected and re-empowered.* "Charlie . . . I could've been *somebody,"* said Brando in a classic scene from *On the Waterfront.*

Two basic strategies are often employed in this self-defeating search for happiness.

In the first approach, the person becomes compulsively driven to achieve in his chosen arena as a way of distinguishing himself—that is, separating himself—from other people. He (or she) defines himself and invests his self-esteem in the outcome of what he does. So, a lot more is at risk than what appears on the surface. It's not just succeeding or failing at a given task—it's being a success or failure *as a person* that's at stake. It's not just winning or losing a race—it's being a winner or a loser. The compulsively driven person's net worth as a human being is always on the line. No wonder the world seems like such a hostile and stressful place. Often such a person may become successful, but the happiness eludes him anyway (it's never enough), leaving frustration, cynicism, and hostility in its place.

In the second approach, the person may strive just as hard to achieve or get what he thinks will bring happiness, but (for whatever reason) is not able to obtain fully what he thinks he needs in order to feel successful, respected, and loveable. Instead, he creates a persona, a mask, an image to make people think that he did indeed achieve it. On one end of a spectrum, the persona has some basis in truth; on the other, it is a pure fabrication.

Athletics was the arena for one of the first patients in our current study, whom I'll call "Sam." He was an accomplished athlete and told us that he was a former Olympic athlete, a world class runner, racewalker, and cyclist.

Sam was one of the most competitive people I had ever met. For him, it wasn't just winning or losing a race; if he won, he was a Winner (at least until the next race), and if he finished second, he was a Loser until proven otherwise, isolated and alone.

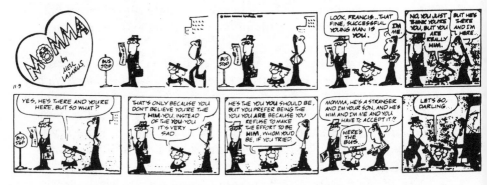

Copyright © 1990 by Mell Lazarus. Reprinted by permission.

At age forty-nine, while racing one day, Sam developed severe chest pain but he still finished the race. Afterward, he consulted his cardiologist, who performed a treadmill test indicating that Sam might have heart disease. Almost apologetically, the doctor told Sam that he would need an angiogram to find out for sure—"Of course, with all the exercise you do, and since you've never smoked, I'm sure it will be normal."

It wasn't. The angiogram revealed that several of Sam's major coronary arteries were severely blocked. He then underwent coronary angioplasty to widen his arteries, and the chest pain went away. He began running races again. Six weeks later, during a race, he again experienced chest pain. He went back to the hospital for another angioplasty, but this time the doctors found that one of the major coronary arteries was completely blocked, so angioplasty could not be repeated.

Sam then entered our study and began changing his lifestyle. He followed our diet, never smoked, and did the stress management techniques in a mechanical way for six weeks, then stopped doing them. I told him that he could exercise as much as he wanted within the limits of the exercise prescription that we gave him, but I asked him not to time himself or compete while he was in the study. For Sam, the stress came not from exercising but from the competitive attitude that he took toward it, because his self-esteem was so invested in the outcome. His net worth as a human being was on the line whenever he raced.

Although he followed the diet and exercise components of our lifestyle program, he refused to discuss his feelings in our group meetings. Like many cardiologists, Sam said, "Feelings don't have anything to do with heart disease. It's really all diet, exercise, and getting your cholesterol down." At first, he blamed his girlfriend for most of their problems, and then he stopped talking in our group sessions, sitting with his arms folded across his chest. On occasion, after another patient would share a personal difficulty, Sam would say, "Well, I *used* to have that problem, but not any more." He refused to meet with Dr. Billings, the clinical psychologist on our research team. At the time, I also was not convinced that it was essential to open up and discuss feelings in a group setting, so I did not emphasize everyone's participation in this part of our program.

Sam followed the diet religiously, and his cholesterol decreased from 249 to 121. As a result, his chest pain decreased considerably— the diet alone provides some benefits, even if you don't discuss your feelings or practice the stress management techniques. Before he entered our study, Sam got chest pain just from walking across the street. After nine months, his exercise capacity increased to the point where he was running and cycling over a hundred miles a week without pain. Symptoms often improve faster than the underlying heart disease process.

Unfortunately, Sam was unable or unwilling to address the more fundamental issues that can lead to heart disease. Although he dreamed of being in the Olympics and worked so hard to accomplish that, in reality he had never made it there. He failed in achieving what he thought would make him special—being in the Olympics— so he just pretended to have been. So, unknown to us until much later, he had created an image, a false persona, a myth that he was a former Olympian.

Again, Sam did this out of a profound feeling of loneliness, of not being good enough, of not measuring up—of not feeling lovable. It was his misguided attempt to feel connected again: "Look at me—I'm special! I'm a former Olympic athlete, a world-class race-walker, part of an elite group. Surely, I'm worthy of your love and respect."

Yet Sam's approach was doubly self-defeating. If he didn't feel loved and respected, then he lost. Even when he did, though, he couldn't really enjoy it because the love and respect were for the *image* he created, not for him. Maintaining this image required a chronic state of vigilance, and he lived in fear that he would be found out and left all alone. This created chronic stress for Sam and made real intimacy very difficult for him. As someone once said, "You're only as sick as your secrets."

The need to maintain this image became so great that Sam began competing secretly while on the program. He began entering racewalking and cycling competitions and started racing on a regular basis.

One evening—the last time Sam came to our group meeting—the stress management teacher asked the research participants to draw a picture of their heart as an aid in visualization (as described in chapter 7). Sam drew a heart surrounded by a black wall, representing the isolation that he felt. But he refused to talk about it with anyone.

Ten months after he entered our study, while greatly exceeding his exercise prescription, Sam died—the only participant in our study who has done so.

He was at a local gymnasium on a special rowing machine that allowed him to compete against a video game of other rowers. The faster he rowed, the quicker his video rowboat would go; when he slowed down, the other video rowboats edged ahead.

After an hour of this, he proudly announced to someone next to him that he had passed over 150 of these video rowboats. He then got up, went to the rest room, collapsed, and died. Although a cardiologist was present, efforts at resuscitation were unsuccessful.

It's a chilling image—he beat the video game but lost his life. For me, the situation was tragically striking—here was someone whose self-esteem required him to compete against a machine. Even the ephemeral video images had the power to define him. Sam gave a machine the power to define him and his self-worth, and, ultimately, to hasten his death.

I went to his autopsy—a painful experience for me because I had known him so well. A large blood clot was present in one of his coronary arteries. Another coronary artery had gone into spasm, causing tearing and bleeding into the lining of the artery (plaque hemorrhage). Both of these were likely caused by the intense stress of competition. The emotional stress, in turn, was caused because Sam reacted to the video game as though it were a life-or-death struggle. Unfortunately, for Sam, it was.

Why did Sam react to the video game as though it were a life-or-death struggle? After all, it's only a game, isn't it?

Sam's death was a tragic but powerful lesson for me. First, I was reminded that *providing someone with health information is not always enough to motivate changes in behavior.* We're all going to die sometime, but if we don't really enjoy living, who cares about changing behavior? When I was a medical student, both the chief of oncology and the chief of pulmonary medicine smoked. It wasn't because they didn't know any better, but they seemed to be very unhappy people. There are many ways to be self-destructive, slowly or rapidly, when life doesn't bring us the happiness we expect.

When a person perceives himself as being isolated and alone, this creates a view of the world that is fundamentally self-defeating and self-destructive. This self-destruction can come in many forms, including compulsive exercise, compulsive working, compulsive sex, smoking, alcoholism, drugs, and the million and one other ways that we have to distance ourselves from other people and from our feelings. And while these temporarily may help blunt the pain, they increase our feelings of isolation, leading to more pain in a vicious circle.

Second, *changing behavior is not always enough for real healing to occur.* We need to address what underlies the behavior. It's not sufficient simply to change behaviors like diet and exercise, because our behaviors are only manifestations of our self-perceptions. We need also to change those perceptions of isolation that can lead to these behaviors. The issue is not only living longer, but also being more free of self-imposed limitations that often lead to suffering.

Third, *when we invest our self-esteem and self-worth in the outcome of an event or in the behavior of another person, then we are giving that event or person power over our lives*—to make us happy or sad, to make us feel good or bad about ourselves, and, ultimately, to live or to die. Sam beat the video images and paid with his life.

Finally, *people only have power over us to the degree that they have something that we think we need.* When we define ourselves as separate, we define ourselves as lacking and as needy. When we choose an arena—in this case, "If only I were a world-class athlete"—then we give our power away. I'll discuss this issue more fully in the next chapter.

In a recent interview, the philosopher Jacob Needleman explained:

Several years ago, I asked one of my classes, "What do you consider to be the major problems of our society?" I got the usual answers: the breakdown of the family, nuclear war, ecology. Then somebody said "loneliness." So I asked, "How many people here feel basically lonely?" Everyone raised their hands. I was astonished. Then I asked another, larger class, which had a much broader spectrum of people, and all but two people raised their hands. So I became interested in loneliness.

Then a thirty-five-year-old student from Nigeria said, "You know, when I first came from Nigeria to England, I didn't understand what people meant when they said they were lonely. It's only now, after I've been living in the United States for two years, that I know what it means to be lonely." In his culture, loneliness simply didn't exist; they didn't even have a word for it. There was plenty of pain, plenty of suffering, plenty of grief, but no loneliness.

So what is this loneliness we're experiencing? People are cut off, not just from each other, but also from some harmonizing force in themselves. It's not just that "I am lonely"; it's that the "I" is lonely. We are lacking an essential harmonious relationship with some universal force. To me, this is why loneliness is an important phenomenon to understand.

So, to summarize, *isolation can lead to illness, whereas intimacy can lead to healing.* Isolation comes in several forms:

- isolation from our feelings, our inner self, and inner peace
- isolation from others
- isolation from a higher force

These are explored more fully in part 2.

All cultures and eras have had difficult problems, and people worried about wars, plagues, famines, and so on. The chronic stress in twentieth-century America is not only from the increased pace of modern life but also from the isolation, loneliness, and lack of love and support that so many people experience.

In summary, stress comes not only from what we do but also from how we *react* to what we do. How we react, in turn, is a function of how we perceive ourselves. When we perceive ourselves only as isolated and alone—apart from the world instead of a part of it—then we are likely to feel chronically stressed. Chronic stress, in turn, can lead to heart disease both in its direct effects on the heart and because of the self-destructive behavior patterns that result. Anything that helps us transcend and transform this perceived isolation can be healing. The rest of this book shows how.

"All I know is I'm losing my mind," Franny said. "I'm just sick of ego, ego, ego. My own and everybody else's. I'm sick of everybody that wants to *get* somewhere, do something distinguished and all, be somebody interesting. It's disgusting—it is, it *is*. I don't care what anybody says. . . . I'm not afraid to compete. It's just the opposite. Don't you see that? I'm afraid I *will* compete—that's what scares me. Just because I'm so horribly conditioned to accept everybody else's values, and just because I like applause and people to rave about me, doesn't make it right. I'm ashamed of it. I'm sick of it. I'm sick of not having the courage to be an absolute nobody. I'm sick of myself and everybody else that wants to make some kind of a splash."

—J. D. Salinger, *Franny and Zooey*

■

"Often the test of courage is not to die but to live."

—Conte Vittorio Alfieri (1749–1803)

■

"I have not failed 10,000 times. I have successfully found 10,000 ways that will not work."

—Thomas A. Edison

■

"And the stars down so close, and sadness and pleasure so close together, really the same thing. . . . The stars are close and dear and I have joined the brotherhood of the worlds. And everything's holy—everything, even me."

—John Steinbeck, *The Grapes of Wrath*

5

"This Is a Weed-Out Course!"

I am often asked, "How did you get interested in doing this research?" One reason that I enjoy working with heart patients is that I'm not very different from them, if at all. For many years, I have struggled with many of the same issues—self-worth, self-esteem, and feelings of isolation.

In my own life, and in the process of conducting this research for fourteen years, I have learned how illness and suffering can be catalysts for transforming some fundamental issues: how we view ourselves and how we relate to the world. For the patients in our study, heart disease has been the catalyst; for me, it was emotional depression.

I feel so passionate about this work because I know how much the program described in this book can help to alleviate suffering, both physical and emotional. It has for me, and I have seen how effective it can be with so many others.

I first became interested in this work in 1972 when I was a premedical student in college. I made allusions to this in my earlier book, but I didn't describe it in much detail. Here's what really happened:

I was studying at a small, extremely competitive university where most of the students acted as though academic success defined one's net worth as a person. Over half the students graduated either first or second in their high school classes, and the university had the highest percentage of National Merit scholars in the country. It also had the highest suicide rate per capita of any school in the country; I later found out why.

When I was a student there, most professors graded on a curve, in which 40 percent of the class received a C, 20 percent received a B or D, and 10 percent received an A or failed. If everyone in the class did exceptionally well (which was often the case), then a person could make a 90 percent on an exam and end up with a C. As a result, many students who never before had made any grade lower than an A suddenly found themselves struggling just to pass. When I was there, most of the students studied almost all the time just to keep up—even bringing textbooks to parties!

I had dreamed of becoming a doctor for many years. In college, I enrolled in organic chemistry because it was required for getting into medical school—admissions committees still consider it to be the single most important course for determining entry. Although organic chemistry is relatively unimportant in the practice of medicine, the course does measure one's ability to memorize vast amounts of often-irrelevant information, which is among the most useful skills to have in medical school.

My organic chemistry teacher seemed like a cross between John Houseman in the movie *The Paper Chase* and Adolf Hitler. On the first day of school, he announced to our class, "This is a weed-out course for medical schools, and I'm going to weed you out! You don't need to know organic chemistry to be a doctor, but you'll never get to be one unless you do well in this course." Great.

He taught the course without a textbook and without a conceptual basis, so to learn the seemingly endless equations required rote memory, something I've never been very good at. In what seemed like one of God's little jokes, my roommate was one of the four brilliant people in the country that year who made a perfect score—1600—on his college admissions tests (SATs). He had a photographic memory, so he never studied very hard, yet always scored 100 percent on exams. I had to struggle just to keep up.

I worried that I wouldn't do well enough in chemistry to be accepted to medical school. I got into a vicious cycle: the more I worried, the harder it became to study, and the harder it was to study, the more I worried. My mind was racing so fast that I couldn't sleep, even when I began taking tranquilizers and drinking some alcohol. I would lie down, watch the hands of the clock go around each hour until morning. At one point, this went on for about ten days in a row.

Becoming that sleep-deprived is enough to make anyone a little crazy, and I got to a point where I couldn't function at all. I believed that I was not going to be accepted to medical school, since I couldn't even read a newspaper headline and remember five minutes later what it said—not an ideal situation for someone trying to memorize organic chemistry equations.

I began to feel extremely stupid, that somehow I had managed to fool people into thinking that I was smart. I thought, "I just *seemed* smart in a public high school because most of the people there weren't that smart either. Now that I'm at a school with *really* smart people, they will soon find out how stupid I really am."

So I decided to see the campus psychiatrist. I walked into his office and said, "I'm really very stupid, and I feel like a fraud. I don't really know anything—somehow, I've just managed to fool people into thinking that I do. I'm impersonating a smart person."

"Of course you're not stupid. You've scored in the upper 5 percent of the standardized tests."

"The tests are wrong. Those tests don't measure intelligence—and if *you* think I'm smart, then you're stupid, too!" And I stormed out.

I wandered around the campus, trying to decide what to do. I walked up to people I didn't even know and asked them what courses I should take, what subject I should major in, what I should do with my life. At that point, I didn't feel capable of doing much of anything. Maybe I could get a menial job someday. Maybe not.

My parents very much wanted me to excel, especially in the academic arena—that's probably why they named me "Dean." Awards, achievements, and appearances were very important in my family. (My older sister's name is "Laurel," as in honor and glory.) I began to feel that I would never measure up and would cause them to be terribly disappointed.

And then, to make matters worse, I had a spiritual revelation in which I realized that nothing could bring me lasting happiness and self-esteem. Unlike the patients in our study described in chapter 4, I knew at that moment that "If only I had _____, then I'd be happy" was a lie.

I thought about what people told me would make me happy: "What if I get into medical school? What if I earn a lot of money? What if I marry a beautiful woman? What if I win a major scientific prize? What if I write a best-selling book? What if I become famous? Will that bring me *lasting* happiness?"

And I realized that I would be happy for a while—about 15 or 20 minutes, maybe even a few days—and then I would think, "Now what?" It would never be enough. Or, "So what?" Big deal. None of these would provide the lasting meaning and self-esteem I thought they would.

It was a bad combination. I thought that I was never going to fulfill my dream of becoming a doctor. And even if I did, it wouldn't matter anyway. So I got more and more depressed.

I remember one day very clearly—I was sitting in the organic chemistry class and it suddenly occurred to me, "I'm in so much emotional pain, I'm so tired, I'll just kill myself and be done with it! I can sleep forever." It seemed so logical and clear—like, "Why didn't I think of this before?" (And in the twisted logic of the moment, part of me replied, "Because you're stupid, that's why!")

I was very depressed and getting increasingly worse. I went back to my apartment and looked around at the material possessions that were supposed to make me happy, and the idea seemed like a cruel joke. I threw my expensive stereo down a flight of stairs.

I lived in a sterile concrete apartment complex across the street from the Houston Oilers football practice field. There was a large oil derrick near the end zone, and I considered jumping off it. Too messy—and everyone would know what I'd done.

Instead, I decided to have a one-car collision—to run into the side of a bridge, as though I'd lost control of the car. That way, people would think that I just wasn't a very good driver—and if you'd ever been in a car that I'd been driving when I was eighteen, you'd know that wasn't so implausible.

I came about as close to killing myself as a person can without actually doing it. What saved me, ironically, was a physical illness—a very bad case of mononucleosis. I was so ill that I didn't even have the energy to get out of bed—which saved my life. It was my first understanding of how the mind can affect the body, in this case for the worse.

My parents finally began to understand that all was not well with their son, so I withdrew from school and went home with them to Dallas to recuperate. I felt like a complete failure. I was very anxious to get well enough to go out and kill myself. . . .

Something else happened instead. Like many college students in 1969, my sister Laurel had been searching for answers in her life, but she was dissatisfied by the easy solutions of that era. In 1970 she began studying yoga and meditation with a man named Swami Satchidananda, an eminent and ecumenical spiritual teacher who had met twice with Pope Paul VI, spoken at the National Institutes of Health, and addressed the United Nations.

She became happier and calmer. She stopped getting migraine headaches. As a gesture of support for her, my parents decided to have a cocktail party for the swami when he was lecturing in Dallas in 1972. This was considered a little strange back then, especially in Texas.

He walked in their front door, looking like a casting agent's idea of a swami: he had a long white beard, with intelligent and peaceful eyes, and he wore long saffron robes. There is an old saying, "When the student is ready, the teacher appears," and that seems to have been true for me. He agreed to give a lecture in our living room.

The swami began by saying, "Nothing will ever bring you *lasting* happiness." Well, I'd already figured that out. When I looked at him, though, he appeared very happy and content, and I thought, "This doesn't make any sense."

He went on to say what now sounds like a New Age cliché, but at that time it began to transform my life. "Nothing can *bring* us lasting happiness, but we have that already if we simply quiet down the mind and body enough to experience more of an *inner* sense of peace, self-worth, and self-esteem, one that comes not from getting or from doing but simply from *being*. And the paradox and the irony is that not being aware of this, we end up running everywhere else looking for this elusive happiness, in the process disturbing the inner joy and peace we could have if we simply quieted down the mind and body enough to experience that."

I was in so much emotional pain that I was willing to try anything. This was the first time I really understood how pain, or illness, or suffering of any kind—whether physical or emotional—could be a catalyst for real transformation, as described in chapter 3.

I began to practice the same techniques described in this book: stretching exercises, breathing techniques, meditation, relaxation techniques, and visualization. Although I grew up in Texas on cheeseburgers and steak, I began to eat a low-fat vegetarian diet. I started exercising and practicing meditation.

I found that, over time, I was able to quiet down my mind enough to experience—only fleetingly at first—an inner sense of well-being. It didn't last very long at the beginning, but I began to understand where it came from.

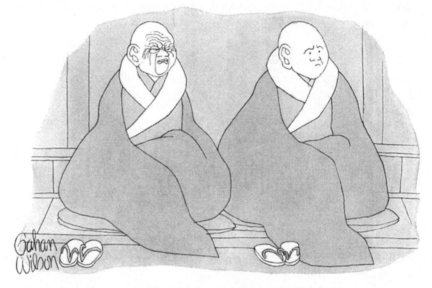

"Nothing happens next. This is it."

Drawing by Gahan Wilson. Copyright © 1980 by The New Yorker Magazine, Inc.

STRESS IS INFORMATION

Once I made the connection between when I felt stressed and why, then stress became my teacher instead of my enemy. When I felt angry, upset, afraid, anxious, or depressed, this suffering and stress reminded me that I was looking in the wrong places for peace and happiness and self-esteem.

I stopped viewing pain—physical and emotional—as punishment and began seeing it as information. The experience reminded me of when I was much younger and realized when I put my hand on a hot stove that there were less painful places to put it. I wasn't being punished by the stove, and I didn't have to blame it for being hot.

In college, I experienced both extremes of a spectrum—how counterproductive it was to be outwardly defined and how empowering it was to be more inwardly defined. When I thought my self-esteem and happiness were dependent on my academic performance—that is, on getting what I thought I needed—I got to a point where I couldn't function at all and I felt like I was going to school at Hell University. I couldn't study, I couldn't sleep, I couldn't even sit still.

When I used the lifestyle program described in this book to start quieting my chattering mind so that I could begin to experience more of an *inner* sense of peace and self-worth, then I was able to perform at the peak of my abilities in the same arena. I went back to college, graduated *summa cum laude,* gave the commencement address, and was accepted into medical school. And I enjoyed the process, not just achieving the goals.

In short, the more inwardly defined I became, the less I needed to succeed and the less stressed I felt. The less I needed success, the easier it came. The less I *had* to get, the more I got. The less I *needed* to acquire power, the more power I realized I already had; before I realized that, I used to give my power away.

These are not new ideas, but they were new to me. Listen to this verse from the *Tao Te Ching,* written over four thousand years ago:

Fill your bowl to the brim
and it will spill
Keep sharpening your knife
and it will blunt.

Chase after money and security
and your heart will never unclench.
Care about people's approval
and you will be their prisoner.

Do your work, then step back.
The only path to serenity.

CHOOSING LIFE AND LETTING GO OF PAIN

When I decided not to die almost twenty years ago, I vowed to live each day fully by choice and not by default. Since then, when I wake up in the morning, I consciously choose to live. My life has been a process of learning to let go of what is unimportant—and the more I let go of, the healthier and stronger I feel. In the final analysis, all I am letting go of is the pain, like letting go of a hot stove.

Likewise, we are always making choices at every moment, even when we don't think of it in those terms. Pain can help us to examine which choices and options we have. What do we want to hold on to and what do we want to let go of? What kind of food do we want to eat? Do we we want to spend time exercising or watching television? How are we defining and limiting ourselves?

Sometimes people tell me, "I know what lifestyle changes I need to make, but it's so hard to begin. What can I do?"

All changes involve some stress at first—the status quo is familiar and comfortable, even when it is killing us. When the pain of the present is worse than the stress of making changes, then it becomes easier to begin.

Illness can be the "big stick" that gets our attention, like the one a Zen meditation teacher uses to rap his students with on the back or head when their attention starts to wander. When we grow tired of being in pain—of banging our head against the wall—then our suffering can be a catalyst for making changes. We can let go of old behavior patterns more easily when we see that they are causing us problems.

Most of us are motivated to make changes either to avoid pain or to gain pleasure. Why give up anything that you like unless what you get back is more than what you give up?

It's easier to see the benefits in some arenas than in others. No one questions the reasons why a prizefighter or a swimmer or a runner spends so many hours a day in grueling training for years to prepare for competition in the Olympics. These athletes often describe the many sacrifices—what they have given up—in order to pursue this goal. Emotional and spiritual goals are more difficult to understand, but the process is also one of making choices and "giving up" or letting go of what is less important.

Learning to let go can even improve athletic performance:

Golfer Mike Reid toured for eleven years, until last October, without winning a tournament. He was the first golfer ever to bank a million dollars and no championships. "I went at it very egocentrically," he says. "I thought everything revolved around me and my ball, as if what the other players did wouldn't matter." For a year or two, he patiently waited his turn. "Then I got to the questioning stage, from there to the changing-everything stage." After a while, the kidding of friends and the kind telegrams from strangers stopped. "In the locker room, the other players didn't know what to say. I could feel their helplessness as much as my own."

Finally, Reid and his wife came to a conclusion. "Both of us had to let go of wanting it so bad," he says. We looked each other in the eye and said, "It's all right if it doesn't happen." You know, it wasn't two weeks later that it did." [*Time* magazine, 6/6/88, p. 74.]

Even in the realm of diet, the choices become clearer. If you choose to eat a low-fat vegetarian diet instead of a cheeseburger, you may do so to avoid pain: not having chest pain is more satisfying than eating meat. Likewise, you may choose a low-fat vegetarian diet to gain pleasure. You'll lose weight. You'll feel better. You'll have more energy. You may need less sleep. And so on.

When the pain becomes intense enough—or when we allow ourselves to experience how much pain we have been feeling—then it becomes easier to let go. Oftentimes we ignore the earlier, minor pains, and we have to wait until we are knocked flat on our backs with a heart attack or similar crisis before we begin to make changes. Even a heart attack may not be enough to motivate some people. I have often seen patients demand a telephone in the coronary care unit "because the business just can't get by without me."

But we don't have to wait for full-blown illnesses; by then, it may be too late. It's better to pay attention to the early warning signals of distress (whether physical or emotional). When a ship is even a few degrees off course, it is easier to reset its path early on; otherwise, the ship can drift thousands of miles out to sea.

PAYING ATTENTION

So the question is: what am I not paying attention to? The function of pain, whether physical or emotional, is to get our attention. We all have an inner teacher, an inner guide, an inner voice that speaks very clearly but usually not very loudly. That information can be drowned out by the chatter of the mind and the pressure of day-to-day events. But if we quiet down the mind, we can begin to hear what we're not paying attention to. We can find out what's right for us.

The stress management techniques described in chapter 7 have several functions. First, of course, they can help us manage stress more effectively. Then, they can help to quiet the mind so we can become more aware of the early warning signs. Finally, when the mind quiets down, we can then begin to hear the information provided by our inner teacher.

EMPOWERING OURSELVES

Studies by Dr. Judith Rodin at Yale and by Dr. Ellen Langer at Harvard have shown that the greatest risks for illness occur when people believe that they have a low amount of control or choice over their work or home environments.

But we always have choices. We always have options. In his book *Man's Search for Meaning,* Victor Frankl wrote about how even in the Nazi concentration camps people responded to the same dire environment in different ways. Those who chose to give meaning to their experiences were more likely to survive. The environment was the same for all of the inmates, but the way they reacted to that situation was different.

Forty years later, Natan Sharansky rediscovered the same truth. In his book *Fear No Evil,* he described how he survived the Russian prison camps by making a conscious choice not to obey his captors.

Knowing that we always have choices can empower us. This way of looking at the world—that is, looking at pain as a teacher instead of an enemy—helps us to see new choices and new possibilities.

Where does real power come from? Where does real happiness come from? Where does inner peace come from?

Many of us believe that power and happiness come from getting more and more and more of our wants and needs fulfilled. As I described in the previous chapter, though, this belief is ultimately self-defeating. Either we don't get the needs and wants fulfilled and we're disappointed and stressed and unhappy and, ultimately, sick, or we do get them fulfilled and find that they don't really bring the lasting meaning and happiness and self-worth that we thought they would.

The other way to have more power and happiness in our lives is to *decrease* our wants and needs, which is where lasting power comes from. The more we can walk away from, the more we can let go of, the more power we have.

Real power is ours already—when we stop giving it away. Real happiness is ours already—when we stop believing it's something we have to get from outside ourselves. Real peace is ours already—when we stop disturbing it. Real freedom is ours already—when we stop limiting ourselves.

We tend to think of power as something we get, not as something we already have. But everything that comes eventually goes. If we get power from outside ourselves, then we can lose it. If someone gives us power, then they can take it away.

Real power is not given to us or even created; real power is realized. It comes from realizing an inner sense of peace, self-worth, and happiness.

No one has power over us unless they have something that we think we need. If we can reduce our needs, then we increase our power. If someone says, "If you don't do what I want, I won't give you this," you can reply, "Fine, I don't need that." And then he or she has less power over you.

The more inwardly defined you are, the less you need. The less you need, the more power you have.

This is often why people become monks and swamis and nuns and other types of renunciates in various religions and cultures. While some may be doing this to avoid the world, the true renunciate understands that the more he or she can let go of, the more joy, power, and peace he or she will maintain.

I'm not advocating that you renounce your physical possessions, move to the Himalayas, live in a cave, and have a begging bowl. You can be just as attached to that begging bowl and just as unhappy. What really frees us is letting go of the idea that these things are going to bring us lasting happiness. When we do, we can enjoy our material possessions without being bound by them.

Paradoxically, the more grounded we are in an inner sense of peace, the more we can accomplish in the external world, and with less stress, anxiety, fear, and worry. We can focus on the task instead of being too concerned with how well we are doing. We don't have to give up our jobs—we can perform them even better.

There is an old Zen proverb: "Before enlightenment, chop wood, carry water; after enlightenment, chop wood, carry water." In other words, our outward actions may not appear very different—we may still go to work every day, raise a family, etc.—but our motivations are different because our perceptions have changed.

That is, to the degree we are inwardly defined and inwardly content, then we do not need to tell ourselves, "If only I had _____, then I'd be happy." We have that already. We can act for the joy of it, not because it's essential to our happiness.

Likewise, to the degree that we perceive ourselves as *a part of* the world rather than *apart from* it—connected and intimate rather than isolated and alone—then we can begin changing the self-destructive perceptions and the resulting behavior patterns that leave us feeling even more lonely.

Of course I can't say I know how you feel, but I know how bad it is to feel alone. I know how painful it is to feel despairing. I know the darkness of feeling suicidal. I know how bleak it is to feel empty—"is that all there is?" I've had those feelings. They may not be exactly the same as yours, but they may be similar. And in that sense we are connected.

I'm not a lot further along than I was; I still make many of the same mistakes I used to, although I catch myself sooner. I still might say to myself, "Oh, if only I can get another grant, if only the patients get better, if only I can do this or that, *then* I'll be happy." But then I start to feel stressed, anxious, worried, or depressed, and my life becomes unhappy.

That emotional stress reminds me that I'm looking in the wrong place for my happiness. I'm digging a hole and falling in it again and then blaming the world for having too many holes—which is about as useful as blaming a stove for being hot.

So it's a gradual process; it's not all or nothing. Just making the connection between when I feel stressed and why made a profound difference in my life—as important as when I realized that putting my hand on a hot stove caused pain and suffering.

But we can make different choices. We can put our hands somewhere else. It becomes easier to let go once we understand where the pain comes from.

In summary, then, chronic emotional stress can lead to heart disease and other illnesses. Stress comes not only from what we do but how we react to the external world. How we react, in turn, is based on how we perceive ourselves in relation to the world. Anything that leads to the perception of isolation causes chronic stress and, in turn, can lead to heart disease or other illnesses. Anything that enhances the perception of intimacy reduces stress, allowing our hearts to begin healing and our lives to become more joyful.

"Anger is short-lived madness."

—Horace (65–8 B.C.),
Epistles

■

"I don't deserve this award, but I have arthritis and I don't deserve that either."

—Jack Benny

■

"As for me, except for an occasional heart attack, I feel as young as I ever did."

—Robert Benchley

■

"If you're going to do something different with your life because you've found out you've got a disease, then you're not living as you should be."

—Arlo Guthrie

6

"A Very Short Fuse"

The program described in this book can transform lives in powerful ways. Although the scientific data are the most convincing to doctors and scientists—angiograms showing the coronary arteries opening, PET scans demonstrating increased blood flow to the heart—I find the personal stories of transformation to be even more gratifying and persuasive. Here are a few. The study participants asked me to use their real names.

"I'm Werner Hebenstreit, and I'm a business consultant. When I first began this program, I had terrible chest pains, tremendous burning pains with even minimal exertion. It was even a problem for me to cross the street against a traffic light, because I couldn't walk fast enough to make it without getting severe chest pain. Pains, pains, pains. Even taking a shower or shaving caused me to have intense chest pain although there's practically no physical effort. I was hardly ever without angina pains.

"After a few weeks on this program, my chest pains began to decrease. After a few months, I had no more pains whatsoever. Now I walk for an hour with no pain. Or I swim an hour a day, fifty lengths in an Olympic-sized pool—no chest pains. I just relax and meditate while I swim. I don't even think about having angina pains any more. And I got off many of the medications that I had been taking, with all their blasted side effects.

"Now, my wife and I can hike four to six hours at a time. Last year, we hiked the whole day at the Grand Teton National Park at six thousand feet high and had no pain.

"My mental well-being has improved as much as my physical well-being. I enjoy life much more than I did before. I was known, I would say, as a man with a very short fuse. I felt attacked very easily.

"I had the tendency to get upset or frustrated about things over which I had no control whatsoever. A newspaper headline could get me into such a bad mood that I couldn't enjoy my breakfast: 'What kind of politician would do this or that?' Waiting for a late bus got me so full of rage that I decided to write letters to the bus company complaining. And so on.

"Then, one day, I recognized it was so stupid to bring up my blood pressure and to get annoyed over things I had no control of. And to illustrate it for myself, I started to write down whenever I got upset in a notebook. On my very 'best' day, I had thirty-three times where I got angry over occurrences over which I had no control whatsoever.

"Now, I don't even carry notebooks around anymore. Whenever I feel frustration coming up, I think of the notebook and I start to smile. I laugh. And I'm much more patient. I take time to analyze, discuss, and to evaluate before I shoot off my mouth, which I used to do. My fuse is much longer now. Some days I am fuseless.

"And from a business point of view, I'm much more successful than before my being sick. The program was a godsend for me. It gave me hope. I faced death, and now I'm facing a second chance at life. Before, I was very negative about things. I thought I would have to be an invalid for the rest of my life. Now I am very positive. I am able to do so many things that were impossible before. Instead of dreading each day, my wife and I look forward to each day. We enjoy each day as it comes.

"After a year, my angiogram showed that the blockages were beginning to reverse. I knew how much better I was feeling, but to have scientific evidence proving that—well, the feeling was just unbelievable.

"When I first heard of this program, I thought it would be too late for me to benefit from it. I mean, I'm seventy-five years old! But, of course, I changed my mind. You're as old as you feel—and I'm getting younger all the time."

"My name is Jim Keith. I'm a carpenter—I own a company that rebuilds and remodels kitchens and bathrooms. I'm fifty-nine years old.

"I began this program over four years ago because I had severe heart disease, diabetes, and terrible chest pains. Now I feel a lot younger. I feel more relaxed than I ever have. I don't have any heart pains like I used to. And I have much more energy than I've had in a long time.

"I lost about fifty pounds, even though I was eating more food than before. I was taking two kinds of insulin injections every day; after six months on the program, I was able to stop one kind and to cut the other in half. I was able to reduce many of my cardiac medications and even get off some of the other ones altogether.

"I started feeling so good, I kind of forgot that I still had a heart problem. So after the first year on the program, I got off it a little. I started eating some fish and chicken, I didn't do the stress management exercises very often, and I stopped swimming regularly. And you know what? A few months later, I started having a few chest pains again.

"So the choice became pretty clear for me. I used to like eating doughnuts, and I still like the taste of meat, but I like feeling this good even more. I feel so much better when I stay on the program. It's definitely worth the effort.

"Before, almost any exertion would bring on the chest pains. I was turning into a real couch potato. I liked to swim, but I could only swim a little before I'd have to quit. One night in the pool, for example, I was swimming about five laps and I started having some bad pain that began in my chest and traveled down my arm, down my side. My wife came out to find out what the matter was. I said,

'Well, I don't feel good swimming tonight.' And she gave me a nitro, and about a minute or so later the pain subsided. I wanted to start swimming again, but she said, 'No, you better not swim any more. You better take it easy the rest of the night.'

"But now, she doesn't tell me that. I can just keep swimming. One night, I swam 165 laps in my pool, and I didn't feel like I wanted to stop! I didn't have any pain, and I felt like I could keep going. But I thought that was enough for one night.

"I felt so great! After I finished swimming, I went to take a hot shower, which used to cause chest pains, but didn't anymore. I felt like I was a young kid again. I had tears coming down from my eyes because I felt so great. I couldn't wait to tell my wife, 'Gee, I feel so *good!*' You can't explain that feeling. It's just something that you have in yourself. You feel like your whole body is lifted up.

"My physical improvements were very important to me, but even more meaningful were the emotional and spiritual changes that occurred. Before I went on the program I was very depressed.

"I didn't care what my business was doing. I didn't care how many jobs I had. I would go to work in the morning around eight, and I was so tired and depressed that by one-thirty in the afternoon I'd go home. I'd just sit on my chair and fall asleep until around four-thirty, when I'd eat something and go to bed. It was a terrible feeling to be that tired and unhappy.

"I didn't care about anything and I didn't want to do anything. I didn't feel like working. I just felt like I wanted to take off and say to heck with it. I didn't care if the jobs were coming in or not.

"I was really disheartened. I felt so bad sometimes that I just wanted to lay down and die. It seemed like there was nothing I could do about it, so I felt helpless, which was even more depressing. And if I died, I thought I wouldn't be missed very much. There was a darkness in my soul and spirit. Nothing mattered. And it was depressing thinking that I'd always feel this bad or worse, that I'd never feel good again. Why bother?

"Then, after I began the program, I learned that there was a *lot* I could do to help myself. So I began to feel less helpless and more hopeful. Soon, I had more energy than before. My mind became clearer. Even my vision improved. I began to feel great.

"And as I started to improve physically, I began to feel much better emotionally, too. I didn't feel depressed most of the time. My communication and relationship with my wife became much better than it was.

"I can accomplish much more in my work than I could before. *Much* more. Now, I work as much as I want to—I start around eight-thirty in the morning and I work straight through until five-thirty or six in the evening. Working hard doesn't bother me anymore. I earned twice as much money the first year on this program than I did the year before, and even more now. Like the guys in the shop said, 'Nice to have you back after all these years.' "

"I'm Bob Finnell. I'm fifty-three. For the past three years I have made substantial lifestyle changes that I thought were impossible for most people and certainly inconceivable for me. But I knew I had to do something: two of my coronary arteries were totally blocked, and the third one was 79 percent blocked. In addition, I had a heart attack without even feeling anything.

"After my angiogram, several cardiologists told me I should have a bypass, but ultimately I refused. I thought there had to be a better way. When I had the opportunity to join Dr. Ornish's program, I did. I was extremely scared, skeptical, and desperate when I began the program. It wasn't difficult to change my lifestyle; the alternative made it imperative that I do so.

"The heart attack was one of the best things that ever happened to me. I could no longer deny that I was seriously ill and that my life was in jeopardy if I continued to live the way I had been. I couldn't pretend that I was misdiagnosed. But at first I didn't understand that this was a tremendous opportunity to lead a more balanced and full life. I just thought that was a cliché.

"And I'm not just talking about the physical level here. I'm learning to react differently and to get rid of extraneous things in my life. Rather than feeling that I've been cheated or whatever, I have a greater sense of inner peace and personal power.

"Sooner or later, most people go down this path. We're all in the same boat. Frequently I pick up the paper and read about someone I knew who had a heart attack and died. But I've been given a second chance.

"I used to be a college professor of literature, and then I was the president of the National Action Council for Minorities in Engineering, a major foundation in New York City. I knew my life was getting out of balance—but, I thought at the time, so what?

"I was often very volatile because of the way I was working. I would always try to keep things under control because so much of my self-esteem was tied up in my work. When you're planning a board meeting or a big project, there can't be any errors or surprises.

"But it's impossible to control everyone and everything, and I was under a lot of stress from trying to do that. At the time, though, I didn't look on that as stressful. I just thought that was part of the job.

"In fact, I was under so much chronic stress that when my first cardiologist asked me if I had any stress in my job, I said, no, I didn't. After I entered this program, I realized that for decades I have had an excessively high amount of stress in my life. Not only because of the external responsibilities I had related to work, family, moving, and traveling, but more importantly from what was going on inside me.

"I also used to try to control my feelings. I didn't show many of my emotions to anyone. I thought I had to have a certain amount of indignation or anger in order to be motivated to get a job done.

"In this program I learned that I can't always control everything. Now, my life is more in balance. I'm learning to let go of a lot of those things that were negative and to experience a greater sense of inner contentment. I don't define who I am by what I do like I used to. And I'm learning how to communicate better, how to speak from my heart instead of only from my head.

"I'm still more comfortable talking about thoughts than emotions, but I can talk about my feelings better than before. I've always been a little afraid of intimacy, of getting too close to someone. So I was frequently in long-distance relationships. When my heart condition was diagnosed, I lived in New York and Marianne lived in San Francisco. If things got too difficult, I knew I would soon be on a plane and flying three thousand miles away. Now things are different—we got married and we're living together for the first time.

"My interactions with people now involve more of a personal interest in them, not just in getting done what *I* want. For example, I'll take a few minutes to talk with the produce man at the fruit and vegetable stand instead of rushing away as soon as I've bought what I need, the way I used to do. Now I take some time to get to know the people I do business with instead of getting it over with as quickly as possible and moving on to something or someone else. It's a different sense of time than I used to have.

"I'm learning to listen better. I'm more interested in what the other person has to say instead of just having my own agenda met.

I'm more patient with the evolution of events. And it's made me more effective.

"More importantly, I'm really positive about leading a moderate life. I don't feel a sense of deprivation. As I become more inwardly defined, I'm not as driven as I used to be. The ironic thing is that now, as a result of the relaxation and stress management and exercise I am doing, I can handle all of that better than when I was younger or even when I had less responsible jobs.

"Before, I thought I didn't have time to exercise or meditate. I would take a taxi to go three blocks in New York because I was always in such a hurry! Now, I usually begin the day by going for a walk and then doing some yoga and meditation for an hour.

"Four years ago, my diet was probably 40 to 50 percent fat. I ate meat two or more times a day. I had large amounts of cheese. I ate lots of desserts. I drank a half bottle or more of vintage wine on the average with the meals I had in the evening. I would say it was the opposite of the kind of diet that one would prescribe for good health.

"Yet it's not hard for me to follow the diet now, even when I travel. I've discovered things that I never had eaten before—squashes, certain beans, and grains—and I love it. I spice it up more than most people.

"My cholesterol was 232 when I started—which I discovered in this program is not only average in America, but average in the intensive care unit. After a few months, my cholesterol decreased to 128, and it's been as low as 95! Without drugs. At the last measure it was 114. I lost about forty pounds in the program during the first six months, and since then my weight has stabilized at 148 pounds, my ideal body weight. I feel stronger, I'm more alert, and my joints aren't stiff. I think all of the things that I did—the diet, the exercise, the relaxation, the meditation—had an impact on it, and I wouldn't want to risk not having done all of it together.

"After a year, my angiogram showed the blockages in my coronary arteries were beginning to reverse. And the PET scan showed that the blood flow to my heart was much better. And not only to my heart—my sex life has improved a lot. And I'm not afraid that something catastrophic will happen to me while I'm making love with my wife as I used to be.

"I started this program over four years ago. Although I showed tremendous improvements during the first year, I noticed even bigger changes between the third and fourth years after starting the program. The tests seem to confirm this—the angiogram and PET scan after four years showed even more improvement than after the first year.

"But it's a mistake to focus too much on the physical changes. I think the mental and the emotional transformations are more important, both in myself and in the others I've been with in this program.

"Personally, the program has meant much more to me than just a health exercise. In my early fifties, I have had an opportunity to reflect on a lot of things that some of my colleagues don't reflect on until they are much older, and it has affected my values and my beliefs. If it were to turn out that it was all a hoax that I had heart disease, I would still continue to follow this program. Because I know now that life is not only about survival, it's about the *quality* of life. These practices have given me a much better life, and probably a much longer one."

"My name is Robert Royall. I'm fifty-four years old. And I'm an Episcopal priest.

"My first angiogram was in 1986, which showed that several of my coronary arteries were partially blocked. I decided to move back to North Carolina for a year—I promised a church there that I would come.

"I made some lifestyle changes during that year—I did what my doctor told me to do. I ate much less red meat and oils, more fish and chicken—and I'd take the skin off the chicken, that kind of thing. But it wasn't easy—being from North Carolina, barbecue was next to ambrosia. Also, I was doing my own type of meditation. And I did some exercise, although the hot weather made it difficult. Living in San Francisco, I had forgotten what hot weather was like, I think. So I gained a lot of weight.

"After about ten or eleven months, I started having a lot more chest pains. And then I had a heart attack also. So I came back to San Francisco and had another angiogram.

"The angiogram showed that in less than a year my coronary artery blockages had gotten much worse. Whatever lifestyle changes I had been making clearly weren't enough. So I joined Dr. Ornish's study.

"When I first entered, I was having angina almost every day.

And the pain was almost constant. I still have a hard time believing it, but after the third or fourth day on the program, I started having much less chest pain. *Much* less. Since then, I've had very few episodes of chest pain. Now I have pain only rarely. And it's always when I'm in a hurry and it's cold and windy outside.

"I talk to a lot of people, and some are beginning to have symptoms that I recognize. Being a disciple of this program now, because I've made so much improvement, I want to tell them, 'Hey, you don't have to suffer like this.' Or, 'You don't have to endure these chest pains.'

"I lost over sixty pounds during the first six months of the program. I must have hit where I'm supposed to be because I haven't gained or lost more than two or three pounds since then. But I haven't been forcing myself to eat less. I'm never hungry on this diet. I find that fruits and vegetables give me the sustenance that I need and they fill me up.

"After a year on the program, I had another angiogram. This time, instead of getting worse like before, I was getting better! The blockages were reversing.

"As a priest, I'm very interested in the psychological and spiritual dimensions of what's been happening to me and to the other study participants in the last year or so. As a theologian, I deal with cosmic questions, but at the same time I also deal with very close personal relationships with people. I think that stopping, taking time, looking at myself, learning how to relax, meditating—all of these things gave me hope and opened different doors to places in myself that I had not been using. Whereas I may have been a little dictatorial in my ministry at times, I find that now I'm much softer and kinder. The program has helped me to see the part I like best about me, and to develop that part.

"Dealing with my own self and my own mortality has helped me begin to look at people in my ministry that I needed to look at very closely. And this is not only the obvious like the homeless, the hungry, and the poor. Coming to grips with my own loneliness and spiritual hunger and fear inside is helping me to empathize with and serve others more effectively.

"Through the deep relaxation and yoga, taking the time to be with me, thinking things through, going through my holy rites, I'm seeing my life in a different light than before. I'm more aware that I'm human and the people I'm working with are human, too. So I look at them a little differently—because all of us have a need, you know, to feed the hungry person deep within us. Somehow that connection needs to be made with all of us. You know, it's the fear that we're just but one step away from oblivion.

"So as I feel more connected within myself, then I feel more connected with other people. Now, it's a more focused compassion rather than a compassion for everything. You know, coming from deep within, I now see each person as someone so unique. I didn't before, because I didn't see it in myself. But as I dug deeper and deeper and meditated a little longer on it, I began to realize even my own uniqueness. That makes me feel better about myself. And I think that any time we feel better about ourselves, then there's going to be healing, deep healing. And any time you reach out for other people, that's healing to you, too.

"So my heart is really opening now. The facades are falling down. And I can reach out and take people into my heart in an easier way than I could a year ago."

PART TWO

THE OPENING YOUR HEART PROGRAM

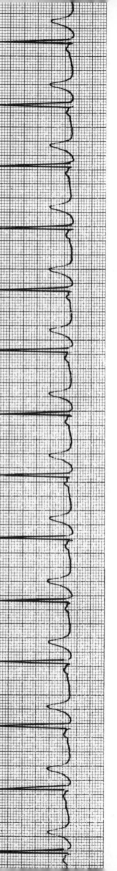

" 'I grew my own body. . . . I may have lost the conscious knowledge of how to grow it . . . but the knowledge is still there. . . . It would take quite a lot of meditation and emptying out to get the whole thing back . . . but you could. If you opened up wide enough.' "

—J. D. Salinger, *Nine Stories*

Introduction to the Opening Your Heart Program

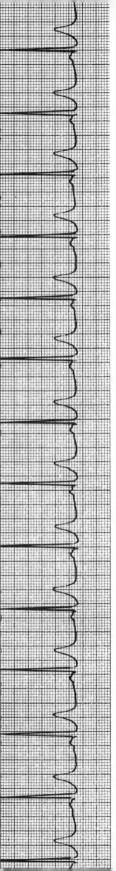

Part 1 described the medical rationale and the scientific evidence for the Opening Your Heart program. I also included a few examples of how powerful this program has been in transforming both my own life and the lives of our study participants.

Part 2, which follows, explains the program in detail and how you can tailor a program that is right for you.

The program has the following components:

- Techniques for increasing intimacy and managing stress more effectively (chapters 7 to 9)
- A diet very low in fat and cholesterol (chapter 10)
- A system to help you stop smoking and to let go of other addictions (chapter 11)
- A program of moderate exercise (chapter 12).

All of these elements are combined to allow healing to begin at the deepest levels.

Here's what our study participants were asked to do each day:

STRESS MANAGEMENT TECHNIQUES

Participants did the following for a total of at least one hour per day:

- 20 minutes for a series of twelve stretches
- 15 minutes for a progressive relaxation technique
- 5 minutes for three breathing techniques
- 15 minutes for meditation
- 5 minutes for directed or receptive imagery

The program also includes communication skills and other techniques for increasing intimacy.

DIET

There are two versions of the diet. The Reversal Diet is for people like our study participants who have heart disease and want to begin reversing it. The Prevention Diet is for people who want optimal health and performance and would like to prevent heart disease.

The Reversal Diet has no animal products at all except egg whites and nonfat dairy products, and no added oils or other concentrated fats. It includes moderate amounts of sugar, alcohol, and salt (if a person has no hypertension, kidney disease, or heart failure), but no caffeine or other stimulants.

The Prevention Diet is somewhat higher in fat and cholesterol than the Reversal Diet. Preventing heart disease probably requires less effort than reversing it. Chapter 10 describes how people without heart disease can customize a diet that is optimal for them.

STOP SMOKING

Chapter 11 describes a number of techniques that our participants used to quit smoking. So can you.

EXERCISE

Participants walked for at least one half hour per day or for one hour three times per week. In chapter 12, I review new research indicating that more exercise than this may not be necessary for a healthy heart and a long life.

One of the most interesting findings of our research was that *the more people did, the better they became.* The more time people spent practicing these stress management techniques and exercising, and the more carefully they stayed on the Reversal Diet, the more their hearts began to heal. In other words, the degree of adherence to the Opening Your Heart program was directly correlated with the amount of reversal in their coronary artery blockages.

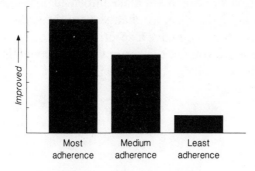

Lifestyle Change Group Only

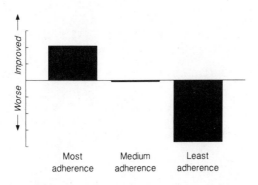

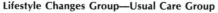

Lifestyle Changes Group—Usual Care Group

**Adherence to the Opening Your Heart Program
and Amount of Reversal of Coronary Artery Blockage**

The more severe your heart disease is, the more closely I would advise you to adhere to the Opening Your Heart program. Over time, as you feel better and if your blockages begin to reverse, you may not need to follow the program as closely. Your doctor may be able to give you more specific guidelines based on your progress.

Our research was designed to determine what is true, not what is easy. You may find that some aspects of the program are easy to adopt; others might be more challenging. For example, the diet may represent a whole new way of eating for you, and it may take some time for your palate to adjust to these new foods. Coronary artery blockages take decades to build up, so reversing this process requires an intensive, comprehensive approach. Preventing heart disease may be easier.

My goal in writing this book is to give you accurate, scientific information that you can use to make informed, intelligent decisions. Whether or not you wish to change your lifestyle, and to what degree, is up to you. You have a spectrum of choices—it's not all or nothing. The more you do, the better you'll feel, whether or not you have heart disease. Here's how to begin.

"Before I built a wall I'd ask to know
What I was walling in or walling out."

—Robert Frost, "Mending Wall"

∎

"And if I have built this fortress around your heart
Encircled you in trenches and barbed wire
Then let me build a bridge
For I cannot fill the chasm
And let me set the battlements on fire."

—Sting, "Fortress Around Your Heart"

∎

"As a man thinketh in his heart, so is he."

—Proverbs 23:7

∎

Luke Skywalker: "I don't believe it!"
Yoda: "That is why you fail."

—George Lucas, *The Empire Strikes Back*

∎

"Like anybody, I would like to live a long life.
Longevity has its place. But I'm not concerned about
that now. I just want to do God's will, and He's
allowed me to go up to the mountain. And I've looked
over. And I've seen the promised land."

—Dr. Martin Luther King, Jr.
(April 3, 1968, his last speech)

∎

"It's very hard to get your heart and head together in
life. In my case, they're not even friendly."

—Woody Allen, *Crimes & Misdemeanors*

7

Opening Your Heart to Your Feelings and to Inner Peace

INTRODUCTION TO THE STRESS MANAGEMENT TECHNIQUES

Back in 1977, when I was a second-year medical student, I asked several cardiologists if they would be willing to refer patients to the first research study I was planning.

"What's the name of your study?" one prominent cardiologist asked me.

"It's entitled, 'Effects of Yoga and a Vegetarian Diet on Coronary Heart Disease.' Would you refer any of your patients to it?"

"Well, Dean, I'd like to support your research, but it sounds too weird. What would I tell my patients—that I'm referring them to a swami?"

"Okay—what if we call it, 'Effects of Stress

Management Techniques and Dietary Changes on Coronary Heart Disease'? Would that be better?"

"Yes, then I'd be delighted to refer patients to your study."

Although that was over thirteen years ago, for some people the words "yoga" and "vegetarian" still conjure up negative images: the sixties counterculture, Hare Krishnas with shaved heads wearing orange robes and chanting and dancing, people selling copies of the *Bhagavad Gita* in airports, and so on. "Meditation" was often confused with TM, or "transcendental meditation," popularized by Maharishi Mahesh Yogi. And where is the land of Vegetaria where vegetarians come from?

It was in the mid-seventies that researchers in various parts of the world began to prove how effective stress management techniques and a low-fat vegetarian diet could be. Studies in Boston, New York, California, England, and in other parts of the world were proving, for example, that meditation can lower blood pressure, decrease the frequency of irregular heart rhythms, reduce cholesterol levels, and so on.

Yet almost all of these techniques ultimately derive from yoga. It's a testimony to the power of these techniques that entire careers have been built around different aspects of yoga, sometimes even renamed after the person who rediscovered that practice.

For example, in the thirties, Dr. Edmund Jacobson, a Harvard physiologist, rediscovered the benefits of deep relaxation (a yoga technique described later in this book). He renamed it "Jacobson Progressive Relaxation" and documented its benefits during the next forty years. (He later wrote a popularized but rather tense book on his work entitled *You Must Relax!*)

More recently, Drs. Janice Kiecolt-Glaser and Ronald Glaser of the Ohio State University College of Medicine found that medical students who practiced relaxation techniques during exams increased their levels of helper cells that defend against infectious diseases. Those who did the relaxation techniques (which were derived from yoga) the most regularly had the strongest immune effects.

Meditation and imagery, too, are also ancient yoga techniques. Herbert Benson, M.D., a well-known cardiologist at the Harvard Medical School, has spent the past two decades conducting pioneering research on the beneficial effects of meditation. He found that regular elicitation of what he terms the relaxation response (in contrast to the fight-or-flight response) can lower blood pressure, decrease premature heartbeats, inhibit gastric acid secretion, and produce other beneficial effects. Jon Kabat-Zinn, Ph.D., director of the Stress Reduction Clinic at the University of Massachusetts Medical School, has found similar results in using yoga techniques with his patients. Carl Simonton, M.D., a radiation oncologist, and his former wife Stephanie Matthews Simonton studied and popularized the importance of visualization and imagery as adjunct therapies in treating cancer. Also, the books of Dr. Mike Samuels, Nancy Samuels, and others have inspired and educated many people about the importance of imagery in healing. Harvard psychologist Mary Jasnoski found that while relaxation alone increased defenses against upper respiratory infections, adding imagery enhanced the effect.

Millions of women have used Lamaze breathing techniques as powerful aids in childbirth. Athletes of all types have found that slow, gentle stretching helps to reduce the risk of injuries, and many are finding that meditation and visualization can improve athletic performance. These techniques also originate from yoga. Others have found that these methods help to slow the physical effects of aging—even Raquel Welch's beauty book is largely a collection of yoga techniques.

The point is simply this: While each of these yoga methods is very powerful even by itself, combining all of these techniques in their original context yields a power even greater than the sum of individual methods. That's because while yoga is a very powerful system of stress management, these techniques were designed for something much greater—as tools for transformation.

The system of yoga was first compiled by Patanjali somewhere between 5,000 B.C. and 300 A.D., although the information had been passed from generation to generation via oral history for many years before then. In his book, *Yoga Sutras,* Patanjali outlined general principles showing step by step how a person can find inner peace and knowledge through yoga.

Patanjali did not limit his instructions to any particular technique, religion, or philosophy, for yoga is not a religion. The methods of yoga are ecumenical and all-encompassing. It is a system that can help broaden a person's present experience of his or her own philosophy, religion, and daily life.

Yoga complements rather than replaces Western approaches and medical care. Knowing the power and limitations of each is very important.

In 1979, during my senior year of medical school, I spent a

month in India and Sri Lanka (Ceylon) with Swami Satchidananda and four other medical students to learn more about the various medical systems there.

I went there expecting to come back with a real enthusiasm for these alternative approaches. I was already convinced of the usefulness of yoga, since it had helped me so much in my own life and I had already conducted my first study on the effects of lifestyle changes (including yoga) on coronary heart disease.

We landed in New Delhi, and one of our first stops was to visit the All India Institute of Medical Sciences, considered the most prestigious Western-style medical school in India. I presented our preliminary research findings there—and found myself in the curious position of being an American lecturing to a very skeptical audience of several hundred Indian doctors about the value of ancient yoga techniques! Most of these Indian physicians viewed yoga as their "illegitimate stepchild," and instead embraced Western medicine to the exclusion of their own heritage and traditions.

After a week traveling around north and south India, I developed a terrible case of dysentery and profound diarrhea. And most of the places we visited were small villages without toilet paper or even toilets—all in all, a bad combination of events. Also, it was August, the temperature was over 100 degrees on most days, and water supplies were scarce.

Partly as a result of my delirium, I decided that this was a wonderful opportunity to try some of the various local remedies to treat myself. So for the next two weeks, whenever we visited a clinic or traveled to a new village, I offered myself as a patient. I tried the Ayurvedic, naturopathic, homeopathic, and yogic remedies, and I just kept losing weight and getting more dehydrated.

Finally, almost apologetically, I decided to take an antibiotic that I'd brought with me. Within twenty-four hours, I was much better, and within two days I was well.

So I came back with a healthier respect for Western medical approaches. But I have also seen the limitations of conventional Western medicine and the power of these ancient yoga techniques. Both are useful; both are important.

Western techniques, such as drugs and surgery, can be very helpful in a crisis, but they are limited, as I described in chapter 1. The stress management techniques derived from yoga address the more fundamental issues that predispose us to illness.

A recurrent theme in this book is that isolation can lead to stress and, ultimately, to illness, whereas intimacy can be healing. Isolation comes in several forms:

- isolation from our feelings, our inner self, and inner peace
- isolation from others
- isolation from a higher force

This chapter focuses on the first type of isolation: how to rediscover and begin healing our inner self. Healing our isolation from others and from a higher force are discussed more fully in the next two chapters.

Although many people think of yoga only as a collection of various stretching exercises and postures to limber up the body, it is more than that. Yoga also includes breathing techniques, meditation, visualization, progressive relaxation practices, self-analysis, and altruism. All of these different methods, though, have a common purpose: to heal our isolation.

The word "yoga" comes from the Sanskrit word meaning "yoke," to bring together, to unite, to make whole. Stated another way, the relaxation techniques and stress management techniques described here are much more than simple strategies to help us cope with or deal with or manage stress. Yoga is a system of powerful tools for achieving union—and healing—with parts of ourselves, with others, and with a higher force.

Awareness is the first step in healing. Unfortunately, we are often more aware of what is going on *around* us than what is going on *inside* us. From the moment the alarm clock or radio jars us awake in the morning until we fall asleep at night while reading or watching television, our attention is drawn outward. We seldom take the time to notice what is going on inside our own body and mind until something goes wrong and we're in pain.

The techniques described in this chapter are designed to increase our awareness of what is happening inside us—physically, emotionally, and spiritually. Increasing our awareness extends our control over what is happening within. As a result, we can notice the effects of stress and make changes before they become full-blown illnesses such as heart disease.

"I used to get terrible back pains," said one of the participants in our research. "Sometimes they were so bad that I had to lie on the floor in the middle of my office. I got so incapacitated that I had three spinal fusions (laminectomies). Each operation would help for a while, but the pain eventually kept coming back.

"Then I tried the yoga techniques that I learned in this program. The stretching exercises helped me loosen up the chronically tensed muscles. The meditation and breathing techniques helped me to become more aware of situations in which I felt stressed and they gave me the tools to do something about it. After a while, I began to realize that I tended to clench my jaw, my neck, and my back muscles throughout the day whenever I felt worried, upset, or angry, which was most of the time.

"Now, when I start to feel a little discomfort in my back or jaw, I use that as a signal to tell me to pay attention to my stress level. I notice the early warning signals of distress better than I used to. During the day, I remind myself to pay attention to what's going on in my back—*before* it starts hurting. Whenever I notice that it's getting a little tight or tense, then I simply allow it to relax. It's much easier to make the necessary corrections before the damage to my back is severe.

"Before, I couldn't even bend over far enough to see my feet. Now, I'm so flexible I can even put my palms on the floor! And I don't ever get severe back pains anymore. Never."

Throughout this chapter, please keep in mind that all of these seemingly different techniques have a common purpose: to help quiet down your mind and body, thus enabling you to experience an inner sense of relaxation, peace, and joy. This is our natural state until we disturb it.

At the end of a stress management session, remind yourself that this feeling of greater peace didn't come from anywhere outside you; it was there already. You simply removed some of the physical and emotional stress that may have kept you from feeling that way all the time.

Relaxation and Lethargy Are Not the Same

There are many, many misconceptions when it comes to yoga and relaxation, some of which I've already discussed. For example, relaxation and lethargy are often confused, but they are really quite different.

Professional athletes make their living from knowing how to increase their performance. They know that when they are relaxed they are working at peak efficiency and performing their best.

Among world-class athletes, such as in the Olympics, there is not much difference in the physical abilities of the various contenders. At that level, the major differences are mental. According to tennis star Boris Becker, "The difference between number one hundred and number one is minimal. About ninety-five percent of it is decided in the head." Athletes describe tensing up as "choking," a vivid image portraying how tension impedes performance.

Edwin Moses is one of the great runners of all time. His string of consecutive victories in the hurdles lasted eight years. Before running a race, he would lie down on the track by his starting blocks and spend a few minutes meditating and visualizing. In the final innings of the 1988 World Series, pitcher Orel Hershiser spent the time between innings with his eyes closed. During the post-game interview, when a reporter asked him what he had been doing, he replied, "I was singing hymns to myself to keep myself relaxed," a form of meditation. He was voted the most valuable player.

Athletes are also beginning to find that increasing flexibility can substantially improve their performance. In general, world-class athletes are more flexible than their less accomplished counterparts.

Bob Prichard is the director of the Somax Posture and Sports clinic in San Rafael, California, where he has been studying and working with gifted athletes for over a decade. In general, he is finding that tense muscles impair performance. For example, he studied Matt Biondi, a swimmer who won seven gold medals at the Seoul Olympics. Although Biondi had measurably less arm power than other swimmers on his college team, he had 70 degrees more range of motion in his shoulders. This greater flexibility gave him the ability to precisely position his arm and hand during swimming, thereby increasing his efficiency. And this enhanced efficiency more than made up for his lack of power.

Similarly, Prichard found that increasing external arm rotation (how much the shoulder rotates back just before hitting a serve) improves tennis performance. His studies show that for every degree that you increase your external arm rotation, you can add a mile per hour to your serve.

In other words, your body and mind function most efficiently and effectively when you are relaxed. Because of this, these yoga techniques can help you to achieve more in the world, not to withdraw from it. By learning to be relaxed, you can perform even better.

Although the ancient swamis and mystics might cringe to hear this, practicing yoga on a regular basis gives you a competitive advantage, whether your arena is in the business world or on the playing field. As I described in chapter 5, this was certainly true in my life when I was in college. When you can manage stress more effectively, then you can accomplish even more.

As I described in chapter 4, there are two basic ways of dealing with stress. One way is to avoid it. Reduce external stressors when you can, but this is not always possible or even desirable. The other way to manage stress is to change how you react to a situation. The circumstances don't change, but *you* do. These stress management techniques can help you react to potentially stressful situations in ways that are more healthful and productive. Your stress threshold increases. In other words, your fuse gets longer.

In the final analysis, all of the techniques described here are restorative. Eventually, if we can learn to maintain a relaxed state even in the midst of our busy lives, eat a healthful diet, and avoid disturbing our health with stimulants, smoking, and so on, then we may not need to spend very much time each day doing these stress management practices. In the meantime, they can be extraordinarily useful.

STRETCHING

The stretching exercises, also known as hatha yoga, are a series of gentle positions designed to limber the body. Actually, "exercises" may not be the best word, for these stretches are performed slowly and gently, with grace and control, as a type of meditation rather than as a form of calisthenics.

"Ha-tha" is translated from Sanskrit to mean "sun and moon." In various cultural traditions, religions, and mythologies, the sun and moon represent the various dualities and cycles of life: day and night, male and female, on and off, conscious and unconscious, rational and irrational, light and dark, breathing in and breathing out, and so on. In digital sound recordings (such as compact discs) and in computers, all sound and information are reduced to a series of on/off switches represented by the duality of ones and zeros.

Hatha yoga is more than just a collection of stretching and breathing techniques. Ultimately, the purpose of hatha yoga is to begin rebalancing these opposing forces and to experience the equilibrium, peace, and common unity that underlie these dualities.

For most of us, the duality of our muscles—contracting and relaxing—is out of balance, for our muscles are chronically tensed and contracted. The first step toward experiencing inner peace and healing is to quiet down and relax the body.

As described in chapter 3, your mind affects your body. It's also true that your body affects your mind.

For example, new research by Dr. Robert Zajonc, a psychologist at the University of Michigan, is uncovering evidence that putting on a sad face or a smile directly produces the feelings that these expressions represent. In other words, facial expressions are not just the visible signs of our emotions, but actually contribute to the feelings themselves. Dr. Paul Ekman, a psychologist at the University of California Medical School at San Francisco, found that when people mimic different emotional expressions, their bodies produce distinct physiological patterns, such as changes in heart rate and breathing rate, for each emotion.

During times of perceived danger, all of your muscles begin to clench and contract as a way of fortifying your "body armor" so that you are more protected during a fight. During times of chronic stress, your muscles may become chronically tensed. After a while, this may lead to neck pain, a sore back, or discomfort in your shoulders. Learning to stretch and lengthen muscles that are chronically contracted helps to rebalance both your body and your mind.

Every yoga teacher has his or her own variations. I like the method taught by Swami Satchidananda because it is comprehensive yet gentle, and the classes include breathing and meditation techniques as well as stretching exercises. Classes in these methods are given at Integral Yoga Institutes, which are located in many cities.

These techniques require no special equipment other than a mat or carpeted floor and some comfortable clothing. The illustrations for the stretches in this section show people who are very flexible. However, the point is not to see how far you can stretch, but rather just to stretch as far as feels comfortable for *you.* You may find that some days you can stretch farther than others, or even that you can stretch farther in the afternoon than in the morning. The point is to pay attention to how you are feeling and to stretch accordingly, not to what you think you "should" be doing. Like the story of the tortoise and the hare, slow but steady wins the race. As you progress, you do not need to learn more advanced positions; just hold these a little longer.

When you stretch chronically tensed muscles, slowly and gently *allow* your body to relax. More vigorous stretching to *force* your muscles to lengthen may actually make matters worse.

Although stretching can be done at any time, it's a good idea to develop a routine. It's better to do a little every day than to wait until you have more time to spend. Many people find that the morning is a good time, before everyone else wakes up. The morning time is often peaceful and there are fewer distractions. And if something unexpected comes up, you can make up a missed morning session in the evening.

The participants in our study practiced the yoga techniques for one hour a day (including the stretching, breathing, meditation, progressive relaxation, and visualization techniques). You may wish to do more or less than this. It's not all or nothing; the more you do, the more benefits you receive. Even five minutes a day is better than nothing. If you don't have much time, just do the twelve-part movement once or twice and a few minutes of meditation (described in chapter 9). If you have a little more time, add the shoulder stand.

Sometimes these yoga stretches are referred to as "poses" rather than stretches as a way of emphasizing that these movements are done very slowly. The movements are unforced and gentle, without bouncing, moving with the control and grace of a dancer rather than a Marine drill instructor. Pay attention to the areas being stretched. The time relaxing in between the poses is as important as the stretches themselves.

Use common sense. If you hurt, stop what you are doing. Hold each stretch only for as long as it feels comfortable for you.

Head Rotations
Many people find that their neck becomes tense and stiff during times of chronic stress. Head rotations are a simple way to begin relaxing the neck and shoulders. And unlike some of the other stretches in this chapter, head rotations can be done anywhere, at any time.

Sit comfortably in a chair or on the floor. (Head rotations can be done while standing, but some people find it hard to keep their balance while doing them.) Inhale. Exhale as you allow gravity to slowly bring your head down as close to your chest as you find to be comfortable. Feel the gentle stretch on the back of your neck and in your shoulders. Bring your head back to the center and relax. Now begin inhaling as you slowly roll your right ear towards your right shoulder. (Try not to bring your shoulder up to your ear, and avoid any sudden or jerking movements.) Continue inhaling as you rotate your head past your right shoulder and allow your head to gently drop backwards. Relax your jaw. Now roll your head around to your left shoulder as you begin to exhale, and continue around to where you began. Do this a few times in each direction.

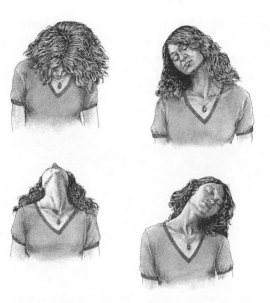

Shoulder Shrugs

Now that your neck is more relaxed, turn your attention to your shoulders, another favorite place for holding in chronic tension. Some people feel like the "weight of the world" is on their shoulders. For the next few minutes, just shrug it off.

Begin by standing or sitting in a comfortable position with your arms hanging loosely by your sides. Then push both shoulders forward and slowly begin to raise them towards your ears. As you continue raising your shoulders, let them rotate back towards your ears. After you reach the top of the rotation, gently push your shoulders back as you begin to lower them to where you started. Each shoulder should make a complete circle. Do this two or three times, then rotate your shoulders in the other direction. If you wish, you can rotate each shoulder individually, alternating one side with the other. Then rest for a few seconds and notice how you feel.

Twists
Stand comfortably with your feet apart. Raise your arms to your sides so they are outstretched and parallel with the floor. Then gently begin swinging your arms as you rotate your hips and torso from one side to the other. Remember to keep breathing while you do this.

Resting Position
You already may be an expert at doing this yoga position.

Lie on your back with your eyes closed, your arms to the side with palms up, and your feet about eighteen inches apart. Allow your arms and legs to relax so that you're not using any muscles to hold them in position.

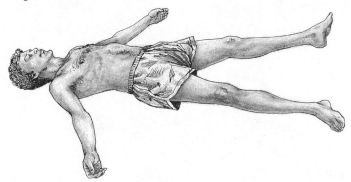

The resting position can also be performed while lying on your abdomen.

Back Stretch (Cobra Pose)
Lie on your abdomen. Place your palms on the floor beneath your shoulders, with your fingers pointing forward and your elbows raised and close to your body, as if you were going to do a push-up. Keep your legs together and your toes pointed. Inhale. Stretch your chin

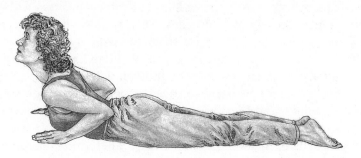

forward and without pushing down on your hands, slowly raise your head, neck, and chest off the floor. Keep your pelvis on the floor. Breathe normally.

At first, hold this position for only a few seconds, repeating it two to four times. Exhale as you slowly roll down, first touching your chin, then your forehead, then your shoulders to the ground. Turn your cheek to the side but leave your hands in place. At your own pace, gradually increase the time you spend in this position (up to a minute) and do it fewer times. The last time you come down, turn your cheek to the side, release your arms and legs, and spend a few seconds in the resting position on your front side.

Leg Lift One (Half Locust Pose)
Lie facedown with your chin on the ground. Push your arms underneath your body, with your elbows close under your body and your palms facing your thighs. Keep your pelvis on your arms. Inhale, straighten your right leg and slowly raise it off the floor as far as you feel comfortable. Hold it in the air for up to ten seconds while breathing normally, then slowly lower it. Do this two times with each leg.

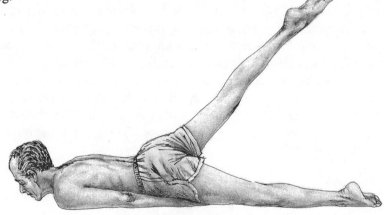

Leg Lift Two (Full Locust Pose)
As above, but this time inhale stiffen the body, keep your chin on the floor, and raise both legs together a comfortable distance without bending your knees. Breathe normally. Repeat two or three times for up to ten seconds each time.

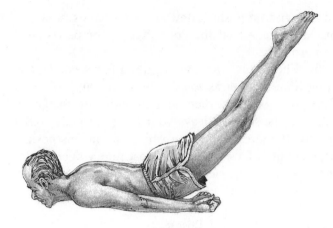

Forward Stretch One (Head-to-Knee Pose)
Sit on the floor and stretch out both of your legs in front of you. Bend your left leg and place the sole of your left foot against the inside of your right thigh. (Keeping your toes curled back will help keep your right knee straight.) Inhale, look up, lock your thumbs, and raise your arms overhead as far as you comfortably can. Exhale, bending forward from the hips, keeping your back straight. Take hold of your foot, calf, or whatever you can comfortably reach. Allow your head to relax. Breathe normally. Hold this position for up to ten seconds, then repeat this with your other leg. Repeat two or three times with each leg. With regular practice, gradually increase the time you spend in this position and do it fewer times. Then relax in the resting position for a while.

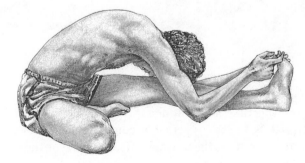

Forward Stretch Two (Forward Bending Pose)
This pose is the same as the one above, but instead of bending one
leg, you stretch out over both legs together. Remember to stretch up
before bending forward.

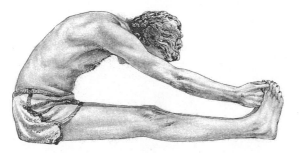

Shoulder Stand
MODIFIED VERSION: Lie on your back and rest your feet on a chair
with your legs elevated. Maintain this position for two to three
minutes, sooner if you become uncomfortable. Do only this modified
version if you have severe high blood pressure, back pain, neck or
shoulder injuries, or if you have had problems so far with any of the
other stretches.

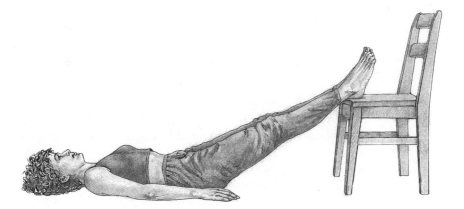

REGULAR VERSION I: Adjust your clothing to loosen any restric-
tions on movement. Lie on your back with your feet together and
your arms alongside your body, palms down. Inhale, straighten your

legs and lift them over your head in a horizontal position as shown
in the illustration. (You may find that you need to bend your knees
in order to raise them over your head.) Begin breathing normally.
Then bring your palms to your lower back for support and gradually
straighten your legs to a vertical position, bringing your chin and
your chest close together.

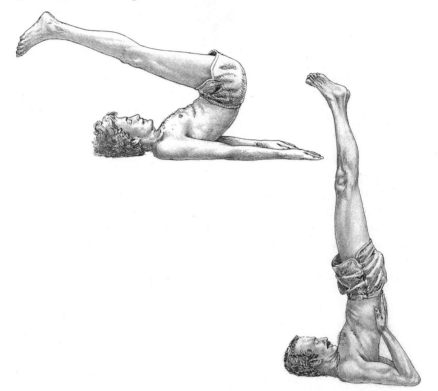

Continue breathing normally. When you're ready, slowly lower
your legs over your head again so they are parallel to the floor,
transfer your forearms to the floor, and bring your trunk down
slowly, then lower your legs to the ground. If your abdomen is not
strong enough to allow this, then just roll down slowly with control
in whatever way is most comfortable for you.

Chest Extension (Fish Pose)
Lie on your back. Bring your legs together and grasp the sides of
your thighs. Resting your weight on your elbows, raise your head
and trunk to a half-seated position. Arch your back, thrusting out
your chest. Lower your head and place the top of your head on the

floor. Your weight should be balanced between your elbows, the top of your head, and your buttocks. Have a slight smile on your face to relax any tension in your jaw. To come down, shift your weight to your elbows, straighten your neck and back, and then lower yourself down to the floor. Whenever you do the shoulder stand, do the fish pose next, as it helps release any tension caused by the shoulder stand.

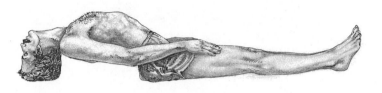

Half Spinal Twist

Sit on the floor and extend your left leg straight out in front of you. Cross your right foot over your left knee, placing the sole of your right foot flat on the floor. Sit up straight. Bring your right knee close to your chest. Now extend your arms in front of you, lock your thumbs, and twist to the right. Unlock your thumbs and place your right hand on the floor behind you, close to your body, with your fingers pointing away from you. Place your left arm between your trunk and your right knee (i.e., on the outside of your right knee), and press your knee to the right. Reach around your right knee with your left hand and take hold of the outside of your left leg or the instep of your right foot. Slowly twist your head and trunk to the right and look over your right shoulder. After 15 to 60 seconds, slowly unwind and do the same pose on the other side.

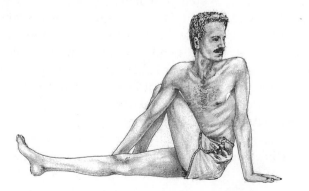

Forward Stretch Three (Yogic Seal)
This is my favorite stretching pose. Sit in a comfortable, cross-legged position, with your eyes closed. Bring both hands behind your back and grasp your right wrist with your left hand.

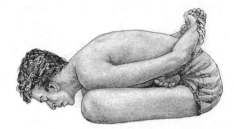

Sit up straight and inhale deeply. Exhale, bending forward from your hips. Come forward as far as it is comfortable. You may wish to spend several minutes relaxing into the position, letting go of tension in your neck, back, and shoulders. To come out of the pose extend your chin, inhale, and come to a seated position.

The Twelve-Part Movement (Sun Salutation)
The Twelve-Part Movement combines many of the benefits of the preceding poses, stretching you both forward and backward. It can be used as a warm-up, as a cool-down, or as a substitute for the other stretching poses when you don't have time for doing all of them.

POSITION ONE: Exhale. Stand up straight with your feet together. Bring your palms together in front of your chest.

POSITION TWO: Inhale. Lock your thumbs. Stretch out your arms in front of you. Watch your hands as you slowly raise your arms overhead. Bend backwards a little from the hips as you stretch.

POSITION THREE: Exhale. Fold forward slowly from your waist.

POSITION FOUR: Inhale. Bend your knees and place your palms alongside your feet. Stretch your left leg back, placing your left knee on the floor. Leave your right foot between your hands and bring your right knee to your chest. Look up.

POSITION FIVE: Exhale. Bring your right foot back to meet your left. Raise your buttocks so that your body now forms a triangle. Stretch your heels toward the floor and look at your feet.

POSITION SIX: Begin to inhale. Lower your knees, chest, and chin to the floor, leaving your pelvis slightly raised. Your palms are now beneath your shoulders, elbows close to your body and pointing upwards.

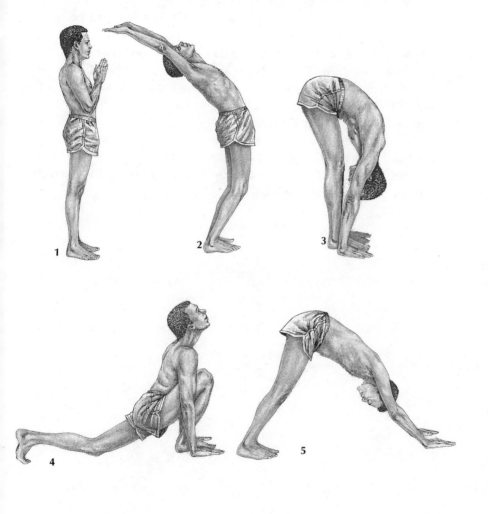

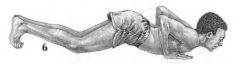

POSITION SEVEN: Continue to inhale as you lower your pelvis to the floor. Stretch up your head, neck, and chest. Keep your elbows slightly bent and in toward your body.

POSITION EIGHT: Exhale. As before, press down on your palms and feet to lift your buttocks forming a triangle.

POSITION NINE: Inhale. Move your left foot forward between your hands, with your left knee touching your chest. The right leg is now stretched back, with your right knee on the floor.

POSITION TEN: Exhale. Bring your right foot forward to meet the left. Bring your feet together and straighten your knees as you stretch forward, as though touching your toes. Bend from your hips only as far as you feel comfortable.

POSITION ELEVEN: Inhale. Again lock your thumbs, stretch up and bend backward slightly, as in position two.

POSITION TWELVE: Exhale. Slowly bring your palms together in front of your chest. Relax.

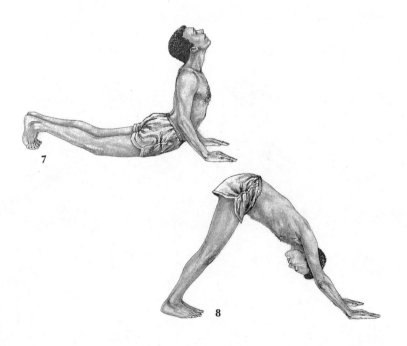

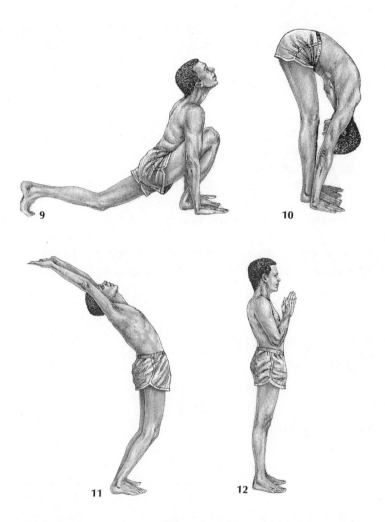

Repeat this two or three times. If you wake up a little sluggish, you may want to do the sun salutation a little faster and more vigorously. If you're feeling a little agitated, try doing it more slowly than usual.

Afterwards, close your eyes and relax for a while in the resting position.

Office Stretches
Working in an office often combines the chronic physical stress of sitting for long periods in front of a computer or hunching over a desk with chronic emotional stress. Taking a few minutes to stretch can help to break the cumulative, chronic stress cycle. Here are some examples and exercises you can do while seated:

- head rotations
- shoulder shrugs
- forward stretches
- spinal twists
- stretching your lower back
- stretching your legs and ankles

Although not part of our program, therapeutic massage is another useful way of relaxing chronically tensed muscle groups.

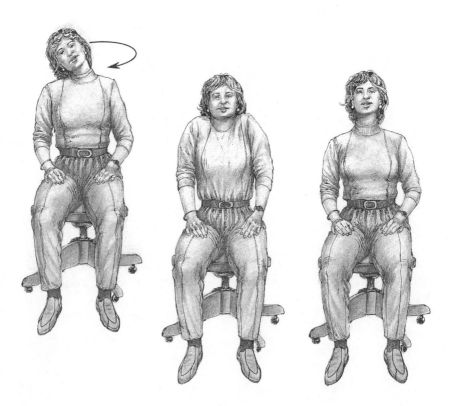

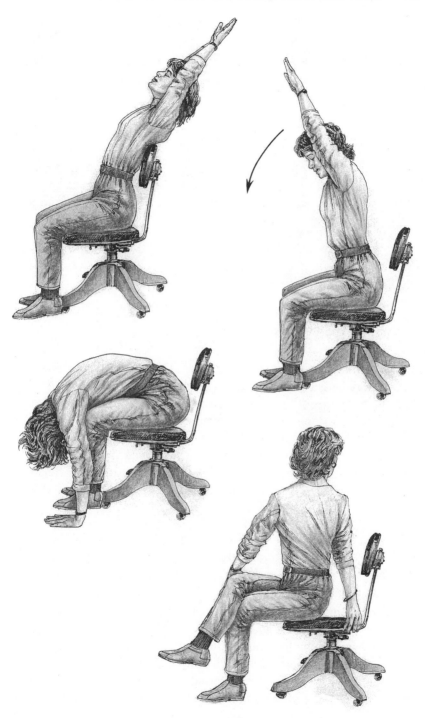

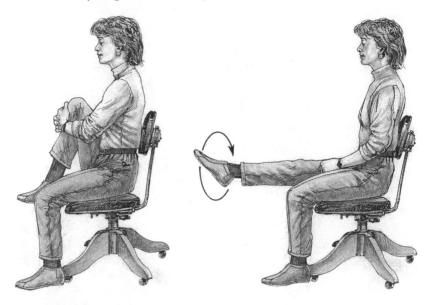

PROGRESSIVE DEEP RELAXATION

For a moment, think of each muscle as if it were a pendulum. The easiest way to get a pendulum to swing over to one side is by first pulling it to the other. Deep relaxation is a simple yet powerful technique based on this phenomenon. A muscle will relax more profoundly if you first tense it.

Lie on your back with your eyes closed. Move around a little until you feel comfortable, then try to lie without moving. Begin by inhaling, tensing your right leg and raising it a few inches off the ground . . . hold it there for a few seconds . . . and then let it drop to the floor as you exhale. Then do the same with your left leg.

Then inhale deeply and contract the muscles of your right arm as you raise it a few inches off the ground, hold it there for about five seconds, and then let it drop to the floor as you exhale. Then do the same with your left arm.

Now inhale deeply and contract the muscles of your buttocks as you raise your pelvis a few inches off the ground, hold it there for about five seconds, and then let it drop to the floor as you exhale.

Then inhale deeply and push your abdomen out like a balloon, hold your breath for about five seconds while contracting your abdomen, and then let your abdomen completely relax as you exhale, through your mouth. Repeat the same sequence with your upper chest.

Leaving your arms relaxed, inhale and bring your shoulders up toward your ears, then bring them together in front of your chest, and then push them toward your feet. Relax.

Gently roll your head from side to side and allow your neck to relax. Inhale and squeeze together all of your facial muscles, including your jaw, mouth, eyes, and forehead. Then relax.

Finally, mentally allow each part of your body to relax even more.

Sometimes the experience of deep relaxation feels profoundly healing on many levels. For example, you may begin to experience more clearly what is happening in your body. Thoughts and feelings that were previously walled off may come to the surface, where they can be reintegrated into your awareness. On a still deeper level, you may even find that you begin to experience being a part of a larger whole, as described in chapter 9.

As your body begins to quiet down, observe what's happening in your mind. Just notice whatever thoughts or feelings come up, but let them pass without trying to judge, suppress, or control them. I'll talk more about these processes in chapter 9.

Then bring your awareness to your breathing. Without trying to change your pattern of breathing, just observe or feel the gentle flow of air as it comes in and out of your nose. After a few minutes, or whenever you wish, gradually allow your inhalations to become a little deeper with each breath. Imagine that you are breathing in light and healing energy as well as oxygen that is revitalizing and recharging your body and mind. Slowly move your fingers and toes, hands and feet. Then gently roll your arms and legs back and forth. When you are ready, slowly roll over onto your side, and then come to a seated position.

After you have practiced the deep relaxation several times, you may be able to get into this state without having to sequentially tense and relax each muscle group. For example, if you are under a lot of time pressure, simply lie down, inhale deeply, and tense *all* of your muscles simultaneously. Hold this for a few seconds, then release everything as you exhale deeply and relax completely.

Bob Finnell, a participant in our study, described it this way after finishing a deep relaxation one evening: "It feels like the beginning of the day instead of the end."

BREATHING TECHNIQUES

Your breath is a bridge between your body and your mind:

Changes in your body affect your breathing. When you exercise, your oxygen requirements go up, and you breathe faster and deeper.

Changes in your mind affect your breathing. When you are anxious, your breathing is rapid and shallow. When you are relaxed, you breathe slower and deeper.

Changes in your breathing affect your body. When a baseball pitcher winds up to throw, he first takes a deep breath. It helps him perform better. When a marksman is taught to shoot a rifle, he or she is told to inhale fully and to pull the trigger while slowly exhaling. Artists who sing opera or popular music and martial artists who practice karate, judo, or aikido also use breathing techniques to improve their performance.

Changes in your breathing affect your mind. When you are a little tired, a deep breath can make you more alert. When you are feeling anxious or worried, a few deep breaths can help to calm you down. To some degree, our language reflects the importance of breathing and its influence on our mind. The term "inspire" means both to inhale deeply and to become energized, creative, or motivated. "Expire," on the other hand, means to die.

Besides connecting your mind and body, breathing is also a bridge between your sympathetic and parasympathetic systems. During times of emotional stress, your sympathetic nervous system becomes stimulated. As a result, as described in chapter 2, your heart rate, blood pressure, and muscular tension all increase. In people who are chronically stressed, the autonomic nervous system is out of balance—that is, the sympathetic nervous system is chronically overstimulated.

The breathing techniques that I'm about to describe can help balance your sympathetic and parasympathetic nervous systems. When practiced regularly, they produce a profound, calming effect on your mind and body and decrease sympathetic nervous system stimulation. And unlike the physical stretches, these breathing techniques can be practiced anywhere, any time.

During my medical training, I was taught only the pathology of breathing—what happens when something goes wrong with the lungs or respiratory system. But in the tradition of yoga, thousands of years have been spent studying the more subtle effects of the breath on the mind and body, and how these can be enhanced for greater power, health, and inner peace.

In this system, we inhale not only oxygen but also energy, or *prana* (pronounced "prah-na"). In Sanskrit, prana means both breath and spirit. In other languages, the words for breath and spirit are similar. In Hebrew, for example, the term is *ruach.* In Latin, it is *spiritus.* The Greek word is *pneuma.*

Breath is the vehicle for prana. This "vital force" may sound a little mystical to a Western physiologist since it cannot be measured using conventional scientific equipment. Yet in our daily language we refer to our "energy level," which is high at some times and low at others. Our experience validates the concept of "energy" even though we can't measure it. Likewise, practicing these breathing techniques may enhance your level of energy. See for yourself.

The breathing techniques described here are called *pranayama,* literally "control of prana." These techniques can expand and balance the availability of energy to you. In meditation, described later, this flow of energy can be focused and intensified. Using visualization, also described later, you can learn to direct this energy to assist in the process of health and healing.

According to this school of thought, we are composed of several "bodies," each more subtle than the other. Your physical or material body is derived from your "pranic" or energy body. Other "bodies," which are not described here, are even more subtle.

Whether or not this is literally true has not been scientifically proven, although it may be experienced. For example, at the end of a deep relaxation, when your physical body is very quiet, you may feel your energy body swaying back and forth as you breathe. Also, when a person's arm or leg is amputated due to injury or disease, he or she often experiences the arm or leg as still being there even after it is gone. Sometimes he or she will even experience pain in the amputated body part, a phenomenon that doctors term "phantom pain." Although part of the physical body is gone, that part of the energy body still remains.

As I described earlier, if we make changes at the psychological and spiritual level, then the physical heart also may begin to improve. We can measure these changes in the physical heart using quantitative coronary angiography, cardiac PET imaging, and other advanced medical imaging technologies. But these changes in the physical body may be partly due to the effects of more subtle changes in the energy body, although these cannot yet be measured. If we attempt to change only the physical body without also working at more subtle and fundamental levels, then the problem may recur in the same form or in a different one. But if the energy pattern is sufficiently changed, then the physical body may change, too.

In other words, your emotional state and your breathing first affect your energy body and then may affect your physical body—for better and for worse. These breathing techniques are simple yet very powerful. In fact, almost all of the yoga books and teachers warn that any breathing techniques more involved than those outlined here should be avoided or, at the very least, performed only under close supervision with an experienced teacher in combination with other physical and spiritual practices.

On a more down-to-earth level, chronic stress can restrict your range of breathing. To measure your breathing range, put a tape measure around your chest and take a deep breath. Measure your chest. Then exhale fully and measure the change in circumference. Bob Prichard, whose research measures range of breathing as well as range of motion, found that people who don't have problems with endurance, who are able to exercise and to go about their daily activities without respiratory distress, have a 10 percent expansion range (range of breathing). The best competitive athletes have as much as a 15 percent range of breathing. For example, Janet Evans won three Olympic gold medals in swimming, even though she competed against women who had 50 percent greater cardiovascular capacity than she did, perhaps because she did not have any restriction in her range of breathing.

In contrast, people with heart disease tend to have markedly diminished ranges of breathing. Their breathing range often may be in the 2 to 5 percent range, significantly lower than the general population. So heart patients, who need more oxygen than the average person, unfortunately receive less.

Why do people have such a tremendous restriction in their range of breathing? One of the ways we respond to stress is by holding our breath. Over time, when stress is chronic, we may develop connective and muscular tissue that cause a decrease in our range of breathing.

Stretching and breathing techniques can help people to improve both their range of breathing and their range of motion. Clearly, this may improve athletic performance. Whether or not this alone can improve or help prevent illnesses like heart disease is not yet proven.

Abdominal Breathing

Abdominal breathing is one of the simplest yet most powerful stress management techniques. Opera singers refer to this as diaphragmatic breathing, and it helps give their voices the power to fill a large concert hall. When I studied karate, I was trained to breathe this way because it can give a person more power to break boards or to fight. Also, breathing from the abdomen lowers your center of gravity and thus increases your stability during sparring. Later, when I studied yoga, I was trained to breathe this way as a way of learning to be more peaceful. Like any form of power, abdominal breathing can be used for violent or peaceful purposes. (Fortunately, the philosophy of my karate teacher was "By knowing how to fight you can choose to be nonviolent.")

Your diaphragm is a large muscle located between your chest and your abdomen. When you contract it, this large muscle is forced downwards, causing a partial vacuum that forces air into your lungs. Diaphragmatic breathing increases the suction pressure in your chest, thereby improving venous return of blood to your heart.

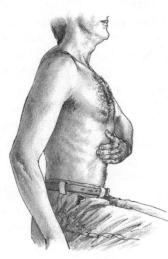

Do you breathe from your chest or your diaphragm? To find out, place your right hand on your chest and your left hand on your abdomen. Inhale. If you right hand rises more than your left hand, then you are breathing from your chest. If your left hand rises more than your right hand, then you are breathing from your diaphragm.

Unfortunately, most people breathe from their chest. What's the matter with that?

- Chest breathing is usually rapid, shallow, and irregular.
- Breathing this way is a manifestation of the fight-or-flight response, and it also can create the stressful feelings associated with that response.
- Although the lower lobes of your lungs receive the greatest amount of blood flow, they are not well oxygenated during chest breathing.

To practice abdominal breathing, sit comfortably with your back straight. If at all possible, always breathe through your nose, which filters and warms the air. Once again, place your right hand on your chest and your left hand on your abdomen. This will help you to be aware of your abdominal muscles as you breathe. Concentrate on contracting your diaphragm and breathing from deep down within your abdomen. As you begin to inhale, your left hand should begin to rise, but your right hand should move very little.

Now exhale as much air as you can, while contracting your abdominal muscles. Once again, your left hand should move in as you exhale but your right hand should move very little.

This is abdominal breathing. While it may feel unnatural at first, breathing from your abdomen will gradually become automatic if you practice it on a regular basis. After a while, you will breathe from your abdomen most of the time, even when you are asleep. When you are able to do this, then you will feel less stressed and more balanced. Eventually, breathing from your chest will feel unnatural—because it is.

If you are having a hard time learning how to breathe from your abdomen, then lie on the floor in the resting position and gently place a telephone book or small, soft weight on your abdomen. Abdominal breathing will cause the book or weight to rise and fall with your respirations.

Deep Breathing

Deep breathing is one of the simplest yet most effective stress management techniques. You can do it anywhere, at any time. It becomes even more effective with practice.

Deep breathing works both to prevent harmful reactions to stress and to help relieve them. If you practice deep breathing for a few minutes each day, you'll find that events don't upset you as much as before. Also, whenever you do feel upset, anxious, or worried, taking a few slow, deep breaths can help break the stress cycle and calm you down. Even when you can't control the situation, you can always control your breathing and thus help to change your reaction to those circumstances.

First, exhale completely through your nose. Place your right hand on your chest and your left hand on your abdomen, as before. Then begin inhaling by filling your abdominal area with air, as described above. As you do this, your left hand should begin to rise but your right hand will not.

After filling your abdomen with air, keep inhaling as you allow more air to rise, filling your lower chest, which should now cause your right hand to rise. Feel your rib cage expand as you inhale.

Keep inhaling and feel the air rising even higher in your chest. As the air reaches the top of your lungs, you will feel your collarbone begin to rise. (At this point, be careful not to draw your abdomen inward.)

To exhale, repeat the same process in reverse—that is, from the top to the bottom. First, exhale and allow some air to escape from the top of your chest, and feel your collarbone lowering as you do so. Next, continue exhaling as you feel the upper and then the lower parts of your chest contracting. Finally, allow the remaining air to be expelled from your abdominal area, and your abdominal muscles to contract, thereby pushing out whatever air remains.

Since exhaling is the most relaxing phase of breathing—aahhh—take longer to exhale than to inhale. Many teachers advise that a 2:1 ratio is ideal—that is, take twice as long to exhale as to inhale. For most people, achieving this ratio takes some practice. If at any time you feel dizzy, short of breath, or light-headed, simply resume normal breathing.

Schedule a few minutes each day to practice deep breathing. Also do it whenever you have some free time or when you're feeling stressed.

Bellows Breathing

This technique is a series of rapid, forceful abdominal exhalations followed by relaxed, natural inhalations. When you're feeling a little tired or sluggish, less than a minute of bellows breathing may be especially helpful to increase your level of energy.

Here's how to do it: Using the abdominal breathing technique, exhale fully, inhale fully, then exhale forcefully a small quantity of air. Move only your abdominal muscles. Increase the frequency of exhalations and inhalations to about two per second. After the fifteenth exhalation or if you experience any discomfort, resume breathing normally. You may wish to repeat this once or twice. End each session with a gentle, full exhalation, inhalation, and exhalation.

Alternate-Nostril Breathing

Your nose is lined with erectile tissue that expands and contracts during the day, causing your nasal mucosa to swell and shrink. Although you probably are not aware of it, the flow of air through your nose shifts from one nostril to the other during the day as the lining of each nostril expands and contracts in a biological rhythm.

For most people, the breath will flow predominantly through one nostril for about two hours, and then the predominance will begin to shift to the other nostril. Although Western physiology does not have much to say about this phenomenon, yoga texts state that this rhythm and alternating pattern is important in maintaining physiological and psychological equilibrium.

I like to think of myself as being reasonably open to new ideas, but this sounded like nonsense to me when I first heard it. And it may be; research has not yet been done to confirm or refute these concepts. We do know, for example, that the two hemispheres of your brain function somewhat differently. Maybe this, in turn, is reflected in your breathing—who knows?

The technique of alternate nostril breathing was developed to "rebalance" the equilibrium of breathing. Whether or not it works for the reasons that yoga teachers believe, alternate nostril breathing is an exceptionally powerful technique for calming and relaxing your mind and body.

Here's how to do it:

- Sit in a comfortable position and close your eyes.
- Exhale fully.
- Close off the right nostril with your thumb and inhale slowly through your left nostril. (Traditional yoga texts instruct a person to make a gentle fist with the right hand, and then open only the thumb and the last two fingers. The side of the thumb is used to close off the right nostril, and the side of the ring

finger is used to close off the left nostril. In practice, though, do whatever is most comfortable for you.)

· Close off the left nostril and exhale through the right nostril.
· Inhale through the right nostril.
· Close off the right nostril and exhale through the left nostril.

Continue this pattern. In other words, change nostrils after each inhalation. If you can do it comfortably, gradually increase the duration of your exhalations until they are about twice as long as your inhalations. Continue doing this for thirty seconds to three minutes. If at any time you feel like you're not getting enough air, simply resume breathing normally.

DIRECTED VISUALIZATION

Your mind may think in words, but your body responds to images as though they were really happening right now. Try it and see.

For example, if you remember an argument that you had with a friend yesterday, your body reacts today as though you were still fighting. Close your eyes and remember the last time you argued with a close friend or loved one, and pay attention to what happens in your body. You may notice that your breathing has become more rapid and shallow, your muscles have tightened, and your heart is beating faster, and you feel anxious or disturbed.

Now, remember the last time that you felt close to a friend or loved one. Or imagine a peaceful scene. Once again, pay attention to what happens in your body. You may notice that your body has begun to relax, your breathing has become deeper and more regular, your heart rate has slowed, and you feel good.

Here's another example. With your eyes closed, imagine that you are holding in your hand an intensely yellow, plump, juicy, ripe lemon. Imagine now that you are dropping it on a table, and "listen" to the thud it makes. Now visualize that you are taking a sharp knife and cutting the lemon in half. Take half of the lemon and (still in your imagination) bring it up to your nose, scratch the surface with your fingernail. Imagine what it smells like. Finally, visualize that you are biting into it. By now, your mouth probably will be salivating as though you really were biting into a ripe lemon.

Your mind talks to your body by using such mental images. This dialogue is going on all the time—sometimes in healing ways, sometimes in harmful ways—although much of the time you may not be consciously aware of it. Likewise, your conscious and unconscious mind communicate with each other by using imagery.

Visualization, also known as imagery, can be done using any of your senses, but it seems to work best when you combine several of them. In the example above, you used all of your senses—sight, sound, touch, smell, and taste.

Many professional athletes find visualization to be a powerful tool to enhance their performance. As baseball legend Yogi Berra (not a yogi) once said, "Ninety percent of the game is mental, and the other half is physical." And according to Dr. Armand Nicholi, a professor of psychiatry at Harvard and one of the team physicians of the New England Patriots, "The best players will use any method to gain a fraction of an edge over the competition. Mind/body techniques like visualization can provide that edge."

A new field, sports psychology, is emerging to study and teach visualization and other mind/body techniques to professional and world-class athletes. The 1988 Olympics marked the first time that a sports psychologist, Dr. Shane Murphy, was assigned by the U.S. Olympic Committee to teach visualization to athletes. More than seventy athletes in different sports requested his services. Here are a few examples of athletes, Olympic and otherwise, who use visualization to improve their skills:

- Mary Lou Retton was the first American woman to win an individual gold medal in gymnastics. In an interview with *The Mind-Body Health Digest*, of the Institute for the Advancement of Health, she said, "Doing mental imagery was always a constant for me. I'd see myself performing in my head, and it really helped tremendously. It gave me confidence. After a workout and dinner, I'd be lying in bed, and I'd review all my moves of the day. I'd see myself in each event. It was especially helpful in the Olympics, which were so important to me. I did all the routines in my head the night before competition. Since I usually had trouble on the balance beam, I'd review that in my mind a lot, picturing myself landing straight on the beam."
- Jerry Rice, star wide receiver of the San Francisco 49ers, caught eleven passes for a record-shattering 215 yards in the 1989 Super Bowl and caught a record three touchdown passes

in the 1990 Super Bowl. "I think my attitude is the reason I'm so successful on the football field. I simply concentrate on the defensive backs all week, study their every move—how each player is going to react when a receiver with a ball comes his way." Then he choreographs his own moves at least three days before the game. "I visualize everything that's going to happen in the football game. I know exactly what I am going to do, how I'm going to run the pattern on each defensive back. I've got it down to the last step."

- Greg Louganis, the Olympic diving champion, visualizes each dive from start to finish, and he believes this is crucial to his performance. He first learned this technique in childhood dance classes.
- Larry Mahan, champion rodeo rider, said: "I try to picture a ride in my mind before I get on the bull. Then I try to go by the picture."
- Dave Stieb, pitcher for the Toronto Blue Jays, said: "My preparation for the game is simple. I visualize first warming up and getting the right movements on my fast ball. Then I think about the first few innings and what I want to do. When I get to the mound, the same thing applies. I see the pitch doing whatever I want it to do and accomplishing whatever I want it to accomplish. Then I just wind up and throw it."
- Elizabeth Manley won a silver medal at the 1988 Winter Olympics. "I used a great deal of imagery. In learning the triple Lutz jump, for example, I would stand at the side of the boards, close my eyes, and picture myself doing the jump perfectly in my mind. Nine out of ten times I would successfully do it by preparing this way. Eventually we captured a couple of perfect jumps on videotape. I watched it over and over until it was engraved on my mind. I would actually see in my mind my entire body, the jump, and the landing position. I was then able to take that image onto the ice with me and picture myself doing the jump perfectly before it came time to perform. I would practice my imagery every night before I went to sleep. I think that training ten minutes this way was equivalent to doing a forty-five-minute session on the ice. I began practicing mind/body techniques intensely two years prior to the 1988 Olympics. Besides visualization, progressive relaxation and breathing exercises helped calm me

down. I believe that mind/body techniques had a lot to do with my success."

Visualization can produce measurable changes in the body. Psychologist Richard Suinn, Ph.D., recorded muscle activity while a skier visualized himself racing downhill. He found that these recordings were similar to those made when someone was actually skiing downhill.

How to Perform Directed Visualization

Visualization can be done using any and all of your senses. Even if you don't "see" mental images in your mind's eye, you might "hear" sounds, "taste" food, "smell" fragrances, or "touch" something or someone. For example, some people visualize detailed scenes in color, whereas others imagine only the rough outlines of a scene in black and white. There is no right or wrong way to visualize, only what works for you.

Close your eyes and relax for a moment. (After you close your eyes, you may want to ask someone to read this section aloud to you.) Imagine that you are in your bedroom, lying comfortably on your mattress. Notice the number of windows, the color of the walls, the texture of the floor or carpeting. If you have a telephone in your bedroom, remember what color it is and how it appears. Now imagine that you hear the telephone ringing. When you answer the phone, notice what it feels like when you pick up the receiver. Hear yourself saying, "Hello," and the voice of a close friend in reply. Pay attention to what your friend's voice sounds like. Remember the last time you were with your companion and what it felt like being with him or her. Visualize what your friend's face looks like.

Now open your eyes. If you were able to do any part of this, then you were visualizing. Practice paying attention to how you feel during each part of a visualization exercise.

To digress a moment, I was lecturing in Moscow in 1988 with a delegation of U.S. scientists and physicians from the Esalen U.S.-Soviet Exchange Program. Dr. Ken Pelletier of the UCSF School of Medicine began leading a similar visualization exercise with a room full of Soviet scientists. He began by asking them to visualize the number of windows in their bedroom, when the group suddenly erupted in laughter. We looked puzzled until the translator explained, "You see, we all live in exactly the same type of government-built apartment, and all of us have only one window in our bedroom."

The Healing Heart Visualization

In chapter 2, I described the various mechanisms that can reduce or shut down the flow of blood to your heart: coronary artery blockages, coronary artery spasm, and blood clots. Each of these mechanisms is influenced and activated by lifestyle factors, including our emotions, for better and for worse.

We know, for example, that emotional stress can cause arteries throughout your body to constrict. When this occurs in the heart, it is known as coronary artery spasm. We also know from research on visualization that having a mental image of blood flow improving to your hands can actually cause blood flow to increase to your hands. An erection is another example of how thoughts can increase blood flow, in this case to the penis. Other studies have demonstrated that visualization can decrease blood flow to your heart if you imagine terrible things happening. So it seems reasonable to assume that visualizing more healing images may improve coronary blood flow by dilating your coronary arteries to some degree. Other evidence suggests that visualization may reduce the number and severity of irregular heartbeats. And while there is not yet scientific evidence that visualization can affect coronary artery blockages, it is possible that visualization may help those as well.

If you have heart disease and if you have had a coronary angiogram, ask your cardiologist for a diagram showing the exact location of each of your coronary artery blockages. This can be helpful in the visualization process.

Even without this information, though, you can simply bring to your mind an image of what your heart may look like. Figure 3.1 (page 51) contains an example of a heart, although for this purpose anatomic accuracy is less important than what you think your heart looks like to *you*.

Make a copy of figure 3.1 and color in the location of your blockages (if you have this information) or where you imagine your coronary artery blockages to be, as I have done as an example in the next illustration. Or draw a picture of your heart the way that you think it may look (see the example in figure 7.1).

Then choose a healing image that incorporates the following:

- Your heart is beating regularly.
- Your heart is pumping a healthy amount of blood with each beat.

Ailing   **Healed**

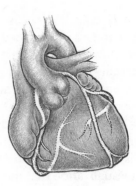

Figure 7.1

- The arteries in your heart are dilating and allowing more blood to flow.
- New blood vessels are growing and supplying oxygen and other nutrients to your heart.
- The blood is flowing smoothly and unobstructed.

If you don't have a known heart problem, then just choose an image in which your heart is healthy.

As with any visualization, adding detail may be useful. You may want to check out some medical books showing various pictures of hearts. Or you may even want to watch a film of a heart during surgery. If you have had an angiogram, you may want to ask your cardiologist to show you the movie of your own heart. Or you may find that you would prefer to imagine without seeing these.

In our current study, for example, one patient visualized a tunneling machine (used in highway construction) burrowing through his blocked arteries and creating new pathways for blood to flow. Another person visualized that he was breathing in white light with each inhalation and that this light traveled from his lungs directly into his coronary arteries and burned up the blockages. When he exhaled, he would breathe out the residue from his previously blocked arteries. One person visualized a gentle solvent that dissolved the coronary artery blockages.

You can visualize your heart improving at any time, but it is most effective when done following meditation, because meditation helps to focus your awareness. (Meditation is described in chapter 9.)

RECEPTIVE VISUALIZATION

In the preceding section we have been using visualization in a *directed* way—that is, using images that may influence directly what is happening in the body. We can also use imagery in a more *receptive* mode—that is, to help us become more consciously aware of previously hidden information that can have a powerful influence on our health and well-being.

Using directed visualization, as we've seen, you can communicate mental images from your conscious mind to your body and to your unconscious mind. You choose a mental image that you want to occur—such as throwing a baseball more accurately or your coronary arteries becoming more open.

Using receptive visualization, you can bring to your conscious awareness useful information that had been unconscious or ignored. Instead of choosing a mental image that you want to occur, you receive images from your mind that arise in response to your questions.

Receptive visualization is based on the idea that you know more about yourself than you may be aware of. In working with many heart patients over the years, I have been amazed at how frequently a similar image appears from a person's unconscious: the image of a wall or fortress around the heart.

There is an emerging field of research in cardiology called silent ischemia. Ischemia ("is-*kee*-mee-ah") is medical jargon for reduced blood flow to the heart. Cardiologists used to believe that chest pain (angina) occurred whenever the heart did not receive enough blood flow. Recent studies have conclusively demonstrated that many people have profound reductions in blood flow to their hearts, yet they don't have any chest pain or other symptoms. Sometimes people even have heart attacks without any symptoms at all.

During the past few years, this syndrome has been well documented, although it is unclear why some people experience chest pain whereas others do not. Recent studies have demonstrated that people with silent ischemia tend to experience *all* forms of pain (and pleasure) less intensely than other people, even though their nervous system and levels of naturally produced painkillers (endorphins) are no different. For example, a recent study in the *Journal of the American College of Cardiology* by Dr. C. Falcone and others reported that 71.2 percent of people with silent ischemia did not experience dental pain, even with intense stimulation, whereas 69.7 percent of people with angina complained of dental pain with only low stimulation.

In my work with heart patients, I have noticed that people who have silent ischemia often have a significant dissociation between their feelings and experiences or between their thoughts and feelings. In other words, their feelings are often walled off—not only from other people but even from themselves. If you ask them what they are *feeling*, usually they will tell you what they are *thinking*. (The importance of being able to distinguish thoughts from feelings is discussed more fully in chapter 8.)

Therefore, a fundamental part of the healing process in our program was to create a place in our group support sessions that felt safe enough to allow our participants to re-experience and, in a sense, re-own and re-integrate those feelings that they had quite literally disowned by walling them out of their experience.

Using imagery, we can often begin a dialogue with these inner walls, as extraordinary as that might seem. At the end of this chapter I will present a few examples, transcribed from actual sessions with the participants in our program. These images are powerful. They almost seem like archetypes, because I see them over and over again in a variety of people, including those with heart disease.

Many people, especially those with heart disease, have experienced great hurt at some time in their lives. As we grow older, we try to protect ourselves from emotional pain. We tend to think that we hurt more as we get older, that we have the capacity to feel more, but I think we probably hurt more when we are younger. We get better at protecting ourselves or defending ourselves as we get older.

In a metaphorical sense, the heart is the organ that is most affected by our feelings. Poets and authors and mystics and priests and rabbis and people throughout the ages have talked about the heart as if it were the seat of the emotions. And in chapter 2, I described how the heart is literally affected by our emotions. To protect ourselves from pain—the slings and arrows from our friends, our enemies, our family, and ourselves—we figuratively protect the heart by building walls (emotional defenses) around it.

In this metaphor, eventually we have a well-fortified fortress around our heart. But it's a double-edged sword, for *the same wall that protects us can also isolate us.* This isolation, in turn, can lead to chronic stress and, in some cases, physical heart disease.

At one stage of our development, these walls may have been

protective, even necessary for our emotional survival. But *what be-gins as protective can itself become destructive if the walls always remain up.* By analogy, the fight-or-flight response, which starts out as being protective and necessary to our survival, can become harm-ful or even lethal to us if the fight-or-flight response is chronically turned on, if we react as though saber-toothed tigers are lurking around every corner.

As we discussed earlier in this section, your body responds to what is happening in your mind as though it were real, because what is happening in your mind *is* real, at least as far as your body is concerned. When you visualized biting into a lemon, your salivary glands responded as though you were.

The mystics might say that what happens in your mind creates what happens around you: "As you think, so you become." What you think about intensely is what you begin to manifest in your life to some degree. What you meditate on or visualize tends to become actualized.

Whether or not this is true, what happens in your mind is happening to at least some degree in your world. If you perceive that you are in danger, you *are* in danger. If you perceive that you live in a world that is dangerous and hostile, then your fight-or-flight mechanisms may be chronically overstimulated to the point of creat-ing danger for you. It becomes a self-fulfilling prophecy and a vicious cycle.

Similarly, fear of being hurt or rejected often causes us to create inner walls around the heart that can keep it isolated and in darkness. It becomes another self-fulfilling prophecy and a vicious cycle. The perception of isolation causes us to feel pain. And the wall says, "See, it's a painful world out there. You really need me." The wall grows stronger, we feel even more pain and isolation, and the cycle contin-ues.

If the world is dangerous, and if the expression of feelings is dangerous, then it may seem easier not to feel at all. You will need to keep the wall around your heart very well fortified to protect you both from other people and from parts of yourself that you may view as threatening.

It would be unwise to walk around in the world defenseless and open all the time. You want to have walls and emotional defenses when you need them. But you pay a big price for having the walls up all the time. *When you put a wall around your heart, when you wall off the ability to feel pain, you also shut down the ability to feel pleasure.* And when the walls become so well fortified that they're always up, then you feel chronically isolated and alone.

In order for us to risk letting down these fortress walls and lowering the drawbridge, then we need to see that there's a reason for doing it. When we understand that these walls can create pain and illness, then that pain, whether physical, emotional, or spiritual, can be a catalyst for allowing the healing process to begin. But even then it may not be enough, because it's so scary to open up. That fortress almost develops a will of its own, where it really believes that it's protecting us even when it's part of the problem. The wall may not believe that its job may not always be necessary.

This is not always a conscious choice. We may not even be aware of this process until we begin doing the imagery exercises. Our pain or illness can get our attention so we can begin looking at those parts of our lives that are making us suffer or become sick.

Sometimes our isolation from others can be so profound that even our pain seems like the only constant we can depend on. One of our study participants had chest pain almost every day, for years. And then after going on our program, the pain went away completely. Although he was glad, he said that in some ways he felt as though he had lost his best friend. His pain had been the only thing in his life that was there for him, that he could depend on, that he had felt connected to, that made him feel alive. At least he was feeling *something* every day. In mythological terms, sometimes our demons seem more dependable and trustworthy than our angels.

If we put up walls to protect the scared child that we may have within ourselves—this child that feels unworthy, not quite good enough or attractive enough to be loved for who we are rather than for what we do—then it's really hard to begin that process of opening up. The wall tells us, "You're going to make a fool of yourself if you show that part of yourself to other people. And they will reject you. So I will protect you from that." Often, the people in our groups who have been the most hostile to other people opening up, like Sam in chapter 3, are the ones who may have felt this most intensely. So talking about those feelings becomes very threatening.

Instead, if we can learn to recognize and even to have a dialogue with both the barriers we've erected and our heart that is hiding inside, we can begin to reintegrate ourselves. This leads not only to greater intimacy between us and other people, but also a more fundamental kind of intimacy with the various aspects of ourselves that we may have walled off or disowned.

When we begin to have the courage to begin looking at those aspects of ourselves which seem so frightening, then amazing things can happen. Here is an example from John Cardozo, one of the participants in our study, the first time he tried to do receptive visualization during one or our group sessions:

JOHN: Well, I just feel blocked right now, like there's some really strong emotion I can feel in my throat, and I'm not sure what it is.

DEAN: Okay—well, why don't you close your eyes and bring your awareness to your throat. If that emotion had a sound, what would it sound like? Is there any sound that wants to come out?

JOHN: It feels like thunder.

DEAN: Can you reproduce it?

JOHN: I can describe it—it's a rolling, very deep thunder.

DEAN: Just stay with that—let it fill you up. [pause] What do you hear?

JOHN: I hear a ringing.

DEAN: Is it loud?

JOHN: Yes.

DEAN: Stay with that sound a little while now. [pause] What's happening?

JOHN: It's filling me up.

DEAN: Let it fill up your whole body with that sound. Tell me if any images also come to mind, or if it remains a sound.

JOHN: It's still a ringing sound.

DEAN: Where do you hear it? Where do you feel it?

JOHN: I feel it here [points to his abdomen/solar plexus] and here [points to his throat].

DEAN: Okay. What's happening now?

JOHN: The sound in my abdomen is rising up into my chest and connecting the two.

DEAN: What does it feel like?

JOHN: Like a straitjacket.

DEAN: Okay. Just stay with that feeling for a minute. [pause] What are you feeling now?

JOHN: Very rigid.

DEAN: Okay. Can you visualize your heart in all of this?

JOHN: It's very small and enclosed.

DEAN: Enclosed in this straitjacket?

JOHN: Yes.

DEAN: And the straitjacket is making the sound?

JOHN: Yes.

DEAN: Okay. What does that straitjacket look like?

JOHN: Like concrete.

DEAN: Please describe it in as much detail as you can. Use as many of your senses as you can.

JOHN: It's round, a wall, solid. It feels thick and hard, like it's made out of stone or granite.

DEAN: Without speaking out loud, silently ask that wall, or straitjacket—whatever you want to call it—if it has a name, or a voice, or if it can identify itself to you in some way you can understand. You may not hear anything in reply, but if you do, you'll know; you're not just making it up. It will speak quietly but clearly, or it may not speak at all.

JOHN: It says it's a safe.

DEAN: Okay.

JOHN: Now it's saying that its name is "Safe."

DEAN: Ask "Safe" what its function is, what its purpose is.

JOHN: To protect me.

DEAN: To protect you from what?

JOHN: From ridicule.

DEAN: Okay—acknowledge it and thank it for protecting you from ridicule. [pause] Does it say anything or communicate with you in any way in response to that acknowledgment?

JOHN: It doesn't communicate verbally, but it's satisfied. It appreciates the acknowledgment.

DEAN: Ask it what else it's protecting you from, if anything.

JOHN: Nothing.

DEAN: When you hear the word, "ridicule," what sort of images does it bring up?

JOHN: Being laughed at when I was younger.

DEAN: Any images come to mind in particular, any episodes when you felt ridiculed?

JOHN: I felt that way most of the time.

DEAN: Can you think of one instance that comes to mind, one image, when you hear the word, "ridicule?"

JOHN: Yeah—when I was eleven or so—I was laughed at by people for throwing snowballs like a girl instead of like a man.

DEAN: Picture in as much detail as you can what that felt like.

JOHN: Like I wanted to be swallowed up and disappear.

DEAN: Stay with that feeling for a second, even though it's unpleasant. [pause] What are you feeling now?

JOHN: Like I'm hiding behind the safe. It's protecting me.

DEAN: Again, thank it for protecting you at a time when you really needed it, and for being there if you ever need it again. You may. For a moment, though, ask it if it would either become transparent, or open up, or choose some image that it's no longer separating you from your heart, and ask the safe, the wall, what it says.

JOHN: [long pause] It says, "Okay."

DEAN: What do you see? What's behind it?

JOHN: A lot of faces.

DEAN: Do you recognize any of them?

JOHN: Yes.

DEAN: Do you feel like sharing what you see?

JOHN: I see a circle of people.

DEAN: Who do you recognize?

JOHN: Everyone in our group. The same circle that's our group tonight.

DEAN: Do you see your heart anywhere?

JOHN: I have trouble seeing my heart. It's not clear.

DEAN: What do you see?

JOHN: I still see it enclosed.

DEAN: That which is enclosing the heart, or protecting it, it may be called "Safe," or it may have another name.

JOHN: It's a little scary.

DEAN: You can stop now if you want.

JOHN: No, I want to continue.

DEAN: Ask the wall that's enclosing your heart what its purpose or function is.

JOHN: It's almost like it's to keep something from going out, to keep something inside my heart rather than to keep something out.

DEAN: Okay, that's a very powerful image. Ask the wall what it's keeping in, and it may tell you.

JOHN: [pause] Tears.

DEAN: Ask it why it's keeping the tears in.

JOHN: [pause] Ridicule. Fear of ridicule.

DEAN: Ask that part of you that's enclosing your heart if it would let the tears come out, knowing that it can come right back and close off if it's too painful. And thank it for protecting you in the past.

JOHN: Okay. [He begins to cry softly. After a short while, he begins to smile.]

DEAN: What are you feeling now, John?

JOHN: Much more relaxed and peaceful.

DEAN: Just enjoy those feelings for a while. [pause] What happened to the thunder—is it still there?

JOHN: No.

DEAN: Do you still have that sensation in your throat?

JOHN: No.

DEAN: Okay. Please open your eyes now. [pause] Anything else?

JOHN: My heart feels more open.

DEAN: Sometimes it's like layers of an onion, or like Chinese boxes—walls within walls within walls within walls. My guess is that when you go back and do this on your own, you'll find more in there. It takes a lot of courage to do what you just did here, and I really appreciate your doing that in front of the group—especially knowing how hard it must be, given what you've been talking about. For someone who's been hurt very badly by being ridiculed, to show that part of yourself in a group of people is about the hardest thing there is—and perhaps one of the most healing as well. [The group members then gave John a lot of support.]

There are many techniques for doing receptive visualization. In general, the main principle is to pay attention to important information that you may be ignoring. To listen for information without preconceptions of what you're "supposed" to be experiencing. Here are a few examples of receptive visualizations that I have found to be useful:

The Inner Teacher Visualization
One way of gaining access to information that you may not be noticing is to visualize your "inner teacher," sometimes called your "inner advisor." This technique has been used for centuries by other

cultures, including American Indians, and more recently by psychologists Carl Jung, Jean Achterberg, and Lenore Lefer, physicians Mike Samuels, Rachel Naomi Remen, and others. It may be unfamiliar and even a little strange to read about this until you try it and see how powerful this technique can be. Your inner teacher is simply a representation of your inner self.

To begin, close your eyes and put yourself in a meditative state. The best time to practice receptive visualization is after a session of stretching, breathing, deep relaxation, and meditation, although it can be done at any time.

Imagine that you are in a place that is peaceful and relaxing. It could be a place that you have actually been to or a place that exists only in your imagination. If possible, visualize this place in as much detail as you can, invoking all of your senses. What do you see? What colors do you notice? What sounds and smells? What tastes? How does the ground feel below your feet when you walk?

Imagine that you are walking through this place, when suddenly you notice that someone or something comes into view. It may be a man, a woman, an animal, or even an inanimate object. It may be an archetype of a wise figure (such as an old man with a long beard or an old woman) or it may be something totally unexpected. In whatever form, you will recognize this wise figure because of its compassion, love, and wisdom. If the figure does not appear to have these qualities, and especially if the figure is predominantly critical or judgmental, then keep walking until you find one that does.

When you come across this wise figure, introduce yourself and wait for a reply. Ask the wise figure if it has a name, and in what way it prefers for you to address it. Once you gain this information, then address the wise figure in that way.

Then ask the wise figure if it has information that may be helpful to you. If so, this information may be communicated to you in words that you can "hear," in images, in sounds, or in some other form that is clearly understandable to you.

If no information is forthcoming, then ask the wise figure what you need to do for it to provide you with information, and listen for the reply. If information is forthcoming, then you might begin by asking, "What information do you have for me that I may not be paying attention to?" Listen to the response.

This information is usually incomplete and may generate a whole new series of questions to this teacher. If you are receiving information and then suddenly no more is forthcoming, you may want to ask this inner teacher to tell you what is getting in the way. In those cases, you may suddenly see a wall, a fence, or some other barrier. If you do, use the same techniques described in the next exercise.

This wall, fence, or barrier may have its own voice. It is usually different from the inner teacher's voice, although it may be the same.

Introduce yourself to this wall or barrier and ask its function. In most cases, the wall's purpose is to keep something out or to keep something in. Usually it is to keep out perceived danger or threat and to keep in feelings that are believed to be dangerous or threatening.

Thank the wall for protecting you—for at some point in your life it *was* protective and perhaps even necessary to your emotional survival. After you have thanked the wall listen for its reply, if any. Sometimes the wall will acknowledge you—saying "Well, it's about time!" or "Thank you" or in some completely different way. Or not at all.

Ask the wall when it first appeared. What was happening in your life at that time? When did the wall become necessary, and why? Listen for the reply, if any. (The reply may come in words, images, sounds, or symbols.)

Then ask the wall if it would be willing to open a little, to part, to become transparent, or in some other way to allow you to see what is on the other side. Explain to the wall that it can come back immediately if you find that experiencing what is on the other side of the wall is too painful. At this point, the wall either will begin to open or it will remain closed. Or it may become even bigger!

If the wall is unwilling to open, then ask it if it might be willing to open at another time, or what it wants you to do first before it would be willing to let you go any farther. Listen for the reply.

If the wall is willing to begin opening, pay attention to what is on the other side and what feelings and images may be contained there. This, in turn, may generate a whole new series of questions and information. Continue this process only for as long as you feel comfortable.

In most cases, what is on the other side of the wall is described as light, love, joy, release, and other happy images, and it becomes clear to you (and even to the wall) that it is no longer needed at this stage of your life. Sometimes, though, the images are painful or frightening. Usually, though, the experience is healing. If the images behind the wall are really too painful for you to experience, then the wall is not likely to open.

Sometimes there are walls within walls, like layers of an onion. If you find other walls, begin this same process again. The new wall may have the same voice as the previous wall, or it may have its own voice.

Once you have gotten past the walls (assuming that you even had any walls to begin with), listen to the information from your inner teacher. In my experience, the wise figure generally does not volunteer very much information; it waits until you ask, as it might in real life. If you ask specific questions, then you are likely to receive specific answers. Each answer, in turn, may lead to another question. If you are uncertain of the meaning of an answer, then ask your inner teacher to clarify it for you.

Sometimes your inner teacher may even refer you to other teachers or resources, whether inner or in the real world. (Sometimes even inner teachers are specialists!) If your inner teacher refers you to a second inner guide, then your inner teacher will provide you with whatever information you need to find the second one.

When you are ready to end your session, ask your inner teacher to tell you the best way for you to reestablish contact with it in the future. It will tell you.

After you open your eyes, you may wish to write down whatever information you have learned from this session.

If you were unable to meet an inner teacher, don't get discouraged—just try it again at another time. In his book *Healing Yourself,* Dr. Martin Rossman provides detailed information on how to use imagery and the following suggestions on what to do until your inner teacher comes:

- Imagine what your advisor would be like if you had one.
- Draw or sculpt what you think your inner advisor might look like.
- Imagine talking with a very good friend.
- Think of a historical or mythological figure that fits your idea of what an inner advisor would be.
- Write a letter to a "wise person." Then imagine that you are that wise person and write yourself a letter back from this perspective.

The Inner Heart Visualization

In contrast to directed visualization, where you were trying to direct healing images towards your heart, in this exercise you receive images *from* your heart or elsewhere as a way of gaining more information and insight.

Visualize your heart in whatever form comes to you. The image of your heart may look like the anatomical drawings used in the directed visualization, or it may look quite different.

Once you have a mental image of your heart, introduce yourself to your heart as if you were meeting a person. You might even begin simply by saying "hello" and seeing if your heart says anything in return. Ask your heart if it has a name, and if so, what it is. If your heart tells you its name, then refer to your heart using this name when you speak to it, much as you would do with a person.

Your heart has its own voice, which may or may not be the same as your inner teacher's voice. Or your heart may communicate by changing images of itself rather than in words or in sounds rather than words.

Once you are able to receive information from your heart, whether in images, sounds, or otherwise, ask your heart what it needs in order to become healed. Begin by asking what it needs for physical healing. After you receive a reply, then ask your heart what it needs for emotional and spiritual healing. It may give you specific advice, such as diet and exercise, it may tell you about relationships or emotions, or it may tell you something completely different from any of these.

Thank your heart for beating continually since you were born, for keeping you alive and so on. Listen for what it says in reply if anything.

You may find that you ask a question to the heart and do not receive a reply. Or you may not even get to the point where the heart tells you its name when you first introduce yourself. If this happens, visualize a wall, barrier, or obstruction that is keeping you from this information, much as you did in the last exercise.

Many people find an image of a wall or even a fortress around their heart, both protecting and isolating it. You may find a similar image, or yours may be completely different. Or you may not even visualize a wall around your heart.

If you do visualize a wall or obstruction in another form, begin a dialogue with this barrier as you did in the last exercise. As before, thank the wall for protecting you for so many years, and listen for the reply. Ask the wall if it would allow you to experience what is on the other side, knowing that the wall can come back instantly if you need it.

When you've finished, thank the heart for providing you this information and for "opening." Allow yourself to feel love for your heart, and to experience the love that your heart has for you. Finally, ask your heart how you can get in touch with it again, and it may tell you.

This type of imagery can be empowering as well as informative, for it provides you with information that came from *you,* not from an "expert" or other authority figure who may or may not know what is best for you. Whatever images or feelings come up, they are *your* images and feelings, and these can help you become more aware of important information.

As you begin to trust your inner information, you will be able to gain access to it more easily. This information complements rather than replaces your rational thinking. It is both diagnostic and therapeutic, as it gives you both the question and the answer.

Here is an example of this type of exercise with Vic Gilbert, one of our research participants, the first time he tried it in one of our group meetings. It was a very emotional experience for all of us.

VIC: I've been feeling very lonely. I can't explain it, I'm in a crowd but I feel lonely. And so today, I tried to get in touch with it. The loneliness and sadness are there because several things are going on. One, I don't like my body. Two, I am very angry with my body for having heart disease.

DEAN: Do you want to do an imagery exercise?

VIC: Yes.

DEAN: Okay. Please close your eyes and put yourself in a meditative state. If at any time you feel like this is not something you want to do, I'll rely on you to tell me that. Begin by visualizing your body. What kind of image do you get?

VIC: Just mounds of flesh. A wall of fat.

DEAN: Imagine that your body has a voice of its own. Tell it hello. Ask it to just say hello to you, just to identify itself. Does it?

VIC: [pause] It says "hello" back. I'm amazed! Its voice is different from mine.

DEAN: Ask it if it has a name.

VIC: It says, "Fat."

DEAN: Ask "Fat" what is its purpose in your life.

VIC: [pause] It says, "To give me support. To shield me. To protect me."

DEAN: Ask it what is it shielding you from?

VIC: It says, "From everyone. I'm your best friend."

DEAN: In what way is it your friend?

VIC: It says, "I've been protecting you."

DEAN: Ask it what has it been protecting you from?

VIC: It says, "You don't have to do a lot of things because you're fat."

DEAN: Ask it if it's protecting you from anything else?

VIC: [pause] Yes. It says it's been protecting me from my feelings.

DEAN: Okay—ask it if it's protecting you from any feelings in particular.

VIC: [pause] It says, "From loneliness."

DEAN: When it says that, do any other images or feelings come to your awareness?

VIC: Somehow I remember getting fat when I was seven. I see myself going into a room feeling like I was all right, and finding out I was not all right. So my life has been about justification. Justification about being all right. Being accepted. So I used food as a friend. My fat says it protects me from feeling bad. I have a lot of resistance to change. I have a lot invested in this fat. And to give it up is like giving up a friend. It's been a barrier but it's also a friend. It's a friend that gets in the way sometimes, but it also serves me really well. But my size limits me in what I want to do now.

DEAN: Stay with those feelings now. Ask "Fat" what it needs from you now.

VIC: [pause] It says that it needs to be told it's all right the way it is.

DEAN: Maybe you could start by thanking it for shielding, protecting you from loneliness all these years.

VIC: [pause] All right.

DEAN: Does the wall say anything in reply?

VIC: It agrees. It says, "It's about time."

DEAN: Good. Now ask if it would be willing to open up, to stop shielding you all the time. If you could find a different way to shield yourself when you need it—one that is easier to open and close.

VIC: A replacement—is that what you are saying?

DEAN: Yes. Something that you could use to shield yourself when you need it, but isn't there all the time when you want to open up. See what it says.

VIC: [pause] It says, "Yes."

DEAN: Ask it what you need to do for it to begin opening up.

VIC: [pause] To get massaged. To be, perhaps, more vulnerable. To allow myself to be touched.

DEAN: What images or feelings come to mind of your body in that way?

VIC: I'd feel freer.

DEAN: How would you look? Ask "Fat," the one that protects you and shields you, if it would give you a different image of your body. How your body would look if you were more open and less shielded all the time.

VIC: Okay.

DEAN: What does it say?

VIC: [pause] If I'm willing, it's willing.

DEAN: Good. What image do you see? You can always go back to the fat image if you need it.

VIC: I see a thinner body.

DEAN: What does it look like?

VIC: It looks thinner. But it looks disfigured. The fat is very disfigured.

DEAN: How so?

VIC: It's full of stretch marks. Saggy skin.

DEAN: Okay. What does that body have to say?

VIC: [pause] To try and attain it anyway. To try to achieve it. That it's okay to have a thinner body that's not perfect.

DEAN: Do any other images or feelings come to your awareness?

VIC: I feel uncomfortable and sad.

DEAN: Stay with that feeling. [pause] What's happening now?

VIC: It's just a lot of feelings.

DEAN: Okay.

VIC: There's a lot of loneliness.

DEAN: What does that feel like?

VIC: It feels bad.

DEAN: Do any images come to mind? Do you see anything or hear anything?

VIC: I see and hear the years of ostracism. It feels like it's been years of repressing these feelings. I feel a lot of anger and rage because of the repression. There's just sort of an abject loneliness, that's all.

DEAN: I know it's very painful, but stay with that lonely feeling for a minute and see where it takes you.

VIC: I have never felt all right. I've never felt completely whole. I've always felt the need to justify myself. Today when I looked in the mirror it was just like all the damage has been done. I just feel this inward anger with myself.

DEAN: Do any images come to mind of people to whom you've justified yourself?

VIC: Countless people, hundreds of people, hundreds and hundreds over the years. You see it in their eyes, you see it in looks, you hear it in their voices, you just hear the discrimination.

DEAN: Of all those hundreds of people, which image comes to mind first?

VIC: All I see is faces of kids when I was little, the high school years which were just an absolute nightmare, the need and the desire and the want to fit in but never being able to, just faces of those people.

DEAN: Do you recognize the faces of the people?

VIC: Yes.

DEAN: Well, choose one of those faces, it really doesn't matter, any one of them. Do you know who it is? You don't have to tell me who it is, but do you recognize the face?

VIC: Yes, I recognize the face.

DEAN: Does that face say anything to you?

VIC: [pause] Yes.

DEAN: What does it say?

VIC: It says, "You are not all right."

DEAN: What else does it say, if anything?

VIC: It says, "You are not acceptable, you are not all right, get out, you don't belong, you can't participate."

DEAN: What do you want to say to the face, if anything?

VIC: "You don't know me. I am all right. Don't discriminate against kids."

DEAN: What is the face doing now?

VIC: It has receded and I don't see it anymore.

DEAN: What do you see or what do you feel?

VIC: I feel very sad and very lonely.

DEAN: Again, as much as you are able to, just stay with that feeling of being sad and lonely just for a few more minutes, and see where it takes you.

VIC: [long pause] I see my heart.

DEAN: What do you see?

VIC: I feel like there is something cutting in it, a squeezing, just squeezing it.

DEAN: What is squeezing your heart?

VIC: Something that's red and bright. It's red and it's bright and it is squeezing it.

DEAN: What else do you see?

VIC: I see faces. A lot of faces looking and a lot of judgment. I want to scream at every one.

DEAN: You can if you want.

VIC: I just feel this rage, endless rage.

DEAN: I know it must be painful, but see if you can allow yourself to experience that rage for a moment.

VIC: Okay. [pause]

DEAN: What's happening now?

VIC: The red light is diminishing.

DEAN: Do you still feel the squeezing?

VIC: Not as severe.

DEAN: Do you still see the faces?

VIC: I still see the faces. I see faces in judgment. Sitting in judgment, causing judgment.

DEAN: What do you want to do or say to those faces?

VIC: "I want to be with you, I want you to know me, don't judge me."

DEAN: What do they say?

VIC: Nothing.

DEAN: What do you see?

VIC: I just see the faces.

DEAN: Still judging?

VIC: Yes.

DEAN: What do you feel?

VIC: Lonely and sad.

DEAN: What do you see in your heart now?

VIC: I see a lighter light. The red is gone.

DEAN: Something still squeezing you?

VIC: No, I feel heavy. I feel a heaviness.

DEAN: Let your heart have a voice now. It may want to talk to you. It may not. Say hello to your heart. What do you hear if anything?

VIC: [pause] It says "Hello." It's a different voice than the body fat had.

DEAN: Do you recognize that voice as your heart's?

VIC: Yes.

DEAN: Express your appreciation to your heart for keeping you alive for so many years.

VIC: Okay. [pause] It says, "Thanks."

DEAN: What do you see when I ask you to imagine your heart?

VIC: I see all these blockages. I feel stuck.

DEAN: Ask your heart what it needs to be healed.

VIC: Love and acceptance.

DEAN: What do you feel now?

VIC: This overpowering grief is all there is.

DEAN: As before, allow yourself to experience that grief without pushing it back down. Let it out. If it gets too painful, then just stop.

VIC: [long pause; some crying]

DEAN: Ask your heart where it is going to get love and acceptance.

VIC: [pause] It says that it has to come from within. And it's going to support me.

DEAN: What's happening now?

VIC: I feel lighter. I feel like I took a brick off my chest. It seems lighter. It *is* lighter. I don't feel as stuffed. I don't feel stuffed back.

DEAN: Ask your heart if it loves you.

VIC: [pause] It says, "Immensely."

DEAN: Allow yourself to experience that love for a few moments.

VIC: [long pause, smiling] I feel so good. I don't have so much rage and grief anymore.

DEAN: Ask your heart what it needs for you to do in the next 24 hours, if anything.

VIC: [pause] To meditate.

DEAN: On what?

VIC: It says, "On white light—to flush out that stuff that is stuck inside."

DEAN: What kind of image comes to mind now that your heart wants you to use?

VIC: [pause] My heart says, "Just let it bathe in white light, flood it with white light."

DEAN: Just your heart or your whole body?

VIC: [pause] It says to start in my heart and then to let it fill up my entire body. This is very strange!

DEAN: Why don't you let that happen right now? Just for a moment. And then we will stop. [pause] Can you feel it?

VIC: I feel very warm and peaceful.

DEAN: Allow it to fill up your whole body beginning with the heart. [long pause] Just stay with that for another minute or so. [pause] Now please open your eyes. How do you feel?

VIC: [smiling] Thank you. I feel a lot lighter and freer. That was incredibly powerful.

DEAN: You look a lot lighter. Do you feel judgment any place? Look around and see.

VIC: No, I see love.

DEAN: Are you embarrassed?

VIC: Somewhat, yes. It was not my intention to talk about myself today, but I'm glad I did. Thank you.

DEAN: Thank you for having the courage to do that. It helps all of us. I would also suggest that you continue this on your own. Although it must be terribly painful, allow yourself to experience whatever feelings and emotions come up that you've been walling off. I also encourage you to continue the dialogue with your heart, because what it needs today may be different from what it needs two weeks from now.

VIC: That sounds a lot better than stuffing down food to stuff down what I've been feeling. I'm going to try screaming instead of eating.

DEAN: At least you can't do both at the same time.

VIC: Anything else before we stop?

DEAN: I want you to feel the love that people have for you.

VIC: I hear it. The love is here. But I've been too blind to see it, usually.

DEAN: Allow yourself to feel the connection with everyone here.

We all know what it is like to feel judged by others and by ourselves. We all know what it feels like not to measure up to what others think we should be or what we think we should be. And we all know how painful it can be to feel judged and rejected. And in these common feelings and experiences we can feel more connected with each other instead of feeling different and separate.

There are many ways we have to shut ourselves off from our feelings with drugs, with alcohol, with obesity, with compulsive working, with movies, with addictions, and so on. We have many ways of not choosing to live. Sometimes the pain gets so bad that it may seem easier to die. And yet each of us here has chosen to continue living at least for this day, as painful as it's been. And perhaps now, we can also choose to heal as well as to live.

In summary, then, the yoga techniques described so far—stretching, deep relaxation, breathing, and visualization techniques—are powerful tools not only for "stress management" but also for helping us learn to open our hearts to our feelings and to inner peace. In the next chapter, I will describe how communication skills and other techniques can help us to begin opening our hearts and healing our isolation from others. Finally, in chapter 9, I will explain how meditation and visualization can be used to help us open our hearts and to transcend and heal our isolation from a higher self.

"Father, forgive them; for they know not what they do."

—Luke 23:34

∎

"Virtue, like gold, is stronger when alloyed with a baser metal."

—Samuel Butler, *The Way of All Flesh*

∎

"Universal responsibility is feeling for other peoples' suffering just as we feel for our own. It is the realization that even our enemy is entirely motivated by the quest for happiness. We must recognize that all human beings want the same thing we want."

—The XIV Dalai Lama

∎

"Honey, if I weren't rich, would you still love me?" "Of course I'd love you—I'd miss you, but I'd love you. . . ."

—as told by Norman Cousins

∎

Lord, make me an instrument of Your peace.
Where there is hatred let me sow love;
Where there is injury, pardon;
Where there is doubt, faith;
Where there is despair, hope;
Where there is darkness, light; and
Where there is sadness, joy.
Oh divine Master, grant that I may not so much
Seek to be consoled as to console;
To be understood as to understand;
To be loved as to love.

—St. Francis of Assisi (1128–1226)

8

Opening Your
Heart to Others

The exercises and techniques in the preceding chapter can help us to become more aware of what's happening in our own body, mind, and heart and to find greater peace within. In this chapter we take the next step: how to begin healing our isolation from others.

Any action has the potential to lead us toward more intimacy or more isolation—at every moment of the day. *It's not only what we're doing, it's how we approach what we're doing that determines if we end up feeling more connected to others or more alone.* Some actions are more intensely charged than others and so have more energy to push us in either direction.

Sex is one example: When two people are deeply in love and feel safe with each other, making love can be a transcendent and ecstatic experience. The lovers lose themselves in each other as the boundaries that separate them begin to fall away. On the other end of the spectrum, rape is perhaps one of the most isolating and destructive experiences. Survivors of rape often experience profound feelings of isolation and report great difficulty in being able to trust again.

I have found similar descriptions in my work with dying patients. Death can be viewed as going into a dark little room, all alone, forever—the ultimate isolating experience. Or it can be a transcendent experience: a return to the source, a return to the light, a raindrop becoming part of the ocean, a soul becoming one with God. This experience is described more fully in the next chapter.

How we approach other people each day in less extreme situations can determine whether we experience isolation, chronic stress, suffering, and illness, or intimacy, relaxation, joy, and health. Of course, touching, hugging, and massage are ways of increasing intimacy. In this chapter, I describe three powerful techniques that can help us to feel more connected to others and to transcend our sense of separateness instead of feeling alone and isolated:

- Communication skills
- Altruism, compassion, and forgiveness
- Group support and sharing secrets

COMMUNICATION SKILLS

We can learn how to talk to each other in ways that allow another person to hear us better. When we feel heard, then we feel more connected. And feeling connected and heard is an important part of the healing process because it reduces the feelings of isolation that lead to stress and illness.

Communication and ventilation are not the same. *Ventilation* is just getting your feelings out; you really don't care whether the person hears you or not. *Communication* is expressing how you feel to someone so that he or she can hear and understand you better. It's a skill that can be learned.

Many people believe that merely ventilating anger is good for you—a catharsis of negative emotions. But is it? In her book *Anger: The Misunderstood Emotion,* Carol Tavris outlines research that questions this assumption. She writes:

The psychological rationales for ventilating anger do not stand up under experimental scrutiny. The weight of evidence indicates precisely the opposite: expressing anger makes you angrier, solidifies an angry attitude, and establishes a hostile habit.

She concludes that ventilating anger usually does more harm than good, since the other person generally feels attacked and then retaliates—a downward spiral that results in both people feeling increasingly isolated from each other.

The same process of attack and counterattack happens between countries as it does between people. One country commits an act of terrorism against another. Country B retaliates. Country A drops a bigger bomb. And so on.

Oftentimes it seems that when we're in a relationship with someone—either a work relationship or a personal one—we have to choose between either holding our feelings in and making ourselves increasingly upset or exploding and making others around us angry. As one of the participants in our study put it, "If I tell her what I think, then she feels attacked and we get in a big fight. She either attacks me back or she withdraws. Either way, I feel more isolated. So I just stuff my feelings in—until I explode. What else can I do? Sometimes it seems like it's easier not to feel at all."

But we have another option: communicating our feelings in ways that are more likely to be heard without causing the other person to feel attacked. Earlier in this book, I explained that we don't have to choose between an interesting, productive life filled with stress or sitting under a tree and watching our lives go by. Because the stress isn't just "out there," it's also in how each of us reacts to the world. Similarly, although we like to blame others for our communication problems—"If only they would change, then we could communicate!"—there is a lot that each of us can do to make a profound improvement in how we communicate, without relying on the other person to change. And when we communicate in this way, it makes it easier for the other person to change, too.

When we're growing up, most of us don't learn how to talk to each other in constructive ways. As we go through school, we learn so much about subjects that have so little to do with our daily lives, and yet most of us don't learn even basic skills in how to communicate with each other, even though this is one of the most important parts of our lives. But we can learn how to communicate in ways that aren't perceived as attacks or judgments or criticisms by the other person.

The basic principle of good communication is that *our feelings help to connect us, whereas thoughts—especially judgments—tend to isolate us.* Our emotions are more likely to be heard by someone than our thoughts. It doesn't always happen that way, but expressing our feelings increases the likelihood that it will. Communicating ideas brings our minds together, whereas communicating emotions unites our hearts—not quite the same experience. The clear expression of genuine feelings, even negative ones, is a gift to both ourselves and to others, for it helps to bring us together. Thoughts connect our heads, feelings join our hearts.

Why?

- *Thoughts are much more likely to be heard as criticisms than are feelings.* If one person says, "I think you're wrong," or "I think you're a jerk," then the other person is likely to feel verbally attacked or criticized. At that point, the walls (emotional defenses) go up, the discussion spirals downward, and no one really wins. Both people may start arguing about feeling attacked rather than whatever was originally bothering them.

- *As soon as we feel criticized by someone, it's very hard to hear anything else he or she has to say.* If I communicate a feeling instead—"I feel hurt by what you did"—then you're less likely to perceive it as an attack. It's easier for you to hear what I'm saying. And being heard and understood is what we really want.

- *Feelings are true statements.* If I say, "I feel sad," or "I feel angry," nobody can argue with the truth of that statement. Instead, if I express a thought—"I think you're wrong"—then we can argue about whether or not that's true: "No, *I'm* not wrong, *you're* wrong." Then we may end up fighting about who's right and who's wrong rather than trying to hear what the other person is saying.

- *Listening is not the same as obeying.* We want to feel listened to, even if we don't get what we're asking for. When you can communicate freely, the other person may not always give you what you want, but at least you'll understand each other better. But when we don't feel heard, then we feel more isolated and powerless. So we often end up fighting more about that than about whatever issue was originally at hand.

- *Expressing feelings seems to make us a little vulnerable, although it really makes us safer.* Part of what makes being in a close relationship with someone feel so scary is that we know each other's soft spots very well. No one else knows how to hurt us quite as effectively. When we're feeling attacked or judged by a friend, family member, or loved one, the human tendency is to want to attack back and go right for the soft underbelly. But when we communicate our feelings, then we're exposing part of ourselves to the other person. And when you make yourself a little more vulnerable, your heart a little more open, then it makes it easier for the other person to respond in kind. It helps both people to feel safer and thus more free.

- *Feelings are more powerful than thoughts at influencing us.* A few years ago, I was asked to appear on a television show that was trying to raise money for a research institute in Washington. The fundraising expert explained that it was much more difficult to raise money for medical research than for children in Ethiopia, even though contributions to both would save lives. Research focuses on ideas, but a hungry child deeply touches our emotions. Similarly, most political campaigns are not based on a rational discussion of the issues.

- *Expressing feelings helps to keep the discussion in the present moment.* Thoughts usually focus on the past or future: "You didn't take out the trash last week, either," "You'll never get there on time," and so on. The present is usually hard enough to deal with without also bringing in events from the months or years past or imagining what might happen in the future. When we begin to argue about things in the past or future, then we begin to argue about arguing. Keeping the discussion in the present by expressing what we feel right now gives both people more freedom to do things differently than they may have done before.

The basic principles of these communication skills are fairly simple, but it takes a lot of practice before they become a habit. At first, the distinction between thoughts and feelings may seem like splitting hairs, but it makes an important difference in how well we communicate. These techniques can be used for expressing—and receiving—positive feelings as well as negative ones.

Step 1: Identify What You Are Feeling
This isn't as easy as it sounds. Many people have a hard time telling the difference between a thought and a feeling. What are some common feelings?

- I'm angry.
- I'm afraid.
- I'm worried.
- I'm thrilled.
- I'm confused.
- I'm happy.
- I'm depressed.
- I'm envious.
- I'm resentful.
- I love you.
- I want __.

What are some common thoughts or judgments?

- I'm right.
- You're wrong.
- You're not listening.
- You did it again.
- You're always late.
- You're a jerk (always a subject for intense debate . . .).
- You forgot.
- You should wear different clothes.

Sometimes thoughts masquerade as feelings:

- I feel that I'm right.
- I feel as if you're wrong.
- I feel you should do it better.
- I feel you ought to be more careful.

Using the words "that," "like," or "as if" after "I feel" is a clue that what follows is probably a thought (a judgment), not a feeling.

Words like "you should," "you ought to," "you never," and "you always" are thoughts and are almost always heard as judgments or criticisms.

The yoga and meditation techniques described in the previous chapter can help us to become more aware of what we *are* feeling rather than what we think we *should* be feeling.

Step 2: Express What You Are Feeling

Say exactly how you feel, but express it as a feeling rather than as a thought or judgment. You don't have to tone it down, make it nice, or pretend. It is as important to express negative feelings as positive ones, but express them as feelings and information rather than as judgments and criticisms.

Communicating your feelings is not a panacea, but it does help to break the vicious cycle of attack, counterattack, and withdrawal. It's not going to solve all your problems, but at least it won't add more problems to the ones you already have. You can begin to focus on the real issues and deal with those instead of arguing about the arguing and fighting about the fighting. As a result, each person is more likely to get what he or she wants.

Step 3: Listen Actively With Empathy and Compassion

Knowing how to listen is as important a communication skill as knowing how to express feelings. Try to hear the feeling in what the other person is saying, even if he or she is not expressing it clearly or is expressing it as a judgment. Remember that the other person wants to feel heard, just as you do. You're not always going to get the other person to agree with you, but at least you'll understand each other better. Opening, listening, and giving one's attention help to bring us together. Compassion and empathy are healing.

Empathy is not the same as sympathy. *Empathy* means listening with compassion—trying to experience and understand what the other person is feeling. *Sympathy* means feeling sorry for someone, a usually well-intentioned gesture that often creates more distance between two people. The unspoken message can be, "You're the one with the problem, not me."

A variant of sympathy is giving unsolicited advice. When we hear someone describing a problem, our tendency is to try to "fix" it by jumping in with our own advice, comments, criticisms, or experiences. Often the other person just wants to feel listened to and understood, which leads to greater intimacy even when the problem is not easily solvable. The unspoken message behind unsolicited advice can be, "I know the answer; how come you don't?", creating more distance and less intimacy. Listening is very often more supportive a response than giving someone advice.

Step 4: Acknowledge What the Other Person Is Saying
Expressing that you understand what the other person is saying is not the same as agreeing with it. For example, you might say, "I understand that you're feeling angry because I got home late. And I'm frustrated because I wanted to be home with you but I had to stay late to finish that report."

It's easier to acknowledge feelings than thoughts or judgments. If someone says to me, "I feel angry," it's a lot easier to acknowledge that feeling than if he says, "You're always late for dinner." And it's easier to apologize when someone expresses hurt or angry feelings than if that person attacks or judges us.

To make this less abstract, here's a real-life example from a group session with Joe and Anita Cecena, tape recorded at one of our research group meetings:

> JOE: You went to the store today and spent too much money, Anita. How come?
>
> DEAN: Is that a thought or a feeling?
>
> JOE: A thought.
>
> DEAN: Anita, how do you feel when he says that?
>
> ANITA: Criticized. Attacked.
>
> DEAN: What would be your natural inclination to do next?
>
> ANITA: To argue and defend myself. Or to attack back. Usually I just ignore him, just tune him out. Sometimes I pretend I don't hear him. Or I'll say, "'Yes, dear," and then do it anyway.
>
> DEAN: Joe, when you feel ignored, how do you respond?
>
> JOE: I feel like I'm losing control. Powerless. Sometimes I feel abandoned. And then I get angry, because I don't like feeling that way.
>
> DEAN: Joe, how else could you express how you feel about Anita's shopping?
>
> JOE: Anita, what did you buy that cost so much?
>
> DEAN: Is that a thought or a feeling?

JOE: A thought, I guess.

DEAN: Anita, do you still feel criticized?

ANITA: Yes—it's a little less harsh than before, but it still leaves me feeling pretty much the same way.

DEAN: OK, Joe, what is the feeling underlying those thoughts?

JOE: That she's a compulsive spender.

DEAN: Is that a thought or a feeling?

JOE: Hmmm . . . a thought.

DEAN: And a judgment.

JOE: What if I say, "I feel like she's a compulsive spender."

DEAN: That's a thought masquerading as a feeling, and I suspect Anita also feels criticized when you say that.

ANITA: Right.

DEAN: When she came back from shopping and told you what she spent, what did you feel? What's the feeling that underlies what you are trying to communicate?

JOE: Anger and frustration. And I'm a little worried that we might not have enough money to pay the rest of our bills. And like I'm losing control over Anita.

DEAN: Anita, when you felt criticized by Joe, how did you feel?

ANITA: Angry and frustrated.

DEAN: So the irony is that both people generally end up feeling the same way—in this example, angry, frustrated, misunderstood, with a loss of control—and yet each thinks the other person doesn't understand what he or she is feeling. Neither person feels listened to or understood. This frequently happens in arguments between two people, yet it's the opposite of what they both want. Joe, try expressing your feelings instead of your thoughts to Anita.

JOE: When you bought those gifts, I felt angry and frustrated, and a little worried.

DEAN: Anita, do you feel attacked now?

ANITA: When he says it that way, no, I don't.

DEAN: Do you want to attack back, withdraw, or argue with him?

ANITA: Not now. And I knew when I spent so much money that he'd feel this way. But I feel that Joe tends to be very domineering and controlling.

DEAN: Joe, when Anita says, "I feel that you tend to be very domineering and controlling," how do you feel?

JOE: I feel attacked and misunderstood. And judged.

DEAN: Just like Anita does. Anita, any time someone says, "I feel that you . . ." it's probably a thought, not a feeling. It may sound like splitting hairs to distinguish between, "I feel that you're dominating me" (a thought) versus "I feel dominated" (a feeling). But there is a world of difference in how the other person hears each.

When we're feeling controlled, then attacking the other person is one way to try to rebalance the power in the relationship. And it does often make the other person feel less in control and more in pain. That may be what we want in the moment, but it's not going to give us what we really want, which is to feel more free and intimate with our partner. So try expressing what you said as a feeling instead of a judgment.

ANITA: Joe, I've been feeling dominated and controlled by you, and I spent the money as a way of trying to feel freer and more independent.

DEAN: This allows both of you to focus on the underlying issues and to address them more directly. Anita, when you said earlier, "You're dominating and controlling me," then you're judging Joe. It puts all of the responsibility and blame on *him.* Instead, when you now said, "I feel dominated and controlled," it reflects how *you're* feeling, which takes into account that you may have misperceived him. For example, you may be sensitive to feeling dominated because of bad experiences in prior relationships. Or Joe may, in fact, be dominating you. But expressing the feeling frees both of you to explore a wider range of possibilities.

JOE: Anita, I want you to tell me when you're feeling controlled or manipulated by me, and I'll try to stop doing it.

Saying "I want" is a clear and direct feeling—no one can argue if it's true or not. And it makes you a little more open and vulnerable, since the other person knows he or she can disappoint you by not giving you what you want. But saying "I want" is something most of us are taught not to express. It sounds too demanding. So we often tiptoe around the issue without saying it directly. In fact, because it is so clear and straightforward, saying "I want" is less likely to make someone else feel manipulated than if you try to get what you want in a more indirect way. And when we feel manipulated or controlled, we don't feel free.

Where does the need to control others come from? When we're not in touch with our inner happiness, then we think it can come only from another person. Then we think we need to get the other person to do something that we want or to be a certain way: "If only he or she would do this, then I'd be happy." This is where control and manipulation begin.

We all want to feel free, but we can't feel that way if we're being manipulated. We resent it. To the degree that we are more aware of our inner well-being, then we don't need another person to provide that for us. We can enjoy others for who they are, not for who we want them to be.

By focusing on our feelings, our communication and our relationships can become less manipulative, leaving both people feeling freer. We don't have to choose between being independent but isolated or being intimate but swallowed up and controlled by another person. We can relate to each other in ways that maintain both our intimacy and autonomy. In her book, *Intimate Partners,* Maggie Scarf describes different exercises that can be used to enhance both intimacy and autonomy.

Here's another example with Phyllis and Hank Ginsberg at one of our group meetings:

PHYLLIS: Last week, Hank said, "I don't feel good," so I told him to call the doctor. He said, "Well, I don't want to call the doctor now, I'll call him in a few days." And he never did. How do you work that kind of thing out?

DEAN: Hank and Phyllis, why don't you recreate what happened last week?

HANK: OK. [to Phyllis]: Phyllis, I don't feel good.

PHYLLIS: I feel that you should call the doctor, Hank.

DEAN: Phyllis, that's a thought and a judgment. Hank, how do you feel when she says that?

HANK: It's like she's saying, "I know better than you do." Like I'm a small child. I mean, don't you think I've thought of that myself, Phyllis? I know the doctor's number and that calling the doctor might be a good idea.

DEAN: OK, now the thoughts are colliding. Should he or shouldn't he call the doctor? It's a great debate that neither of you wins. Phyllis, how else could you express that? Focus on your feelings instead of your thoughts.

PHYLLIS: Hank, I want you to call the doctor. I'm concerned.

DEAN: Hank, how does that leave you feeling?

HANK: I'm not feeling attacked. But I don't think it's necessary at this point to call the doctor. I think I'll know if it's serious enough, I think I know my body well enough.

PHYLLIS: Well, if you feel that way, then don't tell me when you're not feeling good, because then I worry about it.

HANK: Maybe I shouldn't tell you. Next time I'll keep it to myself.

DEAN: All right, let's stop there for a moment. Both of you end up feeling how?

HANK: Lousy.

PHYLLIS: Bad, very bad.

DEAN: So you both end up feeling the same way.

PHYLLIS: I feel frustrated and helpless. I'm frightened that something may be seriously wrong with Hank, so this is the time to deal with it.

DEAN: Issues of power and control are important in almost all relationships. Why do we need to control our partners? Because we need them to act in a certain way, even if they don't want to. When we try to manipulate them to do what we want, then that engenders resentment.

PHYLLIS: Well, Hank's health is a big part of my life. So it's a matter of controlling my life also.

DEAN: Okay, but if you really want control . . . do you feel like you're in control at this moment?

PHYLLIS: No.

DEAN: Were you successful in getting Hank to call the doctor?

PHYLLIS: No.

DEAN: And that's the irony: The more we try to exert our control, the less control we may end up having. What other options do you have? Would you ever say to Hank, "I'm feeling powerless?"

PHYLLIS: No. I called the doctor and asked him to call Hank.

DEAN: Hank, how did you feel when the doctor called and asked if you're feeling all right?

HANK: I think she was overconcerned. That it's a power play.

DEAN: What are the feelings behind those thoughts?

HANK: I'm not even sure.

DEAN: A few moments ago, you said, "Next time, I won't tell Phyllis how I'm feeling." When we have no constructive way of communicating our feelings, then sometimes it becomes easier to wall them off, even from ourselves. So, Hank, close your eyes and meditate for a moment to become more aware of what you were feeling when the doctor called.

HANK: [a few moments later] I was furious, because I knew that Phyllis asked him to call. I felt controlled. Even though both the doctor and Phyllis told me it's for my own good.

DEAN: When we begin to manipulate someone, we can justify it in lots of ways: "It's for your own good." "Do it because it's good for you." "Do it because I know best." "Do it because I said so." All of which leave the other person feeling more powerless and resentful.

HANK: We've been fighting over control for so many years that as soon as she gets more control, I rebel—it's almost automatic.

PHYLLIS: I don't even have to say anything and he gets upset.

DEAN: You're both so predictable to each other. Wouldn't it be interesting if one of you changed? If only one of you changes, it helps free the other person as well. The balance shifts.

When we feel powerless, we try to restore the balance of power. One way is to attack back. Another is to become withholding, sometimes called being passive-aggressive. A third way is to find someone else less powerful to wield power over or even abuse. Dr. Alice Miller, a German psychiatrist, has written several books describing how parents tend to control and abuse their children in the name of helping them. One of her books, *For Your Own Good,* describes how this pattern of emotional or even physical abuse is passed along from generation to generation—she calls it a "poisonous pedagogy." Abused children often grow up to become abusing parents. Children who were controlled by their parents often do the same to their children. Of course, it's not in our genes; it's in our culture and experience, and we can make different choices.

PHYLLIS: But shouldn't I be concerned about Hank's health?

DEAN: Of course. I'm not saying that you shouldn't be concerned about Hank and how he's doing. But your efforts are counterproductive. The harder you push, the more resentment Hank feels and the less likely he is to give you what you want—even if he risks having another heart attack in the process! He may even risk dying in order to feel free. So neither of you get what you want.

HANK: That's why most of the time I don't tell Phyllis if I'm not feeling well. Because I'm afraid she's going to pressure me into doing something that I might not want to do.

DEAN: That's true for many people. Most of the time when I see a patient in the emergency room in the midst of a major heart attack, he's had severe chest pain for at least four hours before he told anyone. And that can be life-threatening, because some of the newer drugs used to help stop a heart attack in progress have to be used within the first few hours after the pain began or it's too late.

When we try to control or manipulate someone, he or she usually resents it. *More than being healthy, we want to feel free, and we can't feel free when we're feeling controlled.* Only if you can truly accept "no" for an answer can the other person freely say "yes." Then the relationship feels freer and less manipulative, and the person is more likely to give you what you want. Both people are more likely to get what they want when they learn to communicate. Instead of both people feeling frustrated, both feel closer to each other. It's a win-win situation.

Phyllis, you might choose to simply voice your feelings and then let go of them. When Hank knows that you are willing to accept that he may choose not to call the doctor, then he feels more free to do it. He still might not, but it's more likely that he will than if you insist that he make the call. Either way, you haven't disrupted the intimacy between the two of you. Otherwise, the added stress increases the likelihood that he *will* need a doctor!

Let's do it again. This time, notice what you're feeling, express the feeling, and try to avoid thoughts and judgments.

HANK: Phyllis, I don't feel very good.

PHYLLIS: I don't feel good either. I feel worried. I'm frightened.

HANK: I'm a little concerned and frightened, too.

PHYLLIS: How bad do you feel?

HANK: I had a little pain, but it's gone now.

PHYLLIS: I want you to call the doctor.

HANK: I understand that you want me to call the doctor, but I don't want to call the doctor yet.

PHYLLIS: I still feel concerned. Let me know if there is anything I can do for you.

DEAN: Does either person feel attacked or blamed or isolated?

HANK: No, I don't.

PHYLLIS: I still wish he'd call the doctor, but at least I feel understood.

DEAN: Both of you expressed your feelings very clearly. Hank acknowledged that he understands Phyllis' concerns, and I suspect he's a lot more likely to call the doctor than he was after your last discussion.

HANK: Absolutely.

DEAN: Whenever there's a power struggle, there's often fear underneath. Expressing the deeper feelings directly—the fear, in this example—allows greater intimacy. And you're both more likely to get what you really want.

These same power issues that Hank and Phyllis struggle with also occur between many doctors and their patients. I've seen many people choose to maintain self-destructive and painful lifestyle behaviors and communication patterns in order to feel free from someone else telling them to do "what's good for them."

For example, people who have had heart attacks often continue to smoke or eat high-fat foods. Approaching behavioral changes only from an intellectual standpoint is not sufficient to motivate most people to make significant changes. Their emotions and feelings also need to be addressed.

Part of the problem is that doctors are not taught communication skills in most medical schools. A recent study found that the average physician spends less than sixty seconds listening to a patient before interrupting him or her.

Even the words that doctors use to assess behavioral changes reveal the power struggle that often occurs between physicians and patients. Doctors refer to a patient's "compliance" with their prescribed medications or lifestyle recommendations, as though the patient is capitulating and surrendering his will and freedom to the doctor.

This goes all the way back to the story of Adam and Eve, when

God told them not to eat the apple. As soon as someone says, "Don't do this," it's only human to respond, "Why not?" or "Watch me!" We will even die to preserve our freedom—as Patrick Henry said, "Give me liberty or give me death!"

So I never tell people that they *have* to change their lifestyle. I used to, but it didn't work. And even when I was successful in getting people to change, it didn't last very long.

Now, I avoid getting into a power struggle with people. I just provide them with information so they know what their options are and they can make informed choices. And I support whatever they choose. I don't presume to have all the answers. It's their life, not mine. When I maintain that attitude, paradoxically, I find that people are much more likely to make meaningful changes and to maintain them. Because they feel free to make their own choices and to live their own life.

The communication skills used by Joe, Anita, Hank, and Phyllis to improve their personal relationships also are effective in making business relationships more pleasant and productive. Imagine, for example, that Mr. Jones is your employer and he wants you to do something that you think is unsafe. Here are two possible replies, exaggerated somewhat to make the point:

> *Reply 1:* "It's dangerous. You're always asking me to take the worst assignments, and you never treat me fairly. Look, as I've told you before many times, that's not the right way to do it anyway. You're wrong, and you should know better by now."
>
> *Reply 2:* "I would not feel safe if I took this assignment, so I prefer not to do it. I want you to consider some other alternatives."

If you were the employer, how would you feel in response to each reply? And which response is more likely to get the employee what he wants?

ALTRUISM, COMPASSION, AND FORGIVENESS

Altruism, compassion, and forgiveness are also potent tools for helping to heal our isolation from others and to empower ourselves. Often we give our power away to the person or people we dislike the most.

In 1977, on the first day of our first study, one of the participants decided that he had an intense hatred for another patient in the study. The two men began shouting at each other and almost began hitting each other—until they both got severe chest pain and doubled over. One man clutched his chest, ran out of the room, and slammed the door while the other reached for his nitroglycerin. I thought this was going to be the end of my very short research career.

After they both calmed down, I met with them individually and pointed out that each was giving his power away—and his health—to the person he liked the least. The chest pain that each was experiencing could be used to remind him to make the connection between when he suffered and why.

I asked them to begin doing tasks to help each other—not to get a gold star, or to go to heaven, or for good karma, or to be a good person, or for any external reward, or to have the other person in his debt, but rather because this is what would help to empower each of them and to help free each one from his pain. So they began doing each other's laundry, running errands for each other, and so on. While they never became close friends, they had no more episodes of chest pain.

Altruism, compassion, and forgiveness—opening your heart— can be powerful means of healing the isolation that leads to stress, suffering, and illness. In other words, altruism, compassion, and forgiveness are in our own, best self-interest, for they help to free us from our limitations and to empower us.

Scientists at the University of Michigan studied 2,754 people in Tecumseh, Michigan, for more than a decade. They interviewed people between 1967 and 1969 and then followed them for the next nine to twelve years. They found that men who did no volunteer work were two and a half times as likely to die during the study as men who volunteered at least once a week. (Compare this magnitude of difference with the studies of cholesterol-lowering drugs described in chapter 2.) These results were independent of age, gender, or health status when they first entered the study. Similarly, in our study, many of the participants performed volunteer work for various causes. Although they did not do it for this reason, they enjoyed how it made them feel.

A recurrent theme of this book is that lasting peace and happiness are not something we get; we have them already until we disturb them. In that sense, then, acting "selflessly" is the most "selfish" way to behave, since it maintains our sense of inner peace and joy.

Compassion and forgiveness are empowering and healing both for the giver and for the recipient. For example, after Pope John Paul recovered from being shot, he later met with his assailant and forgave him. But there is a spectrum of altruism—the benefit comes from the purity of feeling, not from the magnitude of the act.

In 1975, when I was a first-year medical student, I went to a workshop given by Elisabeth Kübler-Ross, M.D., a psychiatrist who is well known for her pioneering work with dying people. I figured this was something I would need to learn, since in a few years I would be working with patients who were severely ill and dying. Also, I had a hidden fascination with death after coming so close to it myself during my first year in college.

I expected a workshop where Dr. Kübler-Ross would talk about "This is how you deal with dying people," step one, step two; a didactic lecture with a blackboard and slides. It turned out to be something very different.

Dr. Kübler-Ross said, "When you deal with people who are suffering and afraid of dying, they bring up your own pain and your own fears of death. Therefore, the real issue is not to learn a particular technique, but rather to get in touch with your own fears and your own suffering and your own concerns about death and work on that. Otherwise, if you walk into the room of someone who is dying or who is in pain, being with that person will bring all of that stuff up in you. And the person is going to know that and sense your discomfort, and they are going to close up to try to protect you. So you won't really be able to help them very much." That made sense.

There were about sixty people there, an odd collection of ministers, psychotherapists, dying people, and a few nurses. I was the only medical student or doctor there.

The technique that Dr. Kübler-Ross used to help people get in touch with their fears and emotional pain—what she called "the dark side"—was to have people hit a mattress and a phone book with a big piece of rubber radiator hose. For the first four days, I sat and watched how these mild-mannered people would go up to the mattress, hold the radiator hose, and turn into Charles Manson before my eyes—helter-skelter. They began hitting the mattress with such fury and anger that it startled and frightened me. Dr. Kübler-Ross sat just a short distance away, calmly allowing that process to happen and encouraging it.

I watched that for the first four days with a degree of detachment, like I was watching a theater performance. It was very dramatic and so very interesting to me, but I remember thinking, "Having survived my spiritual crisis in college, I'm already in touch with my own darkness and my inner demons, so I don't really need to do this."

And then, on the last day, I thought, "Well, you know, Dean, you're never really going to know what this is like unless you try it. You don't know any of these people here and you may not have this opportunity again. It's not going to hurt you, so why not give it a try?" My curiosity got the better of me.

So I went up to the mat, and I took the radiator hose and I started to hit the mat and the telephone book with it. And I just couldn't get into it. I said, "Sorry, Elisabeth, but this is really kind of silly. I don't much feel like hitting this mat." And she replied, "Well look, Dean, you have a good imagination. Why don't you just imagine you are hitting somebody instead of just hitting a mat?" And I said, "Well, I'm not mad at anybody." (And a little halo glowed over my head. . . .) She asked, "Have you ever been angry with anyone—family, friends, teachers?" "Of course." "Then close your eyes and pretend that you're hitting them with this piece of radiator hose. Don't worry—you won't really hurt them; this is only happening in your imagination."

I closed my eyes, and I was surprised to realize that I still had some anger toward various people—my organic chemistry professor from college, a former girlfriend, a college roommate, one of my siblings, and so on. I said to myself, "If you're going to go through with this exercise, don't hold anything back so you can learn as much as possible."

So I imagined that I was hitting people with the radiator hose, one at a time. In each case, the pattern was pretty much the same. I would hit them, and they would first react with astonishment, shock, and disbelief: "What's come over you, what's happening?" Then they would react with anger and they would fight back. In this image, at least, I would eventually overcome them, and they would react by trying to foster guilt: "How can you do this to me?" Then that would be the end of it and I'd move on to the next person. It was all very brutal, and I was shocked and disgusted with myself. (Even now, I find this difficult to write about.) But I kept telling myself, "If you're going to find out anything useful, don't hold anything back."

After about twenty or thirty minutes of doing this, I was drenched with sweat, I had blisters on my hands, I had shredded several phone books, and I still didn't feel any better. Actually, I felt much worse, inside and out. And I thought, "Well, this is very interesting. I learned that *ventilating anger doesn't free me of it, it only feeds and intensifies the anger.* And that's very useful to know." (A few days after the workshop, one of the other participants committed suicide, perhaps a tragic lesson that ventilating anger is not sufficient to make us feel free.)

So I said, "Well, Elisabeth, I think I'm done. Thank you for this experience. I really don't feel very good, but I learned something very important." Dr. Kübler-Ross is very intuitive and she asked, "Are you sure you haven't left anyone out?" I replied, "I've been hitting a mattress for the past thirty minutes. Who could I have possibly left out?" She said, "Think hard."

So I thought about it some more, and I remembered a lecture that Swami Satchidananda had given six months or so earlier in which he told a story of a man who found God through pure *hatred* of God as opposed to pure love of God. I had never heard anything like that in Western traditions, and this made no sense to me at the time. There are lots of Western traditions about how someone's purity of love takes them to God or peace, but not purity of hatred.

The point is that the purity of the feeling—even a negative feeling—has the potential for being transformative if properly guided. The intensity of negative energy can be directed into something more positive. Being indecisive, unclear, and stuck in the middle of the road, neither here nor there, takes you nowhere. When you really hate someone or something, you focus on that—in a sense, you meditate on that. That which you meditate on you begin to manifest in your life. As someone once said, "Choose your enemies carefully, because you tend to become like them."

I thought, "Well, let's see if what the swami said is true." So I visualized the swami standing in front of me. Since I didn't feel very angry toward him, it was very difficult to motivate myself to hit him. I reminded myself that this was only an exercise, that it wasn't really happening, so it was all right.

So I imagined that I was hitting him with the radiator hose while I was actually hitting the mat with it. And it felt real, not like an exercise—in some ways, it felt "realer than real." It was as though he and I were the only people there. First I started hitting him across his legs and his lower body. And it was very curious—unlike the other people who had gone through the various stages of shock and disbelief and fighting back and being overcome, he just stood there, facing me directly with his arms by his sides, and allowed me to hit his body with the radiator hose. I found myself getting enraged that he wasn't fighting back! And then I started getting angry at myself—loathing myself—for hitting him. But I kept doing it. I told myself, "You might as well continue; you're never going to know if this has value unless you see this through to the end of the exercise."

Then I looked up, and I could see tears coming down his face. And I knew that he wasn't crying because I was hurting his body with the radiator hose. The only way I can describe it is that these were tears of pure compassion. And I had never experienced unconditional love and compassion before. Although he wasn't speaking, I could hear him saying very clearly (since this was all in my mind anyway), "You poor, ignorant boy. You just don't know any better." Without a hint of being patronizing. Just pure love and compassion came through.

And at that point, I melted. In an almost mystical, infinitely long moment, a whole series of transformations began to happen. Here, I had shown my darkest side and had only light coming back, the light of love and compassion. I realized in a very deep way that darkness and light can't coexist, something I had never understood before. And the darkness exists only because I am afraid of it and keep it in darkness—a vicious cycle. My fear creates walls that block out the light, even though the light is always there. Like someone who has been living in a dark room, I don't have to create light, just open the window shades or walls and let the sunshine stream in.

I realized that if somebody else can have that kind of compassion for my inner darkness, then maybe I can for myself, too. I can begin opening the window, allowing the inner light to shine in, and realize that it's not dark anymore.

And to the degree I can do that, to the extent that I can have that same compassion for my own ignorance and my own darkness and my own inner demons, then I can begin to have that same compassion and love for other people whenever they display their darkness to me. When I can do that, it helps to free both of us.

I still have my inner demons that whisper to me, "You're worthless. You have just managed to fool people into thinking that you know something, but you don't really know anything, and sooner or later everyone will realize how stupid you really are." Before, I'd argue with them. Or I'd cover my ears and try to shut them out, to wall them off, to pretend that they didn't exist. Or I'd study and work compulsively at achieving, trying to prove to myself and to others that the demons were wrong—"I'm not really stupid, you see. Look what I've accomplished." And I spent so much energy keeping them away from my conscious awareness. Now, instead of trying to keep my demons in darkness, I welcome them: "Hello, demons. We meet again. Nice to see you—how have you been?" And so on. When I can do that, they lose their power to disturb me in the ways they used to do. And when I forget, the anxiety and the terror remind me.

I learned that it's not enough just to get in touch with anger and to express it. In some ways, that only intensifies the feelings and feeds into that darkness. And we can't simply deny, split off, or push down our negative emotions, pretending they're not there, and say, "Oh, I love everyone." That also intensifies the darkness and the power that negativity has over us. Those feelings can't be bypassed, figuratively or literally. But getting in touch with our emotions, including anger and hatred for others or for ourselves, is an important first step toward what really *can* free us, namely love, compassion, and forgiveness.

In real life, the swami might have gotten angry and tried to hit me back. Who knows? The point is that he represented my inner teacher, the true self and peace that we all have within. What he may be like in person is less important. Someone else might look within and find Moses, or Jesus, or Buddha, or an entirely different inner guide. It might be a priest, a rabbi, a wise friend, or a teacher. It can even be an animal or an inanimate object. But all of us have an inner self that guides us. The meditation and imagery techniques described in chapter 9 can help you to find yours.

Different religious traditions have described this experience in various stories. In the Old Testament, Moses loses his temper and strikes a rock; as a result, God tells Moses that he can't enter Israel. I see the story as a metaphor—that is, when we are consumed by anger (hit the rock), it keeps us from entering our natural state of inner peace (Israel). It's not simply that God punishes us; we limit ourselves. And we can make different choices.

In the New Testament, during the crucifixion, Jesus said, "Father forgive them; for they know not what they do." The same compassion that I felt from the inner swami. What better way to teach compassion than by example? The story of Jesus' body rising from the dead, whether or not historically true, may be a metaphor for how compassion frees us by helping us to transcend our sense of isolation and pain.

After finishing medical school, during my residency training, I had many opportunities to put these ideas into practice. When I was working in the emergency room, for example, sometimes patients would come in who had taken an overdose of drugs. After treating them, they would eventually begin to regain consciousness. Sometimes, they expressed their gratitude by throwing up on me or getting violent. And I'd remember the image of the swami's tears to remind me that the patients weren't there to thank me; I was there to serve them. Whenever I expect something in return, then my inner peace gets disturbed. And I expect something in return only when I've forgotten that peace comes from within.

Fear creates inner walls that keep our hearts in darkness—not only on a personal level but also on political and social levels. In his book, *Faces of the Enemy,* Sam Keen describes how we tend to project our "dark side"—those aspects of ourselves that we are most uncomfortable with—onto other people, other countries, other religions, other racial groups, and so on. By projecting our inner darkness onto others, we can pretend that we do not have to deal with those parts of ourselves—until the pain becomes too great.

The ongoing process of learning compassion—for my own darkness and that of others—is what helps to free me from my sense of isolation. That's what frees us, that's what heals us. And, eventually, it may even open our arteries as well as our hearts.

That's what I am trying to convey with the research and in this book. Pain and suffering, whether in the form of physical illnesses like heart disease or emotional diseases like severe depression or spiritual pain like hatred, can be catalysts for helping to transform us in ways that can be profoundly healing. The goal is not simply to reverse the anatomical blockages. None of us is going to live forever, even though both medical care and self-help programs sometimes create an illusion of immortality—"If I just love enough, or if I just eat an optimal diet, then I'll never die."

The real issue for me is how we can feel more free and more joyful. How to open our hearts on psychological levels—to build intimacy—and spiritual levels—to develop compassion. More precisely, we are free already; by remaining compassionate, we can stop binding ourselves and limiting our freedom. We may live longer because of this, but that's not the primary goal. We can live better.

GROUP SUPPORT/SHARING SECRETS

In chapter 3, I described the healing power of social support as a way of healing our isolation from others. In several studies, even being a member of a club, church, or synagogue significantly decreased the risk of premature death and disability from all causes, regardless of a person's genes or risk factors.

Pat Riley is coach of the Los Angeles Lakers, one of the most successful teams in basketball history. When asked, "Why do your players work so hard?" he replied, "The game is about the primal instinct to be a part of something."

Joining some groups, however, is not likely to increase one's longevity. Why are we seeing a rapid increase in gang membership, even though gang members are frequently brutalized or killed? In Walker Percy's book, *The Message in the Bottle,* he wonders why it is that old soldiers like to sit around and fondly reminisce about their wartime experiences when the experiences were so hellish. Why is there such an outpouring of emotion and closeness among those who visit the Vietnam Memorial? And in his book, *The Youngest Science,* why does Dr. Lewis Thomas describe his year of internship as the most wonderful of his life, even though the demands and stresses of his Harvard Medical School internship were extremely intense?

The desire for intimacy, for transcending our feelings of isolation, is so strong that it can even lead us to self-destructive behaviors. Unfortunately, one way to increase intimacy is to find a common enemy.

In gangs or at war, people often find a level of intimacy, structure, and social support not found at home or at school. When people are at war, the survivors on the battlefield feel a tremendous closeness with each other. (Those who survive internship feel much the same way—when I was a medical student, two of the interns committed suicide, so "surviving internship" is more than just a figure of speech.)

This was beautifully described by William Broyles, Jr., a former editor-in-chief of *Newsweek* magazine and an infantry lieutenant in Vietnam. In his book, *Brothers in Arms,* he described returning to Vietnam and meeting his former enemies ten years later:

I am a peace-loving man, fond of children and animals. In high school I was in the history club instead of on the football team. I believe passionately that war should have no place in the affairs of men, and that the existence of nuclear arsenals means that the emotions that lead to wars can no longer be indulged. . . . But a part of me loved war, and at Duy Xuyen I discovered my old enemies felt the same way. . . .

We loved war for many reasons, not all of them good. The best reason we loved war is also its most enduring memory—comradeship. A comrade in war is a man you can trust with anything, because you trust him with your life. Philip Caputo described the emotion in *A Rumor of War:* "[Comradeship] does not demand for its sustenance the reciprocity, the pledges of affection, the endless reassurances required by the love of men and women. It is, unlike marriage, a bond that cannot be broken by a word, by boredom or divorce, or by anything other than death."

Comradeship isn't a particularly selective process. Race, personality, education—anything that would make a difference in peace—count for nothing. It is, simply, brotherly love. War is the only utopian experience most of us ever have. Individual possessions and advantage count for nothing; the group is everything. What you have is shared with your friends. No one is allowed to be alone.

And in war loneliness is the greatest enemy. The military historian S.L.A. Marshall did intensive studies of combat incidents in World War II and Korea and discovered that at most only 25 percent of the men under fire actually fired their weapons. The rest cowered behind cover, terrified and helpless—all systems off. Invariably, those men had felt alone, and to feel alone in combat is to cease to function; it is the terrifying prelude to the final loneliness of death. The men who kept their heads felt connected to other men, a part of something, as if comradeship were a collective life force, the power to face death and stay conscious.

The participants in our study met twice a week to discuss their progress with the program and any problems they wanted to raise. The meetings became a powerful means of achieving intimacy by encouraging the participants to begin letting down their walls and expressing their feelings. We met in San Francisco at Ft. Mason, the area from which troops disembarked during World War II, in a building that was once used to recharge submarine batteries (a nice metaphor for our current use of the building).

We found that many participants would do things for others that they would not ordinarily do for themselves. We learned the power of a group to motivate and sustain major lifestyle changes. People who might not have stayed on a diet "only" for themselves found it easier to do so as a way of supporting the other group members.

Although it did not start out that way, we ended up creating a community. At first, we talked about how to stay on the diet, swapped stories, sometimes even shared feelings, but we were careful not to probe too deeply, especially since Sam (see chapter 3) and a few others said, "I don't think feelings have anything to do with heart disease. I don't want to air my dirty laundry in front of others, and I don't want to hear about yours."

What they were really saying, though, was, "I already feel isolated and lonely, and I'm afraid that you will reject me if you find out who I really am and what I'm *really* like. If you really knew me, if you knew this dark secret about me then I'd be really all alone, and so I have to hide it. If you knew that I'm really not a former Olympic athlete, if you knew that I'm almost bankrupt, if you knew how stupid I often feel, if you knew that I cheated on my wife, if you knew that I'm gay, if you knew that my son uses drugs . . . then I'd be even more isolated, all by myself, and that's too painful."

All of us struggle with issues that in many ways are very different. Yet when we look a little deeper, we find that others' issues are not unlike our own. We have so much in common. Whatever the issue is, the fear is that we'll be rejected. So we often hide it and pretend to be something we're not.

After Sam died, the support groups took on a new focus, and all of us made a conscious effort to create an atmosphere that felt safe enough for people to begin showing who they really were underneath the masks and personas. A place where they could say, "I'm not really————, I've just been pretending to be." I regret that we didn't get to that point earlier in the study because I didn't realize its importance.

We learned that there is another fundamental paradox: When we have the courage to be self-disclosing, to show who *we* really are—warts and all—then other people in the group feel safer to show who *they* really are, too. This allows us to experience new levels of intimacy rather than rejection or isolation.

A similar observation was made in a recent issue of the Harvard Medical School Mental Health Letter: "Often a patient says that the critical therapeutic moment was exposing a 'dangerous' feeling and finding that it did not lead to catastrophic rejection or derision."

Of course, there is a place and time to have masks and defenses and personas. I don't think it's always inappropriate to have an image of who you want people to think you are. If you're going for a job interview, it's probably not a good idea to bare your darkest secrets there. But *if you never have any place that you feel safe enough to show who you really are, anyone with whom you can really be yourself, then I think it's ultimately stressful and isolating.*

Like the fight-or-flight response, the problem is knowing when to turn it on and turn it off. The people who always have their fight-or-flight mechanism on are the ones who get into trouble. The ones who know how to modulate it are the ones who can function at their peak capacity. They're not victims of it. In the same way, if you know that you're showing an image to someone, for whatever reason, that's not the same thing as feeling like you can never get past the image.

Sharing secrets is a little scary, but it can be healing. I have some misgivings about having disclosed some of my own deeply personal experiences in this book, but I'm hoping that it will touch something in you that will allow us to share a common experience or feeling, even though we may never meet.

I know how painful it can be to feel alone, and I know the joy of feeling intimate. I know how painful it can be to feel despairing, and I know the joy of feeling hopeful. I know how painful it can be to feel rejected, and I know the joy of feeling loved. You may have experienced similar feelings at times. My feelings and experiences may not be exactly the same as yours, but they are similar. And in that sense we are connected.

Although there are many different types of psychotherapy, working with a skilled and compassionate therapist is another way to help you re-experience suppressed or repressed emotions without feeling judged. The therapist's compassion for you can allow you to have the same compassion for yourself and, eventually, for others. This process can help you to heal your isolation both from your inner feelings and from others. The experience of insight during psychotherapy—like getting health information—is important but usually not sufficient to motivate someone to change self-destructive patterns. When insight and information are combined with compassion, though, it can be profoundly healing.

In summary, then, here are a few ideas for how to begin opening your heart to others:

- Use the communication skills described here to express feelings from your heart without being judgmental.
- Create a support group, or join an existing one, that feels safe enough for you to let down your walls, take off your masks, and show your true self. Ideally, find an experienced therapist (psychologist, psychiatrist, or social worker) to work with your group.
- Doing good may be good for you, under the right circumstances. Make a point of helping others in ways that *you* choose and that feel comfortable for you. Resist helping others when you are feeling coerced into doing so. And even in helping, don't neglect your own health.

In his book, *Peace, Love and Healing,* Dr. Bernie Siegel writes:

> The pattern common to all these women [who recovered from breast cancer] was that recovery, which the medical profession views as a return to the predisease condition, was in fact a transformation into something new. In my experience, the disease often opens one to a spiritual reality previously unrecognized.
> The sense of our mortality and our reason for being stares us in the face. What is real? How can we do something real before we die?
> In that moment the long trip from head to heart occurs and the intelligent, loving light shines on our path and lights our way. We contact something that goes beyond all our previous experiences and are aware of an order in the universe that includes darkness and disease. However, it is all spiritual and part of life and leads us to a rebirth and reawakening to a new reality. When one reawakens to this potential in each of us the resources that come with this are incredible. We know we can survive events that are full of pain because we have a constant source of renewal.

We can use our pain—emotional or physical—as a catalyst to begin healing, not just curing. To me, "curing" means only getting back to the way we were before we became diseased. "Healing" is when we use our pain or illness as a catalyst to begin transforming our lives—healing our inner pain and our relationships, our hearts and our souls.

"Why does man look for a God? Why does man, in every nation, in every state of society, want a perfect ideal somewhere, either in man, in God, or elsewhere? Because that idea is within you. It was your own heart beating and you did not know; you were mistaking it for something external. It is the God within your own self that is impelling you to seek Him, to realize Him. After long searches here and there, in temples and in churches, on earth and in heaven, at last you come back to your own soul, completing the circle from where you started, and find that He whom you have been seeking all over the world, for whom you have been weeping and praying in churches and temples, on whom you were looking as the mystery of all mysteries, shrouded in the clouds, is the nearest of the near, is your own Self, the reality of your life, body, and soul. . . . By means of spiritual discipline the individual soul ultimately recognizes its oneness with the Universal Soul."

—Swami Vivekananda (1896),
Jnana Yoga

■

"Be still and know that I am God."

—Psalm 43

■

"We shall not cease from exploration
And the end of all our exploring
Will be to arrive where we started
And know the place for the first time."

—T. S. Eliot,
Four Quartets

9

Opening Your Heart to a Higher Self

Most of us have had moments when we felt as if we were a part of something larger than ourselves. Some put this experience in a religious context and call it God; others describe it in more secular terms as consciousness, a "Higher Self," "Witness," spirit, force, or energy.

The point of this book is not to say what your experience of a higher force should be—or even if you should have one. In general, people are most comfortable when they explain their experiences in terms of their own belief system, cultural upbringing, or religious preference.

Whatever allows you to experience a higher force—whether through prayer, meditation, contemplating nature, and so on—can be a powerful means of transcending feelings of isolation. A direct experience of something larger than ourselves can profoundly transform our lives when we realize that we are not isolated and we are never alone.

To summarize what we've discussed so far, chronic stress can lead to heart disease and other illnesses via a number of mechanisms described in chapter 3. Stress is caused not only by our environment: our job, our home life, and so on. Equally important is how we react to these.

If we go a step even farther back, we can ask, "Why do we react in ways that cause us to feel stressed?" We tend to believe that the stress is "out there"—that our environment alone determines our reactions.

Not so. Between the environment and our reactions to it are our perceptions. *Our perceptions determine how we react to a situation and whether or not that reaction is going to be harmful to us.*

Dr. Robert Eliot, a cardiologist, often tells an apocryphal story about two Arabian oil sheiks who were driving in the desert, each in his new Mercedes. Although they were driving the only cars within a hundred-mile radius, they collided with each other. So they jumped out of their cars, ran to each other—and embraced, saying, "Isn't it wonderful that Allah has arranged for us to meet this way!" Closer to home, two cars recently collided on the Golden Gate Bridge, and the drivers started shooting at each other. The point is that even when the actions remain the same, how we interpret and react to these actions can be quite different.

In the final analysis, *the perception of being isolated is a fundamental cause of why we react to the world in ways that cause us to feel stressed.* And this is an empowering realization—because we can't always change the world. We can't always change other people. We can't always change jobs or families. But we *can* change our perceptions and, in turn, how we react to our world.

We all want to be happy. Even when I came close to dying during my first year of college, as described in chapter 4, it was due to the misguided belief that it would make me happy—or at least stop my suffering. When I started to redirect some of my restless energy toward beginning to heal myself instead of making myself miserable, then the world became more of a heaven than a hell. Of course, the world didn't change very much—but *I* did. As Milton wrote in *Paradise Lost,* "The mind is its own place and in itself, can create a Heaven of Hell, a Hell of Heaven. What matter where, if I be still the same."

In what is perhaps the ultimate how-to book, *How to Know God,* based on the *Yoga Sutras of Patanjali,* Swami Prabhavananda and the English playwright Christopher Isherwood wrote in 1953:

> The tyrant who enslaves millions of people, the miser who hoards a thousand times as much money as he could ever need, the traitor who sells his dearest friend, the murderer, the thief, the liar and the addict—all these, in the last analysis, simply want to be safe and happy and at peace. We seek security in the accumulation of possessions by violence or fraud, or by the destruction of our imagined enemies. We seek happiness through sense-gratification, through every kind of vanity and self-delusion. We seek peace through the intoxication of various drugs. And in all these activities we display an energy of heroic proportions. It is tragically misdirected energy. With less effort, we might easily have found union with God, had we not been misled by our ignorance.

FROM COMMUNICATION TO COMMUNION

The "stress management" and yoga techniques described in this book are really tools for transformation. They allow us to feel an inner sense of peace and strength and connection. At the end of a meditation, when you are feeling more peaceful, stronger, and happier, remind yourself that these feelings came not because you got something you thought you needed or because you fooled somebody into thinking that you are worthy of his or her love and affection, but rather because you simply quieted down your mind enough to experience what we all have, all of the time, if we just remember.

These techniques can be used to quiet down the mind and body enough to experience inner peace and the realization that we are not isolated. And when we do, then we can fully enjoy the richness and diversity of life in all its manifestations.

This experience of oneness—of feeling united with your concept of a higher force or with God—is a common theme of most of the world's religions and many secular philosophies. In Judaism, for example, the Shemah, or central prayer, is translated from Hebrew to mean "The Lord is One." In Christianity, Jesus said, "I and my Father are One." Native Americans refer to the "Great Spirit." In Hinduism and Buddhism, the essence of God is to be found within:

"Tat Twam Asi," which is Sanskrit for "Thou art That," or "you are one with God." Atheists and agnostics can simply call it "peace."

In all of these religions, God is described as being omnipresent, omniscient, and omnipotent—that is, God is everywhere, all-knowing, and all-powerful. If God is everywhere, and if there is only one God, then we are not separate from God.

What is it that keeps us from realizing this? Various religions and philosophies describe it in different terms, but the essence is that our minds create separation and isolation between ourselves and others as well as between ourselves and God. Stated more accurately, our minds keep us from seeing that everyone and everything is simply God manifesting in different ways.

This is not just philosophy or mysticism, for God or a higher force can be experienced. By quieting down and removing the disturbances in our mind, we can experience the underlying unity of all creation. And when we do, then we can fully enjoy the richness and diversity of life in all its manifestations.

Most religions and cultural traditions describe people who have had a direct experience of a higher force or God. Abraham, the patriarch of both Christianity and Judaism as well as some of the non-Western traditions, is said to have experienced God directly. So did Moses, Jesus, Buddha, Mohammed, and many others. These people are described as having *realized* God or enlightenment. That is, they did not *get* peace from outside themselves; they realized that they already had it when they simply stopped disturbing it. They did not *become* one with a higher force; they realized that they already were. They had a direct experience that, in the final analysis, we only appear to be isolated. They realized that the higher force or God without is the same as the higher force or God within. So can we.

Even modern physics is developing a remarkably similar view of the universe. Quantum physics is beginning to help us understand that underneath the diversity—the various names and forms—is an essential unity.

Physics and metaphysics (and some physicians) are beginning to find a common ground. The language of physicists and the language of mystics begin to sound very similar. In trying to describe the experience of oneness—"being, not becoming," "a timeless moment," "everything and nothing"—the words sound full of paradox, even meaningless, as people try to describe something that is beyond the limitations of words.

Einstein's famous equation—energy equals mass times the speed of light squared, or $E = MC^2$—demonstrated that energy and matter are interconvertible. In other words, everything in the world is a manifestation of different forms of energy. The forms change, but the underlying essence does not.

There is an intelligence or superconsciousness behind this energy, as Einstein also recognized. "I shall never believe that God plays dice with the world," he once said, echoing the French philosopher Anatole France who wrote in 1894, "Chance is perhaps the pseudonym of God when He did not want to sign."

Classical physics echoed the view of the world that philosopher Rene Descartes outlined in the seventeenth century. Descartes saw the mind as separate from both nature and one's own body. In his view, the body is simply a machine that functions according to mechanical laws—a view of medicine still shared by many doctors. Because of this way of looking at the world, most of modern medical research is focused on drugs or surgery to affect bodily processes, to the neglect of our mind and spirit.

On one level, of course, we *are* limited by time and space, we *are* separate from each other. You're you, and I'm me. And we can celebrate our differences. Though we are separate from each other, we are not *only* separate. On another level, there is a higher force working through each of us, whatever name we give to that, and that force connects us all. We feel isolated only because we believe we are separate and only separate.

By analogy, the light from a movie projector appears on the screen as different characters, situations, and dramas. But behind this diversity is the same light, which equally illuminates the hero and the villain, the powerful and the weak, the lover and the beloved.

We first need well-defined personal boundaries and a strong sense of autonomy before we can transcend them. When we can maintain a "double vision"—enjoying the diversity and richness of life while remaining grounded in a higher force—then we can begin to free ourselves of self-destructive patterns. Then we can go out into the world without being so caught up by it; without being so knocked around by it; without being destroyed by it. We can enjoy the drama without forgetting who we are.

In 1896, a spiritual teacher named Swami Vivekananda gave a series of lectures in London on these ideas:

In one word, this ideal is that you are divine. "Thou art That. . . ." To many this is, no doubt, a terrible ideal, and most of us think that this ideal can never be reached; but it can be realized by everyone. One may be either man or woman or child; one may belong to any race—nothing will stand as a bar to the realization of this ideal, because it is realized already, it is already there. All the powers in the universe are already ours. *It is we who have put our hands before our eyes and cry that it is dark.* Know that there is no darkness around you. Take your hands away and there is the light which was from the beginning.

This experience of oneness, of an expanded Self, has implications on both a cellular level and on a global level. In this context, "Love your neighbor as yourself" is a description of truth, not simply a command. All religions, all forms of worship, all types of prayer or meditation are equally valid—there are many paths to the same ultimate truth. Our higher self is limited only by our capacity to experience it.

I am writing this chapter from the deepest level of my understanding and experience, limited though it may be. I recognize that some people may be interested in the Opening Your Heart program only for reversing coronary artery blockages, not for contemplating universal truths, and I understand that your experiences, beliefs, and understandings may be different from mine. Please adopt whatever is useful and leave the rest.

There are many methods that we can use to open our hearts to a higher self. One approach is through meditation. Another is with prayer and devotion. Selfless service is a different way: seeing ourselves as an instrument of a higher self or God and treating others as incarnations of God ("That which you do to the least of me, you do to me"). Self-analysis is yet another. This chapter focuses on different types of meditation.

MEDITATION

The *concept* of meditation is very simple. Anyone can do it.

Peace—and stress—begin in your mind. Meditation is the process of quieting your mind. When your mind is quiet, you feel peaceful. You lose your sense of separateness and isolation. You may even experience your higher self.

The *practice* of meditation can be very challenging, though, for it is not very easy to quiet one's own mind. Various meditative traditions and teachers often describe the undisciplined mind as a drunken, restless monkey stung by a scorpion and possessed by a demon. In other words, hard to control.

There are many, many ways of calming your mind, both secular and religious. All of them involve increasing your awareness and control over your own mind.

Dr. Herbert Benson and others have conducted pioneering research at Harvard and elsewhere demonstrating that meditation can lower blood pressure, improve productivity, and decrease health care costs. Many other investigators are beginning to prove other health benefits of meditation.

But ancient monks, swamis, and yogis didn't meditate to lower their blood pressure or to increase their effectiveness at business meetings, and yoga was not developed for those reasons. The effects of meditation on lowering blood pressure and improving performance—or even in helping to reverse heart disease—are only side effects or by-products of their primary purpose: to experience inner peace and happiness. This experience of oneness and inner peace begins to heal our isolation.

When we approach heart disease in this way, on emotional and spiritual levels, then the physical level also may begin to improve, as we measured with quantitative coronary angiograms, cardiac PET scans, and so on. But the physical healing is only one manifestation of a more profound healing that begins on emotional and spiritual levels.

The various stretching and relaxation techniques described in chapter 7 were first developed for the purpose of enabling people to sit for long periods of time in meditation. It's easier to gain control over your body than your mind, so these physical stretches are a good place to begin. But the real challenge—and the most benefit— comes from learning to control your own mind. As you gain more control over your mind, it begins to quiet down.

You cannot force your mind to be quiet, any more than you can smooth out the waves in a tray of water by running your hand across its surface. And if you look at your reflection in a disturbed tray of water, then your face looks distorted. You don't have to do anything to smooth out the waves other than to stop disturbing them. When you do, then you can see your true self more clearly in the reflection.

Similarly, meditation doesn't smooth out the disturbances in your life, as a tranquilizer might. Meditation allows you to go deeper, to where the disturbances begin. It helps you become more aware of how your mind becomes agitated and gives you more control to stop these disturbances. It doesn't *bring* you peace, for the peace is already there once you stop disturbing it.

There are many misconceptions regarding meditation. A common one is that the process of meditation is austere. Another is that meditation is boring. Sometimes meditating is viewed as passive, a withdrawal from the world, for wimps, not productive people. Exercise, in contrast, is seen as active, macho, getting out there and really *doing* something.

In fact, meditation can allow us to engage the world more fully and to increase our awareness. Most of the time, unfortunately, we are not very aware of what we are doing or experiencing. In the terminology of Dr. Jim Billings, we are on "automatic pilot" mode.

Have you ever eaten a meal without really tasting your food? Have you ever driven from one place to another without really paying attention to your driving or what you passed along the way?

When you're on automatic pilot, it's not only difficult to appreciate life; it's also hard to change your lifestyle habits. For example, if you don't notice what you're eating, and if you don't experience the effects of this food on your body, then it's very difficult to change your diet. Or to stop smoking. Or to relax.

The first step of every approach to meditation is paying attention. Paying attention, or increasing awareness, is the beginning of healing. After all, how can we change a problem if we're not aware of it?

Where is our attention when our mind is on automatic pilot? Usually in the past or future. Worrying about something we have to do, daydreaming about a nice experience we had in the past, feeling anxious about an upcoming event, and so on. When we pay attention to our thoughts, we realize how much of the time we dwell on the past or future.

Meditation keeps us in present tense:

• *The present moment is peaceful.* Anxiety, fear, worry, and depression are concerns about past and future events. When we're in the present moment, with full concentration, then even life or death situations need not cause us to feel intensely stressed. For example, great heart surgeons are often at their most relaxed in the midst of performing major surgery. They become completely absorbed in what they are doing, and their work becomes a form of meditation. Other people might find performing heart surgery to be rather stressful. Same situation, different reactions. It is primarily the mind that determines whether or not a circumstance is stressful or joyful. Of course, we need to make plans for the future and to learn from the past—but we don't need to spend most of our time there.

• *The present moment is productive.* Meditation is a process of learning to train the mind so we can do what we want more effectively. It's the opposite of what I experienced in college, when my mind was racing out of control and I couldn't function at all. As I described in chapter 4, when I was worried about getting accepted to medical school, the anxiety kept me from being able to study. When I learned to meditate, I was able to focus better on the task at hand rather than worrying about the future.

When you take care of the present moment, the future tends to take care of itself as well. When you worry about the future, then you lose twice: You may miss the joy of the present moment, and you decrease the chances of future success. Plan for the future, but don't live there.

• *The present moment is joyful.* Often we miss the full benefit of even the most wonderful moments—a sunset, a concert, or even a kiss—when our attention wanders to the past or future. If I'm at a concert and hear some music I enjoy, I might find myself thinking about the last time I heard that song, or whom I was with when I heard it, or what happened after that concert, and so on. While I'm thinking about events in the past, I'm missing the enjoyment of the present music.

• *The present moment is sensual.* Paying attention enhances all sensual experiences. When you meditate regularly, your ability to keep your attention focused begins to increase. And when you really focus on what you are experiencing—eating good food, making love, listening to music, smelling the roses—the pleasure is magnified.

Try it and see. Take a piece of your favorite ripe fruit or a spoonful of your favorite dessert. Pay attention to it. Examine it closely. Close your eyes and bring it up to your nose; notice how it smells. If your attention wanders, keep bringing it back to what you are doing. Take a bite and chew it slowly, noticing the amazing array of subtle and overt flavors and textures as it rolls around your tongue and mouth. Finally, swallow it and notice how it feels going down your throat.

One benefit of this approach is that it takes less stimulation to feel satisfied. I love eating chocolate, for example. When I was much younger, I might consume a pint of chocolate ice cream without really enjoying it very much. I'd often eat while reading or watching television, so I wasn't really paying attention to the food. Now, when I want to treat myself, I'll have only a spoonful of the richest, deepest, darkest, most chocolatey chocolate I can find. If I close my eyes and really pay attention to what I'm eating, then it's exquisitely enjoyable. After all, the first bite and the last bite are usually the best. And if you're only having one bite, then you really pay attention, so it's very, very good.

• *The present moment is liberating.* Our lifestyle choices, such as diet, are the product of years of habit. Since meditation helps to keep us more in the present, we are less influenced by our habits of the past. It becomes easier to make new choices.

Meditation begins with concentration. "Focusing your awareness," "paying attention," and "one-pointedness" are other ways of describing the process of concentrating your mind.

Whenever you concentrate energy, you gain power. Meditation brings strength. In fact, most of the yoga texts emphasize that one should begin meditation only in the context of other spiritual disciplines designed to increase compassion and altruism. Increasing power without discipline can be dangerous. Meditation brings increased power but not necessarily the wisdom to use it properly. Power can be healing or it can be destructive, depending on how it is used.

By analogy, an ordinary light bulb emits light of different frequencies, much as your brain may be thinking about a number of different thoughts. In contrast, a laser emits light of only one frequency and it focuses it—as if you were meditating on only one thought or sound—thereby gaining tremendous power. This power can be used to heal—to weld a detached retina back in place, to operate without a scalpel—or to harm, as the military is beginning to develop laser weapons.

So when you meditate, you gain power. The increased mental power that meditation gives you can be used to study more effectively, to work more productively, and so on. Like lowering your blood pressure, though, these are really by-products of meditation, not the primary goals.

Some people become anxious when they first learn to meditate. In part, as discussed earlier, the mind does not want to relinquish its control over you, so it rebels and wanders. Also, when you begin to meditate, you are focusing your awareness inward for one of the few times during the day, so your anxieties and worries may emerge.

This is normal, so don't get discouraged. When this happens, just notice what you are feeling and return to observing your breath or repeating a sound, as described below. If you find that these feelings become too intrusive, then stop and try again later. Later in this chapter, I will describe a different approach to meditation in which you pay attention to these thoughts instead of focusing on your breathing or a sound.

Meditation does not create unpleasant feelings, but quieting your mind may make you more aware of ones that are already there. This awareness can be an important step in healing these feelings, so you may want to consult a health professional if you experience any disturbing emotions. Yoga and meditation are not substitutes for the various systems of psychotherapy that are available. A good therapist can be very helpful.

How to Meditate
There are many types of meditation. Here are some of the most simple yet powerful:

- Focusing on your breathing
- Focusing on a sound (religious or secular)
- Mindfulness
- Self-analysis
- Prayer or devotion

Further instruction on these techniques is available from Integral Yoga Institutes, located in many cities, or in books such as *The Meditative Mind,* by Daniel Goleman. Also, I am preparing audio and video cassettes demonstrating these techniques, available by writing to me at 1001 Bridgeway, Box 305, Sausalito, California, 94965. And there are many good books on meditation.

You can meditate anywhere, at any time. Many people find it beneficial, especially at first, to meditate twice daily for at least five to thirty minutes, once in the morning and once in the evening. Twenty minutes twice a day seems about right for many people. Some teachers advise that dawn and dusk are the ideal times for meditation, but what's most important is that you find a time that fits your daily routine. It's better to meditate for only a few minutes on a regular basis than to do it for longer on an irregular basis.

If possible, set aside a special room or at least an area within a room used only for meditation. After a while, you will associate that area with meditation, and you will begin to feel more peaceful just being there.

With practice, you'll find that meditation is no longer only something that you do twice a day for a few minutes. You can bring that state of enhanced awareness to everything you do.

FOCUSING ON YOUR BREATHING   Begin by assuming a comfortable position in a quiet place and closing your eyes. Sit still. Without changing how you breathe, simply observe the air coming in and going out.

Notice how the air feels as it comes in and goes out. Then observe the pauses between each inhalation and exhalation.

If you prefer, you can mentally count your breaths. When you exhale, count "one." The next time you exhale, count "two," and so on. After your fifth exhalation, start over again and count "one," "two," back up to five. Only count when you exhale. (If you find yourself counting higher than five, then you know your mind is wandering.) Another approach is to allow your body to relax each time you exhale.

That's all there is to it—in theory. The goal is not to stop all thoughts; it is to focus on only one thing, in this case, your breathing. But as I mentioned earlier, the concept is simple but the practice is not. Be prepared for the mind's tricks.

After a while—only a few seconds at first—your mind may wander, and you will find yourself thinking about something other than your breathing. Usually you will be thinking about an event in the past or future. Or you may start asking yourself questions like, "Why am I sitting here observing my breathing when I have so many other things to do? I could be doing something that I enjoy a lot more!" This is your mind in action, trying to control you.

While meditating, you may have an urge to scratch your nose. Or your leg may begin to ache. Or you may start to experience what seem like a thousand other distractions that weren't there before.

By analogy, meditation teachers sometimes describe the mind as a small child or animal that runs here and there as it chooses, never doing one thing for very long, but being reasonably well behaved. As soon as you start to discipline the mind, though, it becomes unruly.

Therefore, don't be surprised when your mind wanders. This is to be expected, and it is part of the process of learning to meditate. So avoid judging or criticizing yourself when this happens. Also, tell your body that you are not going to move any part of it until you finish the meditation. If you mean it, then the distractions will tend to subside. If you still find it difficult to sit still, then move a little and resume meditating.

This constant process of learning concentration—bringing the mind back again and again—is called *dharana* in Sanskrit. With practice, you will gain progressively more control over your mind and it will begin to quiet down. The more time you spend in this process, the longer will be the intervals before your mind wanders. Once your mind is able to spend more than a few seconds before getting distracted, you will begin to experience more fully the profound relaxation of the meditative state, known as *dhyana*. This state is even more restorative than sleeping. Finally, over time, your mind may remain focused long enough to experience your higher self. Sometimes this is referred to as "pure awareness." In this state, called *samadhi,* you realize and experience that you are not isolated or separate.

FOCUSING ON SOUND   Sounds are powerful. In a biblical story, the walls at Jericho "came tumbling down" when the trumpets blared. Closer to home, anyone who has attended a rock concert knows how sound can influence our emotions.

Different sounds can alter our state of mind in powerful ways. Some sounds, like military music on the battlefield or the chants led by cheerleaders at football games, make us agitated or aggressive. Other sounds, like a waterfall or lullaby, are relaxing. These sounds influence us even when there is no word or literal meaning associated with them.

A time-honored way of focusing the mind is to meditate by repeating a sound over and over. The sound can be secular (for example, repeating the word "one") or religious. Choose a sound that is comfortable and is consistent with your own belief system.

The most basic sound is humming. During times of deep meditation, when your body is relaxed and your mind is very quiet and still, you can hear a low-pitched, continuous humming sound. According to meditative tradition, all sounds are derived from this one.

By analogy, a sculptor may make different types of statues, but all of them are made from the same clay. In the mystical traditions of different religions, the universe was created from this sound: "In the beginning was the Word. The Word was with God. The Word was God." That is, this sound is the manifestation of the essential unity that underlies the diversity of life.

This humming sound is very peaceful. I find it very interesting that these sounds are found in virtually every culture and religious tradition as part of prayers or other meditative rituals. Sometimes these words are literally translated to mean "peace," such as *"om"* in Sanskrit, *"shalom"* in Hebrew, *"salaam"* in Arabic, *"amen"* in English, *"ameen"* in the Muslim tradition, and so on.

When you meditate, you may want to choose a word that incorporates one of these sounds. In any event, use a word, sound, or phrase that is consistent with your own beliefs and values.

For example, an Orthodox Jew may be more comfortable meditating on the word *"shalom"* than the word *"om,"* even though the words sound very similar. A Protestant may prefer to repeat the word *"amen"* over and over rather than *"ameen."* Someone else may prefer a word without religious connotation, such as the word "one." A devout Catholic may wish to repeat "Hail Mary, Full of Grace" or a similar word or phrase with each breath, perhaps even using rosary beads to enhance concentration, whereas someone else may prefer to repeat the Sanskrit phrases *"om shanti"* or *"hari om."* A member of the Greek Orthodox Church may prefer to repeat, "Lord Jesus, have mercy on me" continuously. Neutral meditative words include "peace," "relax," "love," and so on.

Do what is most comfortable for you. Choose a phrase that is short enough to be repeated in its entirety while exhaling.

According to meditation teachers, repeating one of these sounds over and over has a double benefit. First, it focuses your awareness. Also, the sound creates a peaceful state, like tuning a radio.

While this may sound like mumbo jumbo, we know from quantum physics that electrons and other subatomic particles are continually vibrating between different energy levels. Even when it appears solid, all matter is vibrating, even if we cannot fully perceive or hear it. These vibrational states are affected by the energy in the surrounding environment. For example, in magnetic resonance imaging (a new medical imaging technology), a powerful magnetic field can cause your vibrating electrons to become aligned. In a more subtle way, meditation may increase coherence.

When you meditate, sit in a comfortable position in a quiet place and close your eyes. Inhale, then repeat the word, sound, or phrase as you exhale. There is no "right" way to do this; find a tempo and tone that leave you feeling calm and comfortable. When your mind wanders, gently bring it back to repeating the word or phrase. Since it is perfectly normal for your mind to wander, don't get upset when this happens. When you notice that you're thinking about something other than the sound, just bring it back to the sound. Over and over again.

After you have spent a while repeating this sound or phrase out loud, then begin repeating it silently. The effect is more subtle yet in many ways even more powerful when you repeat a sound or phrase silently, although your mind may tend to wander more than when saying it out loud. Also, you can meditate silently anywhere: on the bus, on the train, while waiting in line, and so on.

MINDFULNESS   "Mindfulness" is the process of paying attention to *everything* that you do. In that sense, your life becomes a continual meditation, not simply the fifteen or twenty minutes that you spend observing your breathing or repeating a sound.

I was a photographer for many years before I went to medical school. When I was thirteen, I began as an apprentice to Thomas D'Aquino, an accomplished color portrait photographer. He was a master at making people look much better than they really were, through careful lighting, posing, and retouching.

Because he was very good at what he did, as well as being a genuinely warm person, he had more clients than he had time for. Two years after I began working for him, he sold me some of his equipment, encouraged me to open a portrait studio of my own, and began referring people to me.

Later, in college, I began studying a different type of photography with Garry Winogrand, Walker Evans, Russell Lee, and other exceptionally gifted photographers. Instead of trying to make photographs in which people appeared the way I thought they were "supposed" to look like, they taught me the importance of learning to see and photograph the world as it really is, with fewer preconceptions.

To see without preconceptions and to share this vision is the essence of art. We value artists because they can show us the world in new ways. When this happens, our world expands.

Art helps us to focus our attention. When we see a photograph or a painting in a museum, the artist has chosen to share with us that particular slice of space and time, so we pay attention to it in a way that we might miss otherwise. For example, we might notice the lighting, color, and texture of a painting of a bowl of fruit more than of a real bowl of fruit. The same is true when we go to a movie or watch a play: We may notice more details in the lives of these fictional characters than we pay attention to in our own lives.

The more I began to understand how preconceptions limited my experience, and how paying attention without expectations could expand my awareness, the less photography equipment I needed. So instead of carrying a lot of studio lighting and large-format camera equipment to help make people fit my preconceived images of what portraits were supposed to look like, I began carrying only a small 35-millimeter camera to begin seeing and photographing people more as they really were.

At first, it was very difficult. Either I would try to pose them, or I found myself taking photographs that looked like my teachers' pictures. I was going from one set of preconceptions to another.

Eventually, though, I began to rediscover a sense of wonder that I had lost somewhere along the way (probably in organic chemistry class). I began seeing the world in new ways, with fresh eyes. In those moments when I can see with fewer preconceptions, the world becomes much more vivid and beautiful, more interesting than anything I can imagine.

Children naturally see with this sense of wonder. They haven't yet been told what the world is supposed to be like, so they have no preconceptions to keep them from experiencing the world in its fullness. That is, until we say, "What a stupid question!" or "Because I say so, that's why!" or "Can't you just sit and watch television and leave me alone?"

Preconceptions limit our world and increase our sense of isolation. In some ways, this is useful, because it gives us a sense of order. The universe is infinitely vast and complex, and we would be overwhelmed if we always experienced it in all its fullness. The problem comes when we *always* limit the world and thus never experience its fullness. Life becomes dreary and boring, and we begin to wonder, "Is that all there is?"

In his classic book, *The Structure of Scientific Revolutions,* Thomas Kuhn describes how our preconceptions, or what he calls "paradigms" or "world views," provide a sense of order to the universe. They reduce the universe to a more manageable size. Along with this sense of order, though, these world views also limit our experience of life's fullness and can keep us from knowing the way things really are.

It's like the story of the blind man and the elephant—when he touches the trunk, the elephant seems like a snake. When he touches the ears, the elephant seems like a wing. And when he touches the elephant's leg, it seems like a tree. All of these views are partially true, but no single view or experience is adequate to provide a completely true description.

For over a thousand years, for example, Aristotle and the Church agreed that the earth was the center of the universe. In the sixteenth century, though, the Italian philosopher Giordano Bruno argued that the sun, not the earth, was really the center of the universe. Because he challenged the prevailing world view, he threatened the prevailing order. He was burned at the stake for his heresy.

Later, in the seventeenth century, the Italian scientist Galileo turned his new invention—the telescope—to the heavens and saw that Bruno was right. Although the authorities later forced Galileo to recant his discovery, by then it was too late. He had shown people *a way that they could see for themselves* that the old preconceptions did not fully explain what could now be observed. Eventually, because of this, everyone's concept of the universe changed.

Besides limiting our understanding of the world, preconceptions cause us to judge our experiences, causing emotional stress and disturbance. In contrast, the essence of mindfulness is to pay attention without judging and without preconceptions.

- *Judging increases isolation and separation, because it emphasizes our differences rather than our similarities.* Whether you judge yourself or others as being inferior or superior, better or worse, smarter or dumber, prettier or uglier, stronger or weaker, fatter or thinner, richer or poorer, you still feel separate.
- *Judging reinforces our preconceptions and thus limits our experiences.* Most of us are constantly judging our experiences, and this keeps us from fully experiencing them.
- *When you become the judge, you also may become the jury and executioner.* That is, you may find ways to sentence and punish yourself.

Judging is not wrong or bad, and I'm not asking you to throw your critical thinking out the window. Judging, like the fight-or-flight response, has survival value. And like the fight-or-flight response, it becomes a problem and even a threat to your survival only when you're *always* judging and thinking critically.

Another name for your higher self is the "witness." Beyond the moment-to-moment changes in your body and mind is the witness, or higher self, which always remains peaceful and is unaffected by the turbulence around it. The witness observes and pays attention without judging.

Earlier in this chapter, I mentioned Descartes, the seventeenth century philosopher whose views helped to define our prevailing world view. It was Descartes who said, "I think, therefore I am." So if we stop thinking—and judging—the mind fears that it may cease to exist. But when we stop judging, we do not stop existing; we stop limiting our existence and experiences so that we can live more fully.

Here is an example of mindfulness meditation:

Take a moment and allow yourself to experience whatever it is that you're feeling, without judging it or suppressing it, or even sharing it. Just observe it. And then take it from the realm of "I'm feeling this way" to "He's feeling this way." In other words, go from first person to third person. Take the observer point of view for a moment.

Keeping your eyes closed, bring your awareness to your thoughts. Without trying to control or direct them, just observe each thought as it comes into your mind—as if you were watching a movie entitled, "Thoughts." In other words, you are taking the point of view of the inner witness, observing without preconceptions or judgments.

If you find yourself judging your thoughts as being "good thoughts," "bad thoughts," "pleasurable thoughts," "painful thoughts," and so on, then resume being a witness and just observe yourself judging. You don't have to stop doing it, just be aware of it happening. Otherwise, you may start judging yourself for judging, which quickly becomes a downward spiral. When you simply observe yourself judging, then the judging will stop.

And then go down another level—where it is peaceful and quiet and radiant and healthy. And remind yourself, again, that ultimately everything that we're doing here is to help us find that place again. And that place in you is the same as that place in me, and in that place we can be connected—we are connected already. We can just re-experience that again.

In his book *Full Catastrophe Living,* Jon Kabat-Zinn, Ph.D., discusses this type of meditation in great detail. *Mindfulness,* a book by Ellen Langer, Ph.D., gives other examples of how our preconceptions can limit our experiences.

SELF-ANALYSIS   Self-analysis can also allow us to discriminate what is real from what is not.

In a collection of dialogues entitled *The Spiritual Teachings of Ramana Maharshi,* Ramana describes the process of self-analysis:

STUDENT: How can I attain Self-realization?

MAHARSHI: Realization is nothing to be gained afresh; it is already there. All that is necessary is to get rid of the thought, "I have not realized." Stillness or Peace is Realization.

STUDENT: How shall I reach the Self?

MAHARSHI: There is no reaching the Self. If the Self were to be reached, it would mean that the Self is not here and now but that it is yet to be obtained. You are the Self; you are already That.

In medical school, I was struck by the similarity of the vocabulary used both by immunologists and by mystics. The words that immunologists use are exactly the same as the vocabulary of mystics—"self" and "not-self."

The immune system is based on the body's ability to distinguish what is self from not-self—that is, to attack and destroy everything foreign that invades the body. The spiritual or mystical experience is based on the realization that everything is a form of the Self. If God is omniscient, omnipresent, and omnipotent, then God is everywhere and in everything. Everyone and everything is God in disguise, in different forms.

Sometimes the body gets confused and thinks parts of itself are not-self. As a result, the body begins to attack itself. The resulting illnesses, called autoimmune diseases, can affect any part of the body. Rheumatoid arthritis is an example of an autoimmune disease in which the body begins to attack the joints. Lupus is an autoimmune disease in which the body begins to attack the skin, nervous system, heart, and other organs.

Autoimmune diseases are particularly difficult to treat. Patients are often given steroids and other powerful drugs to suppress their entire immune system. Unfortunately, though, suppressing the immune system with these drugs causes the person to become susceptible to a variety of infections—just as giving drugs that interfere with blood clotting can lead to bleeding, as I described in chapter 2. Neither approach deals with the more fundamental causes of the problem, so the treatments are both beneficial and harmful.

Although there is a genetic component to autoimmune diseases (as with most illnesses), I have often wondered if autoimmune diseases result when a person's sense of self becomes too constricted, causing him to misidentify part of himself as being not-self and then attacking it.

I wondered: If a person's sense of self could be expanded, would that modify the course of an autoimmune disease? If a person directly experiences that "double vision"—seeing himself not only as a separate person, *apart from* everyone and everything else, but also having the awareness of being *a part of* the universe—would that be healing? In short, if that person were to experience everything as simply the Self disguised in different forms, then what would be left to attack?

Although most of my research efforts have been spent in studying heart disease, I have tried the Opening Your Heart program with several patients who had autoimmune diseases of various types. In some cases, people were able to use the yoga and meditation techniques to experience a more expanded sense of self. As a result, they felt better, were able to resume their normal activities, and needed fewer medications. In some cases, even their laboratory studies showed some objective improvements.

An emerging field of research, called psychoneuroimmunology, is beginning to ask similar questions. (In this context, perhaps our research could be called "psychoneurocardiology.") Scientists are beginning to gain a greater understanding of how the mind affects the body via the nervous system. These are explained in Dr. Joan Borysenko's book *Minding the Body, Mending the Mind,* Dr. Stephen Locke's *The Healer Within,* and others.

When we realize that everything is our Self in different forms, in that moment we experience that there is nothing to fear, including death. When Ramana Maharshi developed cancer (even saints and sages can get cancer and heart disease), he was surrounded by his students who pleaded, "Please don't die, please don't leave us." And he replied, "Where would I go?"

PRAYER OR DEVOTION   In his book *The Golden Present,* Swami Satchidananda describes the processes of prayer, devotion, and selfless service:

> Don't think that you can do everything just by your own capacity alone. Know that there is a higher power, a grace, to help you; but you have to sincerely ask for it. Unless you ask, you won't receive it. Just by asking, you are opening yourself to that power. It's not that God is waiting for you to ask; God is not miserly. He is already giving, but we do not always receive.
>
> The process of asking is itself opening; you cannot even ask without opening. So open your heart. Even if you can't open your heart to people, open your heart to God; then you will know how to open your heart to people also. Pray sincerely and trust in a higher power, trust in God. Many, many more things are wrought by prayer than the world dreams of.
>
> You might have the entire world at your feet, all the money, all the material things, all the friends, all the name, all the fame, all the crowns; but unless you have peace you don't have a worryless life. What is the use of having all these things around you? Without that peace, nothing is going to make you happy. If you have peace, even without having anything else, you will be happy. That's what you call contentment. Accept God's will: "Whatever has to come will come. What will not come, will not come. Why should I worry about it?"
>
> Enjoy the coming. Enjoy the going. Enjoy the profit, enjoy the loss. . . . If you are going to enjoy by getting things, you are going to be depressed by losing things. True joy doesn't come from anywhere. Nothing *brings* you joy. No person *brings* you joy. You yourself are joyful always. So enjoy that.
>
> I know some of you might say, "Then should I not do anything?" You should do something, yes. And if you allow yourself to be handled in that way, you will have plenty to do. You'll be doing much more than anyone else. At the same time, you'll be totally relaxed. Don't think that relaxation or peace comes by not doing anything. No. You'll be put to even greater use.
>
> This is the essence of all spiritual teachings and practices, no matter what the label. One can be a Catholic, a Protestant, a Jew, a Hindu, a Buddhist, Moslem, or of any religion. Even if you don't have faith at all or don't believe in any organized religion, it doesn't matter. That is not the criterion to have this realization. All you have to accomplish is to see that all selfishness goes away.

. . . If the mind gets completely purified, then it's no longer an obstruction to your experience of the Truth. When it is clean and clear, the mind doesn't color the appearance of the pure Self. It becomes a pure reflector of the Self to see its own true nature. That is the essence of spirituality.

More recently, a cardiologist conducted an interesting research study giving more evidence of our interconnectedness and prayer's influence. Dr. Randy Byrd conducted a double-blind randomized study of 393 patients at San Francisco General Hospital who were admitted to the coronary care unit during a ten-month period. He arranged for people to pray for 192 of the patients but not for the 201 others. These two groups were comparable in terms of age and disease severity.

Dr. Byrd recruited people from around the country to pray for each of the 192 patients. He asked each person to pray every day in whatever form he or she wished. Each patient in the experimental group received daily prayers from five to seven people, although these patients were unaware of this.

He found that the prayed-for patients suffered fewer complications in three areas. First, only three required antibiotics, compared to sixteen in the control group. Second, only six had pulmonary edema (fluid in the lungs), compared to eighteen in the control group. Finally, none of the prayed-for patients required intubation (artificial respiration), while twelve of the others did. While this study is small (and twenty-three other disease measures showed no response to prayer), it suggests that we may be more interconnected than we often realize.

In summary, then, your mind, body, and spirit are all intimately interconnected. Because of this, coronary heart disease occurs on emotional and spiritual levels as well as physical ones. The Opening Your Heart program is designed to address *all* of these levels, not just the physical ones.

If we limit our treatments only to the physical heart, then the disease tends to come back again and again—or the treatments may be worse than the illness. If we also address the emotional and spiritual dimensions, then the physical heart often begins to heal as well.

You can use the techniques in this book to open your heart in emotional and spiritual ways that can help transform your life for the better. Although we have the technology to evaluate the physical improvements that result from this program, medical science has not yet found a way to objectively measure the emotional and spiritual healing that can occur on this program. But you can experience it for yourself.

"The best doctors in the world are Doctor Diet, Doctor Quiet, and Doctor Merryman."

—Jonathan Swift (1738),
Polite Conversation

■

"Persons living very entirely on vegetables are seldom of a plump and succulent habit."

—William Cullen (1710–1790),
First Lines of the Practice of Physic

■

"But I am a great eater of beef, and I believe that does harm to my wit."

—William Shakespeare,
Twelfth Night

■

"Vegetarianism is harmless enough though it is apt to fill a man with wind and self-righteousness."

—Sir Robert Hutchinson, in a 1930 address to the British Medical Association

10

The Reversal and Prevention Diets

What should I eat? This section of the book will show you how to design a diet that is right for you.

You have a range of choices. A central theme of this book is learning how we can feel more free—from physical pain, emotional distress, and spiritual isolation. But it's hard to feel free when someone says, "Don't eat this" or "You can't eat that." When that happens to me, I feel restricted. As I described in chapter 8, when someone says, "Thou Shalt Not!" it's only human to respond, "I Will!"

So instead of asking you to follow a long list of "do's" and "do not's," you have a spectrum of choices based on your specific needs. If you have coronary heart disease, then your intake of fat and cholesterol needs to be very low in order to increase the likelihood that reversal will begin to occur. If you don't have a heart problem, then you may be able to eat somewhat more fat and cholesterol.

This chapter describes two diet programs. the Reversal Diet, the one followed by the participants in our study, is for those who have coronary heart disease and want to reverse it. the Prevention Diet is for those who want to keep from getting it.

Both diets will also substantially reduce your risk of developing other degenerative diseases, including obesity, high blood pressure, stroke, osteoporosis, diabetes, gallstones, and cancers of the colon, breast, and prostate. (The Surgeon General's recent *Report on Nutrition and Health* confirms this.) Equally important, both diets can help you to feel more energetic, think more clearly, and improve your physical performance—in other words, to enjoy life more.

These are not diets of austerity or deprivation, although they do require you to make choices. There is no point in "depriving" yourself of foods you enjoy eating unless the benefits that come from choosing not to eat certain foods are greater than the enjoyment of eating everything.

For example, let's say you want to lose some weight. Most diets rely on counting calories and restricting portion sizes. Instead, the Reversal Diet allows you to eat almost as much food as you want and yet still lose weight! In our research studies, most of the people continued to lose pounds until they reached their ideal body weight (often for the first time since they were in high school or college). Take Don Vaupel, for example:

"After my first heart attack, I decided on my own to cut back on fat. And I lost about 25 pounds (from 265 down to 240) by just avoiding anything that had more than a few grams of fat listed on the box or package. Before, my favorite meal had been french fries and mayonnaise.

"Later on, after I began the Reversal Diet in June 1988, I lost about 80 pounds during the first six months on the program. I'm about 5'10", so that's about right for me. I lost twelve inches around my waist—my waist went from 45" to 33". Altogether, I've lost over one hundred pounds—from 265 down to 162! And it was virtually effortless. The weight just fell off. Unlike every other diet I've been on, the weight has stayed off. And I don't count calories.

"I've tried so many other diets—Weight Watchers, Overeaters Anonymous, you name it. But whenever I lost some weight, I'd gain it back plus ten or twenty pounds more.

"Now I eat more food than ever, and my meals are more balanced. The food tastes great. It's the first time in my life I'm not feeling hungry all the time. And when I get hungry, I eat just about as much as I want to of the food that's on the Reversal Diet."

FAT, PROTEIN, CARBOHYDRATE, AND CHOLESTEROL

How is this possible? All foods are composed of three constituents: fat, protein, and carbohydrate. Most people consume about 40 to 50 percent of their calories as fat. Although people often believe that carbohydrates (starches) make you fat, it's really not so.

Eating fat makes you fat (and also gives you heart disease). It's not the baked potato that is high in fat and calories, it's the sour cream and butter you put on it. It's not the pasta that's fattening, it's the cream sauce and olive oil you add to it.

Each gram of fat contains nine calories, whereas protein and carbohydrate have only four calories per gram—less than half as much. Instead of being 40 to 50 percent fat, the Reversal Diet has less than 10 percent of calories as fat. So if you eat the same amount of food on the Reversal Diet, you'll be eating far fewer calories. Said another way, you can eat substantially more food on the Reversal Diet without consuming any more calories.

Although the Reversal Diet is not restricted in calories, most people on the Reversal Diet consume fewer calories than the average American. Studies by Dr. Roy Walford at UCLA, Dr. Edward Masoro at the University of Texas, and others are finding that animals who consume fewer calories can extend their life span by 50 percent or more. Also, a diet lower in calories greatly retards most forms of cancer and forestalls many signs of aging in animals. Rats on restricted diets often fail to develop tumors even when they are exposed to cancer-causing substances. They have far less diabetes and cataracts, and they are able to run mazes more successfully than well-fed rats. Why this is so is not fully understood, and whether or not this applies to humans has not yet been proven. In simple terms, when you don't overload your body's systems for digesting excessive food and the resulting waste products, then it may be able to metabolize and remove these from your body more completely. So eat whenever you feel hungry, but it's best to wait until you *do* feel hungry.

In summary, the Reversal Diet:

- is very low in fat and has almost no cholesterol
- has less than 10 percent of calories from fat, and little of it is saturated
- excludes foods high in saturated fat (such as avocados, nuts, and seeds)
- is high in fiber
- allows but does not encourage moderate alcohol consumption (less than 2 ounces per day)
- excludes all oils and all animal products except nonfat milk and yogurt
- allows egg whites
- excludes caffeine, other stimulants, and MSG
- allows moderate use of salt and sugar
- is not restricted in calories

Most diets don't work for long because people get tired of feeling hungry and deprived. So instead of limiting the *amount* of food you eat, the Reversal Diet asks you to watch the *type* of food that you eat, and to select only from vegetarian sources. And there are so many different types of food you can choose from!

In our research study, people have the benefit of meeting two evenings a week to help support each other on the diet and lifestyle program. While this is helpful, many people in other parts of the country have been on the Reversal Diet for several years and plan to continue it indefinitely, even without group support.

Joseph Forgione, for example, had the misfortune of having a cholesterol level as high as 558. At the young age of thirty-nine, he began having chest pains. Shortly thereafter, he underwent coronary artery bypass surgery.

After recovering from surgery, he began to follow the Reversal Diet and the rest of the program with his wife in New Jersey, far from our research in San Francisco. Within six months, his cholesterol level had decreased to 107. "And I feel better than I have in years."

On the Reversal Diet, you eat until you are satisfied. And you can eat whenever you get hungry again. Because the fat content is so low, people on the Reversal Diet often get hungry before the next main meal. As a result, many of the people in our study snack in-between meals, what they affectionately call "grazing." But even though they are eating more often, they still lose excess weight and their cholesterol decreases substantially.

The typical American diet is:
    40 to 50% fat (mostly saturated)
    25 to 35% carbohydrate
    25% protein
    400 to 500 milligrams cholesterol per day

The Reversal Diet is:
    10% fat (mostly polyunsaturated or monounsaturated)
    70 to 75% carbohydrate
    15 to 20% protein
    5 milligrams cholesterol per day

In making this comparison, two things become clear:

First, the Reversal Diet consists primarily of *complex carbohydrates*, also known as starches. Vegetarian foods in their natural form are primarily complex carbohydrates—for example, grains, beans, vegetables, fruits, and so on. Complex carbohydrates are very filling. In contrast, *simple carbohydrates*, such as alcohol, honey, and sugar, are "empty" calories—that is, calories without any nutritional value—so it's easy to eat a lot of calories without being aware of it. Because of this, the Reversal Diet asks you to modify (but not eliminate) the use of sugar and alcohol. Sugar is not very strongly linked with coronary heart disease; the real culprits are saturated fat and cholesterol. The problem is that sugar is often found in the company of foods that are high in saturated fat and cholesterol, such as cake and ice cream—guilt by association.

Besides being more filling than simple sugars and lower in calories than fat, complex carbohydrates are hard for your body to convert into fat. In contrast, it is very easy for your body to convert dietary fat into body fat. Studies by K. J. Acheson at the University of Lausanne in Switzerland and by others have demonstrated that very little of the complex carbohydrates a person eats is converted into body fat. Also, it takes many more calories for your body to digest and metabolize complex carbohydrates than it does to digest and metabolize dietary fat.

A more recent study, directed by Darlene M. Dreon at Stanford, found more evidence that the type of food you eat is more important

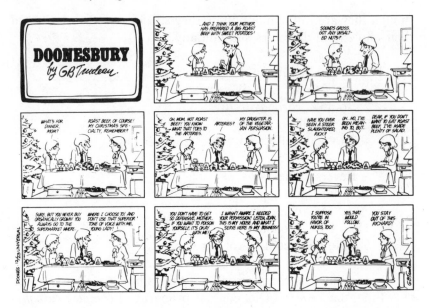

Doonesbury copyright © 1979 by G. B. Trudeau. Reprinted by permission of Universal Press Syndicate. All rights reserved.

than the amount of food you consume. The percentage of body fat in the study participants was directly related to the proportion of their daily calories that came from fat, but not to their total intake of calories or to the number or size of the meals they consumed.

A study from Harvard Medical School came to the same conclusion. The investigators studied 141 women, ages thirty-four to fifty-nine. There was virtually no correlation between calorie intake and body weight, even after adjusting for age, physical activity, alcohol, and smoking. The degree of excess weight was linked to fat consumption (especially saturated fat), *independent of calorie intake.*

In contrast, diets that rely on restricting calories usually cause a "yo-yo" effect. At the University of Pennsylvania School of Medicine, Dr. Kelly Brownell found that after animals gained weight they had lost when they were placed on a low-calorie diet, it took them more than twice as long to lose it the second time around, even though the number of calories they were fed on the weight-loss diet was the same. And it took less than one third of the time to gain it back.

Why? Because losing weight by depriving yourself of calories causes your metabolic rate to slow down—because your body thinks you're starving. A slower metabolic rate makes it harder to lose weight. In contrast, on the Reversal Diet, you consume fewer calories but your metabolic rate may increase rather than decrease.

Thus, eating a lot of fat gives you a "quintuple whammy":

· Each gram of fat that you eat has over twice as many calories as each gram of carbohydrate
· Each of those fat calories is harder to burn off than the same amount of calories from carbohydrates
· Dietary fat is easily converted into body fat, whereas very little of the complex carbohydrates in your diet are converted into body fat
· Saturated fat increases your blood cholesterol level
· Foods high in saturated fat often are high in cholesterol, too

Second, the Reversal Diet has somewhat less protein than the typical American diet. Is this bad?

No—quite the contrary. All of us have been taught the importance of getting enough protein, often equating it with good nutrition. But in the United States, most people (rich or poor) eat too much of it—at least twice as much protein as they need. Assuming you consume an adequate number of non-sugar calories, it is very difficult to eat too little protein. (This is not always true for pregnant or nursing women, small children, and post-surgical or burn patients whose protein requirements may be increased.)

Too much protein, like too little protein, can be harmful for you. Animals that are fed high-protein diets die sooner than animals given the same number of calories but with less protein. Excess protein also can lead to bone demineralization and osteoporosis. And in animal studies, even a low-fat diet that is high in protein can promote the formation of coronary artery blockages.

Protein is formed from building blocks called amino acids. There are approximately twenty-two different kind of amino acids that can combine to form literally billions of varieties of proteins, just as the twenty-six letters in the alphabet can form an endless number of words.

Your body can make thirteen of these amino acids. The other nine are called "essential amino acids," since they must be supplied in the diet. Of these, only three—lysine, tryptophan, and methionine—are critical, since the others are plentiful in most foods.

The amino acids that come from plant foods are exactly the

same as the amino acids that come from animal foods. When you eat protein, whether from a T-bone steak or from a meal of rice and beans, that protein is digested into the individual amino acid building blocks. Your body then takes these amino acids and builds whatever proteins you need. In other words, the protein that comes from eating a T-bone steak is exactly the same quality as the protein that comes from a meal of rice and beans. But when you eat a steak, you're also consuming excessive saturated fat and cholesterol.

Unlike animal products, though, no single plant source contains all of the essential amino acids. Fortunately, though, plant-based foods contain the three critical amino acids in different proportions. By eating a variety of foods, you will obtain all of these necessary amino acids.

Legumes (beans, for example) are high in lysine but low in tryptophan and methionine. Grains (rice, for example) are low in lysine but high in tryptophan and methionine. A meal of rice and beans, therefore, provides a complete protein, no different from the protein found in eggs or meat.

You don't have to be a scientist or a nutritionist to combine foods properly. It's easy: *just eat any grains and any legumes sometime during the same day.* That's all, folks! (Grains and legumes are listed on pages 443–460.) The ideal proportion is two-thirds grains and one-third legumes, but this is not critically important. As long as you consume enough non-sugar calories to maintain your ideal body weight, then you will likely be eating enough protein.

Here are some examples of a complete protein:

rice and beans
tacos with beans
tofu with rice
pasta e fagioli (pasta and beans)
hopping John (black-eyed peas) and rice
boston baked beans and brown bread

Another way to make a complete protein is to *combine any grains or legumes with small amounts of skim milk or nonfat yogurt.* For example:

oatmeal with milk or yogurt
any breakfast cereal with milk or yogurt

pancakes made with nonfat milk or yogurt
meatless chili topped with a dab of yogurt

Egg whites are also a complete protein, and these are allowed on the Reversal Diet. Most of the protein in an egg is in the white; *all* of the cholesterol is in the yolk. (When baking, substitute two egg whites for one egg yolk.)

Consuming a cup of *nonfat* milk or yogurt each day will also help meet your requirements for vitamins B_{12} and D. While milk or yogurt are not essential, they can help insure the intake of adequate protein for people who aren't eating a varied diet.

The terminology can be confusing. Milk rates second only to beef as the largest source of saturated fat in the American diet. "Whole milk" is sometimes called "3.5 percent fat," which doesn't sound too bad—until you realize that it's 3.5 percent of the total weight, and most of the weight is water. Almost 50 percent of the calories of whole milk are from fat.

Likewise, "low-fat" milk, also called "2 percent fat," actually has 38 percent of calories as fat. Nonfat milk, also called skim milk, has less than 2.5 percent of calories as fat.

The Reversal Diet is a very low-fat vegetarian diet, with no animal products except egg whites and nonfat dairy. This is what the patients in our study consumed, whose coronary heart disease began to reverse. I am convinced that this is the world's healthiest diet for most adults, whether or not they have heart disease.

One of the patients in our study is Leslie Peller, whose mother, Clara Peller, became famous for her "Where's the beef?" hamburger ads. When Leslie first entered our study, he asked me the same question!

The American Dietetic Association is the main professional organization of registered dietitians. In 1988, The American Dietetic Association issued a position paper that stated:

A considerable body of scientific data suggests positive relationships between vegetarian lifestyles and risk reduction for several chronic degenerative diseases and conditions, such as obesity, coronary artery disease, hypertension, diabetes mellitus, colon cancer, and others. . . . Vegetarians also have lower rates of osteoporosis, lung cancer, breast cancer, kidney stones, gallstones, and diverticular disease.

Although vegetarian diets usually meet or exceed requirements for protein, they typically provide less protein than nonvegetarian diets. This lower protein intake may be beneficial, however, and may be associated with a lower risk of osteoporosis in vegetarians and improved kidney function in individuals with prior kidney damage. Further, a lower protein intake generally translates into a lower fat diet, with its inherent advantages, since foods high in protein are frequently also high in fat.

It is the position of The American Dietetic Association that vegetarian diets are healthful and nutritionally adequate when appropriately planned.

The Reversal Diet is vegetarian for the simple reason that cholesterol is only found in animal products, including meats, poultry, fish, and dairy. Animal products also tend to be high in saturated fats, which your liver converts into cholesterol. Vegetarian foods are cholesterol-free and, with only rare exceptions, are low in saturated fat. Exceptions include avocados, olives, coconut, nuts, seeds, and cocoa products, such as chocolate.

Halfway measures aren't enough to reverse coronary heart disease for the majority of people. As described earlier, most of the people in the control group of our research and two others were eating a 30 percent fat "low-fat, low-cholesterol" diet along the guidelines of the American Heart Association or National Cholesterol Education Project—less red meat, more fish, chicken with the skin removed, etc.—yet the majority of these patients got *worse,* not better.

The Reversal Diet is also the most effective diet for lowering cholesterol and preventing heart disease. Only a diet almost entirely free of animal fat, oil, and cholesterol will significantly lower blood cholesterol levels reliably in just about everyone. In our research participants, we measured larger drops in blood cholesterol levels than have ever been reported without using drugs.

Your blood cholesterol comes from two places: you eat cholesterol when you consume animal products, and your body manufactures cholesterol from saturated fat in your diet.

Besides increasing your blood cholesterol level, new evidence from both human and animal studies indicates that dietary cholesterol has an independent effect on the risk of dying of coronary heart disease and all cardiovascular diseases, over and above its effect on blood cholesterol. In other words, the more cholesterol you eat, the greater your risk of developing coronary heart disease, even if your blood cholesterol level does not increase much.

In a recent major report, Dr. Jeremiah Stamler at Northwestern University and Dr. Richard Shekelle at the University of Texas studied 1,824 middle-aged men in Chicago who were followed for twenty-five years. In this group of men, dietary cholesterol intake was associated with increased risk of death from coronary heart disease, from other cardiovascular diseases combined (including stroke), and from all causes of death combined. Dr. Stamler said, "Cholesterol-rich foods promote heart disease even in people with low blood cholesterol. And that's why eating less cholesterol must be of concern to all people, irrespective of their blood cholesterol level."

Likewise, the less cholesterol you eat, the lower your risk of developing coronary heart disease. And since the Reversal Diet contains almost no cholesterol—about 100 times less than the average American consumes—eating this way may begin to reverse coronary heart disease even if your blood cholesterol level does not decrease very much.

In another study, Dr. Stamler and his colleagues studied over 350,000 men who were thirty-five to fifty-seven years old. They found that men whose blood cholesterol levels were above 180 had an increased mortality from heart disease. Over a six-year period, cholesterol readings between 182 and 202 increased the mortality rate by 29 percent; levels between 203 and 220 increased the rate by 73 percent; levels of 221 to 244 raised it by 121 percent, and levels of 245 or above increased it by 242 percent.

Despite all the bad press, cholesterol isn't really "bad." Cholesterol forms the building block of some important hormones in the body, including sex hormones such as testosterone and estrogen. It is also an important component of cell membranes.

Your body makes all the cholesterol it needs, even if you don't eat any cholesterol in your diet and even if you reduce your saturated fat intake. In fact, three fourths of the cholesterol in your blood is made by your body. It's the *excessive* amounts of cholesterol and saturated fat in the diet that lead to coronary heart disease.

With rare exceptions, your body makes exactly the right amount of cholesterol to meet your needs. You have exquisitely sensitive feedback mechanisms that tell your liver to increase or decrease the amount of cholesterol it manufactures as needed. (It is not yet clear if cholesterol-lowering drugs may cause long-term problems by artificially reducing your body's ability to manufacture cholesterol.) Within limits, when you eat more cholesterol, your body makes less of it. But when you eat a large amount of cholesterol, you overwhelm your body's ability to handle it. Also, your body manufactures more cholesterol when you are feeling emotionally stressed.

Fat is not "bad" either; we just eat too much of it. The average person needs to consume less than fourteen grams of fat to meet the daily requirements of essential fatty acids, which your body needs to synthesize a variety of important substances. Unfortunately, the average American consumes at least eight times that amount. Over time, this extra fat builds up in the arteries.

All fat is comprised of three components in varying proportions: saturated fat, polyunsaturated fat, and monounsaturated fat. Saturated fat raises your blood cholesterol level, whereas polyunsaturated fat and monounsaturated fat do not. However, monounsaturated fat and polyunsaturated fat *do not* lower your blood cholesterol level.

All oils are 100 percent fat—in other words, *oils are liquid fat.* One tablespoon of any oil contains almost fourteen grams of total fat, with different proportions of saturated fat, polyunsaturated fat, and monounsaturated fat. Here are a few examples of the proportion of fats in one tablespoon of oil, along with some other common sources of fat for comparison:

TYPE OF FAT	SATURATED	MONOUNSATURATED	POLYUNSATURATED
corn oil	1.7 grams	3.4 grams	7.9 grams
olive oil	1.9	9.8	1.2
coconut oil	11.7	0.8	0.2
safflower oil	1.3	1.7	10.0
peanut oil	2.6	6.2	4.1
sunflower oil	1.4	2.8	8.7
canola (Puritan) oil	0.8	8.4	4.4
soybean oil	2.0	3.1	7.8
cottonseed oil	3.6	2.6	6.9
Crisco	3.8	6.0	3.8
chicken fat	4.2	6.4	3.0
lard	5.6	6.4	1.6
beef fat	7.1	6.0	0.5
butterfat	9.0	4.1	0.6

Although many people believe that adding olive oil or safflower oil to their food will lower their cholesterol levels, this is, unfortunately, simply not true. *Adding any oil to your food will raise your cholesterol level.*

The reason for this is simple. While some oils are higher in saturated fat than others, *all oils contain some saturated fat.* So the more oil you eat, the more saturated fat you consume. Olive oil, for example, contains 1.9 grams of saturated fat per tablespoon (about 14 percent saturated fat). So if you add olive oil to your food, you are adding saturated fat to your food—and the more you add, the more your cholesterol level will increase.

The same is true for safflower oil, which has 1.3 grams of saturated fat per tablespoon. The more safflower oil you add to your food, the more saturated fat you are adding to your food, thus the higher your cholesterol level will rise. Even canola oil has some saturated fat. In contrast, coconut oil (found in many prepackaged foods) is a whopping 92 percent saturated fat.

Where did this misconception come from? Several studies have shown that *replacing* oils high in saturated fats (like coconut oil) with oils high in monounsaturated fat (like olive oil) or oils high in polyunsaturated fat (such as safflower oil) will, in fact, lower cholesterol levels. This is because olive oil and safflower oil contain less saturated fat, not because they contain more monounsaturated or polyunsaturated fat. In other words, olive oil and safflower oil are not "good" for you; they are less "bad" for you.

When you read food labels, you may often see a reference to "partially hydrogenated" oils. "Hydrogenation" is the process of making a fat more saturated, so a partially hydrogenated oil contains more saturated fat.

Why would anyone want to do this, since saturated fat is harmful? Because hydrogenation extends the supermarket shelf life of products. Unfortunately, a longer life for the product may mean a shorter life for you. Other labeling can also be confusing. Lately, more and more foods are advertised as being "cholesterol-free," yet they are often laden with saturated fat. And eating saturated fat will raise your blood cholesterol level even more than eating cholesterol.

Oils that are high in polyunsaturated fats are harmful for two reasons. First, as just discussed, these oils also contain some saturated fat. Second, diets high in the kinds of polyunsaturated fat prominent in corn, safflower, and soybean oils disrupt the immune system. (These fatty acids are also called n-6 or omega-6 fatty acids, in contrast to the n-3 or omega-3 fatty acids found in whole grains and in fish oil.) This impairment of immune system function may increase the risk of developing infections or even cancer. According to Dr. John Kinsella, a lipid biochemist at Cornell University, high levels of dietary polyunsaturated fat may foster the growth of tumors, at least in animals. This may help explain the finding in several large clinical studies that diets high in polyunsaturated fats decreased rates of heart attack but *increased* the death rates due to cancer and other causes.

Canola oil (also given the unfortunate name rapeseed oil, and sold under the brand name Puritan) is the oil lowest in saturated fat. Also, canola oil is the highest in omega-3 fatty acids, described later in this chapter. While all oils are excluded on the Reversal Diet, small amounts of oils are allowed on the Prevention Diet. If you use any oil, canola oil should be your choice.

What do other research studies tell us about the effects of dietary cholesterol and saturated fat? Epidemiology is the study of populations. In epidemiological studies, scientists observe large groups of people, often for many years, without giving them any type of treatment. In interventional studies, physicians and scientists treat people with drugs, surgery, or lifestyle interventions and then measure what happens.

What do the epidemiological research studies conducted to date tell us?

- In general, the more cholesterol and saturated fat you eat, the higher will be your blood cholesterol level and your blood pressure
- High blood cholesterol levels and high blood pressure increase the risk of coronary heart disease
- The more cholesterol and saturated fat you eat, the greater your risk of coronary heart disease, even if your blood cholesterol level and blood pressure do not rise very much
- People who eat a low-fat, low-cholesterol vegetarian diet (in other countries or in subgroups in the United States) have low blood pressure and low blood cholesterol levels in childhood that remain low as they get older, and they have very low rates of coronary heart disease
- People who eat a typical American diet have low blood pres-

sure and low blood cholesterol levels in childhood that tend
to increase as they get older, and they have high rates of
coronary heart disease

In summary, we have learned from these epidemiological studies that people both in this country and in other parts of the world
who eat a low-fat vegetarian diet have low blood pressure, low blood
cholesterol levels, and low rates of heart disease. People in most of
the less-industrialized countries of the world eat this way, and coronary heart disease is as rare there as malaria is here. They also have
low blood pressure and low blood cholesterol levels, not because they
are on medications but because of how they live. Unless they suc-
cumb to infectious diseases or accidents, their life span is about the
same as ours despite the lack of modern medical care. The exceptions
are found in the upper-class members of these countries who tend to
eat and live like Americans and who develop coronary heart disease
at rates similar to those in this country. Yet almost all of the major
interventional studies in this country have been conducted using
cholesterol-lowering drugs or surgical interventions.

Only a few major studies have been conducted that research the
effect of diet without drugs on heart disease, and these investigators
used nonvegetarian diets much higher in fat and cholesterol than the
Reversal Diet. Researchers have assumed that people are not willing
to change their lifestyles and eat a low-fat vegetarian or near-vegetar-
ian diet, even though this is how two thirds of the world has been
eating for centuries.

Many anthropologists believe that our ancestors were primarily
vegetarians, despite the popular image of the caveman as a hunter.
For example, our teeth are designed primarily for plant-based foods,
and our intestinal tract is long to allow for the slow digestion of
high-fiber plant foods, rather than the short digestive tract needed to
process meat and dispose of the resulting toxic wastes quickly. In
Jane Brody's Good Food Book, she describes other evidence to support this theory. (One reason why high-fiber foods can help to reduce
the incidence of colon cancer is by decreasing the time that it takes
to digest animal products so that the toxic wastes remain in your
colon for a shorter period of time.)

Even as early as 1900, two thirds of the protein in the typical
American diet came from plant foods, whereas today two thirds of
our protein comes from animal foods. Because of increasing prosper-

ity and the availability of refrigerators and freezers, the consumption of animal foods has increased—and with it, the incidence of coronary heart disease and other illnesses.

Some of the best epidemiological evidence linking diet with heart disease comes from the Framingham Heart Study. Framingham, Massachusetts, is a moderate-sized town near Boston. In 1948, scientists began studying half of the town's 10,000 residents to determine the risk factors for coronary heart disease. These people have been examined and checked every two years since then.

The doctors there said, "Let's measure everything that might be related to heart disease. We'll keep track of who gets a heart attack during the next several decades and see if there is any correlation between these factors and the risk of heart disease." During the next forty years, the Framingham Heart Study gave us the most conclusive evidence showing that high blood pressure, cholesterol, smoking, obesity, and diabetes increase the risk of developing coronary heart disease. They found that for every 1 percent that blood cholesterol levels rise above 150, the chance of developing coronary heart disease increases by about 2 percent.

Dr. William Castelli is medical director of the Framingham Heart Study. According to him, one of their more interesting findings is that *no one in the Framingham study has ever had a heart attack whose total blood cholesterol level was less than 150.* For most adults, a blood cholesterol level this low is achievable only on a low-fat vegetarian diet—that is, the Reversal Diet.

Besides the effect on heart disease, a diet low in animal products decreases the risk of many types of cancer. Drs. T. Colin Campbell of Cornell University and Dr. Richard Peto of Oxford University have been conducting research in China for many years. In a landmark study of 6,500 people living in China, Dr. Campbell and his associates found that reducing dietary fat to 30 percent of calories (less red meat, more fish, chicken with the skin removed, fewer eggs, and so on) is not enough to curb the risk of heart disease and cancer. According to Dr. Campbell, "We're basically a vegetarian species and should be eating a wide variety of plant foods and minimizing our intake of animal foods. The higher the intake of animal products, the higher the risk of cancer. For example, most people who get lung cancer are smokers, but not all smokers get lung cancer. Among smokers, animal products appear to raise the risk of cancer, and fruits and vegetables lower it." In China, this also appears to be true for liver cancer as well. And although the Chinese consume 20 percent more calories than Americans, there is little obesity in China, since the average Chinese diet is less than 15 percent fat.

Like many scientists, Dr. Campbell views the development of cancer as a multi-step process. A carcinogen is thought to initiate cancer, causing biochemical changes that allow tumors to start to form. Then, agents called promotors encourage their growth. Dr. Campbell believes that dietary animal protein is a promotor. He has conducted animal studies for over twenty years finding that animals who consume a lot of animal protein have more tumors than animals that do not. Similarly, a study from Stockholm reported that the higher your blood cholesterol level, the greater your risk of colon cancer.

The Good, the Bad, and the Ugly

Your total cholesterol level is comprised of different components, including LDL (for low-density lipoprotein) and HDL (high-density lipoprotein). Your body stores fat in the form of a substance called triglycerides, ugly yellow fat globules that appear in your blood-stream about an hour after you eat a high-fat meal. By now, many people have heard that HDL is often called "good cholesterol" and LDL is frequently referred to as "bad cholesterol."

These classifications of HDL and LDL are based on studies of people who eat a typical American diet. For those people, a low HDL level increases the risk of coronary heart disease as much as a high LDL does. Likewise, high triglycerides increase the risk of coronary heart disease in people who eat a high-fat, high-cholesterol diet.

For people who eat a low-fat vegetarian diet, though, these guidelines may no longer remain true. Vegetarians have low levels of total cholesterol, very low LDL levels, and very low rates of coronary heart disease *even though their HDL levels tend to be low and their triglyceride levels tend to be high.* In our research, for example, we found that triglycerides often increased, sometimes sub-stantially, and that HDL sometimes decreased in people who were on the Reversal Diet. Despite this, though, most of our participants showed some reversal of their coronary heart disease, in part because their LDL decreased much more than their HDL.

The main function of HDL is to remove excess cholesterol from your bloodstream. It helps transport LDL out of cells, into the bile, and out of your body. When your total cholesterol intake is low, then not much HDL is required to remove cholesterol from your blood, so your body makes less of it. As a result, your HDL level will probably decrease on the Reversal Diet, although your LDL will decrease even more. Therefore, on the Reversal Diet, your HDL level becomes much less important because your intake of saturated fat and cholesterol is so low.

In the Framingham Heart Study, Dr. Castelli and his colleagues found that the ratio of total cholesterol to HDL was a better predictor of coronary heart disease risk than either the total cholesterol or HDL alone in people who eat a typical American diet. To find your ratio, simply divide your total cholesterol by your HDL. For example, if your total cholesterol is 200, and your HDL is 50, then your total cholesterol/HDL ratio is 200/50, or 4.0. An ideal ratio would be less than 3.0. A ratio of 5.0 will put you at "average risk" (remember that the average American gets heart disease), a ratio of 9.5 puts you at twice the average risk, and a ratio over 23.0 places you in the highest risk category (greater than three times the average risk).

In an article reported in *The New England Journal of Medicine,* Dr. Castelli and his colleagues estimated the relative risk of various groups of people based on the total cholesterol/HDL data from the Framingham Heart Study. Long-term vegetarians had the lowest risk of any identifiable group, much lower even than Boston marathon runners, with a total cholesterol/HDL ratio of only 2.8.

Exercise raises HDL, whereas smoking lowers it. Stress management training will lower LDL independent of diet. So the best combination for reversing heart disease is to exercise, stop smoking, eat a vegetarian diet, and practice stress management techniques—in other words, to follow the program described in this book.

In 1985, Dr. Castelli, Dr. Frank Sacks, and I studied a group of vegetarians living near Putnam, Connecticut. We found that the ratio of total cholesterol to HDL was very low in these people, but it tended to increase (worsen) as they added dairy, eggs, or fish to their diet. (This article was published in the *Journal of the American Medical Association* in 1985.) Similar data were found in Oxford, England, by Dr. Thorogood, published in the *British Medical Journal* in 1987.

Even fish that eat a vegetarian diet have lower cholesterol levels than fish that eat other fish. Since oysters and clams are not very mobile, they eat whatever plants and plankton stream past them.

Because of this "vegetarian diet," oysters and clams are somewhat lower in cholesterol than other seafood. Or as Dr. Castelli likes to say, "If you can't be a vegetarian yourself, then eat a vegetarian."

In summary, then, a vegetarian diet will lower HDL, but it lowers LDL even more, and heart disease is rare in people who eat this way. Drugs can lower LDL and raise HDL, but there is little evidence that this is as beneficial as making comprehensive lifestyle changes. Rather than using drugs to lower LDL or raise HDL, though, putting much less cholesterol and saturated fat into your body in the first place makes a lot more sense to me than a lifetime of taking drugs which interfere with the metabolism and absorption of dietary cholesterol and saturated fat.

What are some of the other dietary considerations on the Reversal Diet or the Prevention Diet?

SALT

Salt is not as big a health problem as many people believe. Several cookbooks professing to be "heart-healthy" have appeared with recipes that, while low in salt, include seven or eight egg yolks and a half-pound of butter!

Salt affects your health only to the degree that it causes your blood pressure to increase. Less than one fourth of people who have high blood pressure are "salt-sensitive." If you don't have high blood pressure, then you don't have to limit your salt intake drastically.

Your body maintains a precise concentration of salt, so *when you eat salt, your body tends to retain water* in order to dilute the salt to keep it at a constant concentration. All other things being equal, when you increase the amount of volume (water) in a closed system (your body), the pressure increases. Because salt causes water retention, it was once thought that eating salt would cause everyone's blood pressure to increase. Most people, though, are able to excrete the extra salt and water in their urine, unless they have congestive heart failure or kidney disease. If you do, then you will benefit from restricting your salt intake. And if you have high blood pressure, you might try decreasing your salt intake to see if it helps to bring your blood pressure down. If so, then you are a "salt-sensitive" person. (Some evidence suggests that blacks may be more salt-sensitive than whites.) Otherwise, you can add a little to your food.

Most of us would benefit from reducing the salt content of our diet, at least to some extent. A little salt helps to bring out the flavor of foods and makes a lowfat diet much more palatable, but a lot tends to mask it. Better to add a little salt to your food so it tastes good than to add fat.

Recent evidence indicates that other forms of sodium, such as sodium bicarbonate (baking soda), monosodium glutamate, and so on, have little effect on blood pressure even in salt-sensitive individuals. It appears that salt, not sodium, is the main culprit.

However, monosodium glutamate, or MSG, which is used widely (especially in some Chinese restaurants) as a flavor enhancer, may have other ill effects. While MSG has no effect on heart disease, some research suggests that MSG may be harmful to your health.

MSG may cause the "Chinese restaurant syndrome," the brief symptoms of flushing, sweating, dizziness, or headache that 15 to 25 percent of diners feel after eating food that contains MSG. Of greater concern is that researchers have found that the amino acid contained in MSG, called glutamate, may be dangerous to your brain when consumed in excess. The potential hazards of MSG in children have been cited by Liane Reif-Lehrer, a Harvard Medical School researcher, in a report in *The New England Journal of Medicine.* She noted three cases of infants and children who suffered intense headaches and severe vomiting after eating foods containing MSG. Other studies by Dr. John Olney at Washington University and Dr. Dennis Choi at Stanford University suggest that MSG causes brain damage in animals, although other studies have not confirmed this.

Although the National Academy of Sciences, the World Health Organization, and the U.S. Food and Drug Administration have not regulated MSG, I think it would be prudent to avoid it until more information is available.

STIMULANTS

Caffeine is excluded on the Reversal Diet for the reasons described in chapter 2. Although we sometimes believe that caffeine *gives* us energy, it only *borrows* energy from the future.

When you drink a cup of coffee, the caffeine chemically stimulates your sympathetic nervous system. As a result, your level of adrenalin and other stress hormones quickly begins to rise (see figure 10.1).

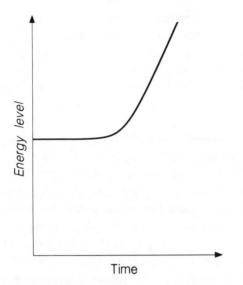

Figure 10.1

You don't get something for nothing, unfortunately, and so later in the day your energy level begins to fall even lower than it was when you started (see figure 10.2).

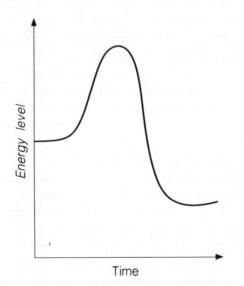

Figure 10.2

There is a good cure for that low feeling—another cup of coffee. And this is one reason why stimulants are so addictive.

This cycle of addiction is seen in much more exaggerated ways with other stimulants, including nicotine, cocaine, and amphetamines, and in its most extreme forms when cocaine ("crack") or methamphetamine ("speed" or "ice") are smoked or injected. The highs are much higher, and the lows are much lower. Again, there is a temporary remedy for the low feeling: another cigarette. Or another line of cocaine. Or a shot of speed. This is the cycle of addiction that makes it so hard for people to stop.

Because of this, most drug users don't put cocaine away for a rainy day—"leftover cocaine" is a contradiction in terms. Sometimes people become intensely depressed or sleep for days after smoking cocaine or methamphetamine because they have borrowed so much energy from the future. And if you don't think you're addicted to coffee or cigarettes, just say no to these for a few days and see how you feel when your body starts to go through withdrawal. So powerful is this addictive cycle that monkeys who are allowed to push a lever giving them injections of cocaine or nicotine instead of food will continue to do so until they die of starvation.

Thus, stimulants are excluded from the Reversal Diet for four reasons. First, stimulants increase the risk of coronary heart disease. However, the link between coffee and coronary heart disease is much weaker than the link between fat or cholesterol and heart disease. A study from Dr. Andrea LaCroix of the Johns Hopkins Medical School reported in 1986 that a person who drinks five or more cups of coffee a day is two to three times as likely to develop heart problems as a person who drinks no coffee at all. However, other studies, such as the Framingham Heart Study, have not confirmed this. But the link between smoking and coronary heart disease or between cocaine or amphetamines and coronary heart disease is unquestioned.

Second, caffeine and other stimulants can increase the frequency and severity of irregular heartbeats. This is true for both the harmless and the life-threatening types of arrhythmias.

Third, caffeine and other stimulants potentiate the stress response. In other words, they make your fuse shorter. After you have gone through the withdrawal period from caffeine, you'll find that your energy level is more constant and your mood is more even. It's easier to maintain your inner equanimity when you don't drink caffeine.

Fourth, your body becomes more sensitive to the effects of

caffeine (and medications) on the Reversal Diet. The opposite is true for people who smoke—that is, they are less sensitive to the effects of caffeine and other drugs. Studies have demonstrated that cigarette smokers require twice as much caffeine as nonsmokers to achieve the same effect.

Caffeine is found not only in coffee but also in colas, chocolate and other cocoa products, regular teas (but not in most herbal teas), and in many over-the-counter medications (for example, Excedrin, diet pills, and many others). Decaffeinated coffees, teas, and soft drinks are a major improvement, but these do contain some caffeine. If you are currently drinking beverages that contain caffeine, you may want to begin by switching to decaffeinated drinks and then slowly wean yourself off these, too. Regular teas (Lipton, Earl Grey, and so on) contain not only caffeine but also theophylline and other stimulants.

Besides herbal teas, a variety of grain "coffees" are available in many stores. These include Bambu (my favorite), Pero, Postum, Cafix, Inka, and others. If you look on these as coffee *substitutes,* then you may be disappointed. If you see these as interesting beverages in their own right, then most of them taste quite good.

Most people find when they stop drinking coffee that they go through withdrawal: they feel tired, think fuzzily, get headaches, and become a little depressed and low on energy. After three or four days of this, though, you'll notice a new calmness. When you wake up in the morning, for example, you won't need a cup of coffee to get you going. Even more important, your "fuse" will get longer, and you won't find yourself feeling as tired later in the day.

SUGAR

Eating refined sugar causes your blood sugar level to rise rapidly. In response, your pancreas begins to churn out insulin, causing your blood sugar level to fall rapidly. As your blood sugar level begins to fall, the pancreas begins to stop secreting insulin, but not fast enough, so your blood sugar level may dip even lower than it was when you started (see figure 10.3). When this happens, you may start to feel tired and run down. There is a good remedy for that feeling—more sugar. The cycle is very similar to the addiction cycle of stimulants I described earlier.

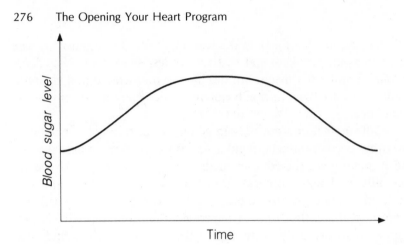

Figure 10.3

Unlike simple sugars, the sugars found in complex carbohy-drates ("starches") are absorbed much more slowly into the blood-stream (see figure 10.4). As a result, your energy level remains more constant.

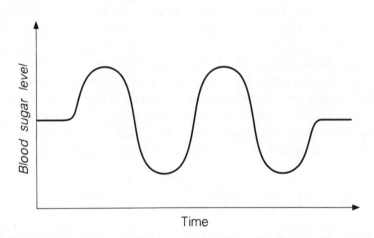

Figure 10.4

At the Royal Infirmary in Bristol, England, scientists gave nor-mal subjects meals of apples, applesauce, or apple juice, each con-taining the same amount of glucose and carbohydrate. This study published in *The Lancet* found three important facts:

- The juice could be consumed eleven times faster than the apples and four times faster than the applesauce

· Given the same amount of calories, the apple was much more filling and thus more satisfying than the applesauce and the applesauce, in turn, was more filling and satisfying than the apple juice
· Participants' blood sugar levels rose to similar levels after all three meals; however, there was a striking rebound fall after drinking the juice, and to a lesser extent after eating the applesauce, which was not seen after eating the whole apples

The same phenomenon is seen with other concentrated simple sugars: honey, maple syrup, corn syrup, fructose, apple juice concentrate, and so on. The only advantage to honey or maple syrup is that these have a built-in "warning" system. That is, if you eat too much honey, after a while you begin to feel a little queasy. With refined sugar, though, all of the warning signals have been refined away, so it's possible to eat large quantities without even being aware of it.

Sugar is linked very weakly to heart disease, if at all. The problem with sugar, as I mentioned earlier, is that it is often found in the company of fat: cakes, pies, and so on. Sugar also provides "empty calories," and it promotes tooth decay.

Therefore, the use of sugar is allowed but not encouraged on the Reversal Diet. Better to eat sugar than fat, but only in limited amounts. You'll feel better if you reduce your consumption of sugar. A little goes a long way.

ALCOHOL

What about alcohol? Several studies have shown that people who drink one to two ounces of alcohol per day tend to live longer than people who drink more than this amount or who don't drink at all. (One ounce of alcohol is equivalent to one glass of wine, one can of beer, or one mixed drink.)

Based on these findings, some physicians even began to encourage their patients to drink "moderately." Participants in our study, while encouraged not to drink, were allowed up to two ounces of alcohol per day. Since people generally become more sensitive to the effects of all drugs on the Reversal Diet, most people in our study decreased their alcohol consumption or stopped drinking altogether. As one participant said, "I used to drink a lot. I enjoyed it. But as

I began feeling so much better on the Reversal Diet, I began noticing how I didn't feel as good after drinking—so I stopped."

While alcohol is not excluded from the Reversal Diet, I do not recommend its daily use. Why not?

First, subsequent, more careful analyses of the studies cited above revealed that many of the people who didn't drink at all chose not to drink because a number of them were in ill health or were recovering alcoholics. They did not die sooner due to an "alcohol deficiency"; they died sooner because they were sicker to begin with.

Second, one reason why people who drink "moderately" may live longer is that they often have more social support than others who do not drink. In our culture, "Happy Hour" is a socially accept- able way to take a break from work and spend time relaxing with friends or spouses. I suspect that the same benefits would result from having social support in activities not centered around alcohol.

Third, alcohol has a direct, toxic effect on the muscle of the heart. Over time, this can cause the heart to beat less effectively, a condition known as an alcohol cardiomyopathy. And alcohol is toxic to a number of other organ systems, especially your liver. Heavy drinking is linked to cirrhosis, pancreatitis, fetal alcohol syndrome, hypertension, cardiomyopathy, cardiac arrhythmias, and malnutri- tion. Drinking less than one drink per day has been found to double the risk for hemorrhagic stroke when compared with not drinking at all. A study of 87,526 female nurses found that women who consumed three to nine drinks per week had 3.7 times the risk of bleeding into their brains as nondrinkers.

Fourth, alcohol is a major factor in most accidents at work and at home. Somewhere between 50 and 80 percent of all fatal traffic accidents are alcohol related.

Fifth, although alcohol does raise your HDL ("good choles- terol"), this is only half the story. There are two types of HDL: HDL_2 and HDL_3. HDL_2 helps to protect against coronary heart disease, but HDL_3 does not. Alcohol raises HDL_3.

Sixth, alcohol provides a lot of extra calories but no nutrition.

Seventh, a study of 7,188 women twenty-five to seventy-four years of age found that moderate alcohol consumption was as- sociated with a 50 to 100 percent elevation in the risk of breast cancer.

OMEGA-3 FATTY ACIDS

During the past ten years, there has been increasing interest in the potential beneficial effects of what have been called omega-3 fatty acids, also known as EPA's or n-3 fatty acids. These are believed to help protect blood vessel walls from the harmful effects of LDL-cholesterol.

As described earlier, LDL is the most harmful type of cholesterol. When LDL is combined with oxygen ("oxidized"), it becomes even more injurious. A high-fat diet tends to promote oxidation of LDL. Omega-3 fatty acids tend to prevent this from happening.

Omega-3 fatty acids also influence other factors that cause atherosclerosis. They help to prevent blood clots and coronary artery spasm by decreasing production of thromboxane and increasing production of prostacyclin and tissue plasminogen activator. They decrease the amount or activity of other substances that lead to atherosclerosis, including leukotrienes, fibrinogen, platelet activating factor, platelet derived growth factor, interleukin-1, tumor necrosis factor, and other terrible-sounding names. They increase the amount of EDRF, or endothelial derived relaxation factor (see chapter 2). Some studies show that omega-3 fatty acids given to animals on a high-fat diet help to prevent the development of coronary artery blockages.

Omega-3 fatty acids are found in fish oils, but they are also found in whole grains, beans, seaweed, and soybean products. Purslane, one of the vegetables eaten extensively in soups and salads in Greece, Lebanon, and other parts of the Mediterranean, is particularly high in omega-3 fatty acids. I recommend the vegetarian sources of omega-3 fatty acids for the following reasons:

- Fish contain saturated fat and cholesterol, so fish and fish oils tend to cause LDL levels to *increase*
- Fish oils are higher in omega-3 fatty acids than whole grains and soybean products; this may increase the risk of hemorrhagic stroke, as described in chapter 3
- In people with diabetes, fish oils may cause insulin resistance and elevation of blood glucose levels
- Fish caught in coastal waters may be contaminated with pesticides, chlorinated hydrocarbons, and heavy metals
- Fish oils are prone to oxidation and spoilage

In our research, we did not study the effects of fish or fish oil. It may be possible that on the Prevention Diet two to three servings of fish each week may be acceptable if your blood cholesterol level is low, although no one knows for sure. (It may even be possible that reversal of coronary artery blockages may occur on a diet that includes some fish or fish oil, but we did not test this in our research.) Studies of animals and humans indicate that omega-3 fatty acids can decrease the likelihood of lethal cardiac irregular heartbeats (ventricular fibrillation).

A recent study from Wales published in *The Lancet* found a 29 percent reduction in mortality in men who ate fish three times per week following a heart attack. The incidence of heart attacks, though, did not change. Does eating more fish or forgoing high-fat beef meals reduce risk? We don't know.

If you already have coronary heart disease, I recommend that you follow the Reversal Diet without adding any fish or fish oil. You will receive all of the omega-3 fatty acids you need in the Reversal Diet. If you don't have heart disease, then eating fish is a better source of omega-3 fatty acids than taking fish oil pills.

FIBER

Fiber is the nondigestible part of plants, comprised mostly of complex carbohydrates. Fiber is found in all whole grains, legumes, fruits, and vegetables. Refined foods remove much of the fiber—for example, white flour has much less fiber than whole wheat flour because the wheat bran has been removed. Animal products contain no fiber.

Dietary fiber consists of soluble and insoluble forms. The Reversal Diet is high in both types.

Insoluble fibers increase stool bulk and substantially decrease the amount of time it takes for food to pass through your intestines. The increase in stool bulk will cure constipation for many people and will decrease the likelihood of hemorrhoids, appendicitis, diverticular disease, and irritable bowel syndrome. Because food passes through your body more quickly, your colon is exposed to carcinogens for a shorter period of time; this may be one reason why the risk of colon cancer is lower on a high-fiber diet. Wheat bran is a major source of insoluble fiber.

Soluble fibers form gels that delay the absorption of certain foods, including cholesterol. Oat bran is only one of many types of soluble fibers that may lower blood cholesterol levels. Others include rice bran, rolled oats, carrots, pectins (found in fruits), psyllium (Metamucil), and guar gum (found in beans). Soluble fibers also increase the excretion of cholesterol in the bile.

Soluble fibers also slow the absorption of carbohydrates, so blood sugar levels remain more constant. (This is one reason why the Reversal Diet often allows diabetics under a doctor's supervision to decrease or even discontinue insulin injections.) In one interesting study, researchers found that cholesterol levels decreased significantly when people were fed exactly the same food in several smaller meals during the day rather than in two or three large meals, mimicking the effects of slow absorption of carbohydrates through soluble fiber.

To digress a little—I was a freelance writer and photographer when I was in college, and in 1972 I was asked to do an article for *Esquire* magazine on a man who installed and serviced condom machines in the restrooms of small-town Texas gas stations. (This was before concern about AIDS caused condoms to become widely available in most convenience stores and corner markets.)

When I finally tracked him down (which is another story), he told me that in some of the smaller towns, a few people would leave money on top of the condom vending machines. He didn't understand why. At first he was puzzled: maybe they just didn't know you were supposed to put a quarter in and turn the handle to get a condom. Later, he found out that they would have sex with someone without using a condom, and the next day they would leave money on top of the vending machine as if it were an offering on the altar of an infertility god. Some people use oat bran in much the same way: after the fact to somehow magically protect them. A bowl of Quaker Oats is an ideal breakfast, but it won't undo the effects of a ham and cheese omelette on the side.

So what can you eat on the Reversal Diet? Here are some examples:

ANIMAL PRODUCTS:
egg whites
nonfat milk or yogurt (1 cup
    per day)

WHOLE GRAINS:
amaranth
barley
buckwheat

bulgur
corn
millet
oats
quinoa
rice
rye
sorghum
triticale
wheat

VEGETABLES:
artichokes
asparagus
bamboo shoots
beets
broccoli
Brussels sprouts
cabbage (all types)
carrots
cauliflower
celery
chili peppers
collards
cucumbers
eggplants
escarole
garlic
gingerroot
Jerusalem artichoke
kale
leeks
lettuce (all types)
mushrooms
mustard greens
okra
onions
parsley
potatoes
pumpkin

radishes
rutabagas
scallions
shallots
sorrel
spinach
sprouts (all kinds)
squashes (all kinds)
sweet potatoes
Swiss chard
turnips and greens
watercress
yams
zucchini

FRUITS:
apples
apricots
bananas
blackberries
blueberries
cantaloupes
casaba melons
cherries
cranberries
currants
dates
figs
grapefruit
grapes
guava
honeydew melons
kiwi fruit
kumquats
lemons
limes
loganberries
mangoes
nectarines
oranges

papayas
peaches
pears
pineapples
plantains
plums
pomegranates
prunes
raisins
raspberries
strawberries
tangelos
tangerines
tomatoes
watermelon

LEGUMES:
azuki beans
black beans
black-eyed peas
brown beans
chick-peas (garbanzos)

Great Northern beans
kidney beans
lentils
mung beans
navy beans
peas
pinto beans
red Mexican beans
soybeans (including miso,
    tempeh, and tofu)
split peas

BEVERAGES
club soda
decaffeinated tea or coffee
    (Prevention Diet only)
fruit juices (all kinds)
grain coffees
herbal teas
mineral water
vegetable juices (all kinds)

What foods are not included on the Reversal Diet?

All animal products (with the exception of nonfat milk, nonfat yogurt, egg whites, or products made from these). That is, meats, poultry, seafood, and egg yolks are not included on the Reversal Diet. Also excluded are vegetarian foods that are high in fat: all oils (except in very small quantities), nuts, seeds, avocados, chocolate and other cocoa products, olives, and coconut. Some of the foods excluded on the Reversal Diet are allowed on the Prevention Diet, which is explained later in this chapter.

There are other reasons to consider the Reversal Diet besides the beneficial effects on your heart. Athletes are finding that a diet high in complex carbohydrates and low in saturated fat improves their performance. Football teams from the New York Jets to the San Francisco 49ers are forgoing the traditional pregame steaks for foods high in complex carbohydrates. According to *The New York Times,* "Janet Horowitz, the Jets' nutritionist, has declared that fat is out and healthy eating is in." Jerry Attaway, the 49ers' trainer, likes to tell about a classic experiment:

> You bring one of our football players in and put them on a stationary exercise bicycle and tell them to work as hard as they can for as long as they can, and you'll time them. Say the guy lasts for eight minutes, and then he's just exhausted. Then for three days you put him on a high-fat diet. He comes back in, goes on the bike and he'll last probably only six minutes. He's lost that much strength.
>
> Then put him on a high carbohydrate, low-fat diet for only three days, and he'll probably go up to 12 minutes. It makes that much difference.

To an athlete, of course, that's important. Tennis star Martina Navratilova credits her low-fat, high-complex-carbohydrate diet for her phenomenal success on the court.

Other athletes are discovering the benefits of a vegetarian diet: as mentioned in chapter 7, Olympic champion Edwin Moses was undefeated in eight years of running the 400 meter hurdles. Dave Scott was a six-time winner of the Ironman Triathalon.

I grew up in Texas on double cheeseburgers with hickory sauce, chili, fried chicken, T-bone steaks, and eggs. Many people report that they lose the taste for animal foods after eating a vegetarian diet for a while, but it hasn't fully happened to me. I still enjoy the way animal foods taste and smell, but I usually don't eat them.

Why not? Because I like the way I feel when I don't eat these foods so much more than the pleasure I used to get from eating them. I have much more energy, I need less sleep, I feel calmer, I can maintain an ideal body weight without worrying about how much I eat, and I can think more clearly (although some might debate the last point).

I began making these dietary and lifestyle changes during my second year of college and have been eating this way ever since. I wasn't worried about coronary heart disease at age nineteen—my cholesterol level then was only 125 (and it still is). I began feeling better after I started eating this way, so I continue to do so. Eating this diet probably will help me to live longer, but it's not my primary motivation. Feeling better is.

In my clinical experience, I often find that fear may be enough motivation for some people to begin a diet, but it's usually not enough to sustain it. As I've said earlier, who wants to live longer if you're not enjoying life?

Since I began making these dietary changes in 1972, eating this way has become increasingly accepted. Beans and grains are becoming, believe it or not, high-status foods. A recent article in *The New York Times* said:

> Although people don't usually rhapsodize at cocktail parties about great bean dishes they have enjoyed lately, that is beginning to change. As new varieties of dried beans arrive on the market, and research unveils ever greater nutritional properties, beans are finding passionate advocates among culinarians. When properly cooked, beans have a satisfying, sensual texture and tastes that range from buttery to tomatoey. Stylish restaurants are offering far more bean dishes than they did a few years ago, and the choices have expanded far beyond the basic white, black, and red beans to varieties with variegated patterns and striking colors.

Fat does taste good, but as you decrease the amount of fat in your diet, your palate will begin to readjust. After a while, you'll find that the food in the Reversal Diet tastes delicious, even though it contains much less fat, and the food that used to taste so good will begin to seem too rich or oily. I may not have completely lost my taste for meat, but I really have lost my taste for excessive fat. The same is true of salt—as you begin to decrease the amount you consume, your taste buds will readjust, and the food you used to eat will begin to taste too salty.

But I don't want to minimize the fact that, for most people, the Reversal Diet is a big change. The transition period may be stressful until you become acquainted with it. But it's worth it, and you can have a lot of fun experimenting with new tastes and textures, as you'll see in the recipe section in Part 3.

Fenton "Pete" Talbott is a managing director of The First Boston Corporation in New York. At age forty-four, he underwent coronary angioplasty. A few months later, the arteries closed up again, and he needed another one. This happened again two more times—a total of four angioplasties. Says Talbott,

> Then I began following this program, including the Reversal Diet. My cholesterol decreased from 307 to 130, and I lost over sixty

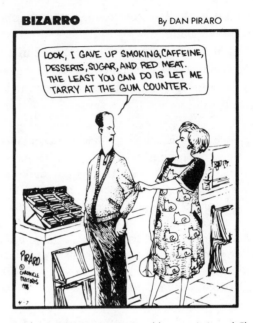

The "Bizarro" cartoons by Dan Piraro are reprinted by permission of Chronicle Features, San Francisco.

pounds, from 238 to 175 pounds. My weight has now stablized at about 185. I went back and found an old high school football program that listed me as 6'2", 185 pounds.

During my first year of college, I gained forty pounds when I began throwing the javelin. For the next twenty years, I carried all of this extra weight and kidded myself that I was in good shape since that's what I weighed in college. Now that I've lost all that extra weight, I feel great!

After seeing how much I've improved, many of my colleagues are beginning to do what I've been doing. Once I became convinced that this program was scientifically sound and that it worked, then I decided just to do it. You don't have to wait for anyone else to change. It would be easier for me if everyone else ate this way, but why should I have another heart attack waiting for them to get the message?

People say all the time, "Well, how do you live without eating cheeseburgers or this or that?" and I say, "You just don't. It's not even an option." It's not that hard once you get on it.

The most difficult parts for me are the social aspects of eating. For example, hamburgers were hard to do without at first because I identified eating them with fun times—sitting on the floor with the kids watching television, or in a fun place with people sitting around laughing, drinking beer and eating burgers.

It's the same at a tailgate picnic at a football game. It was hard—not because of the foods there, but because of the social factors. But once you understand that, then you can say, "I can enjoy the social part without having to eat that food." It's more what you're doing than the food itself.

My wife Judy has been extremely supportive, and that makes it much easier. I've seen some wives even encourage their husbands to get off the diet, but Judy is even more disciplined than I am. And my angioplasties have stayed open.

GETTING STARTED ON THE REVERSAL DIET

Although you won't need to count calories on the Reversal Diet, you do need to keep track of the fat you consume if you eat any commercially prepared products. How much cholesterol and fat can you eat on the Reversal Diet?

Foods on the Reversal Diet have no cholesterol, so you don't have to calculate your cholesterol intake. It's easy—there isn't any. The only exception is nonfat milk or yogurt, and these contribute less than five milligrams of cholesterol per cup, a minimal amount.

On the Reversal Diet, most people will be able to eat somewhere between 15 and 35 grams of total fat per day, or between 5 and 12 grams of saturated fat per day. (Most Americans eat over 100 grams of fat per day.) You probably don't know how much fat you consume, but it's easy to find out. Although it is saturated fat that we're primarily concerned about, it's easier to figure out how much total fat is in a given food item.

Almost all packaged and processed food manufacturers list on the label the amount of total fat per serving the food contains, but they generally do not specifically list the amount of saturated fat. (New FDA guidelines recommend that manufacturers change their labels to include the amount of saturated fat, so this information may be available in the near future.) Since none of the foods on the Reversal Diet is high in saturated fat, calculating the total fat is a good enough estimate.

For example, the label on a package of Crisco shortening proudly touts, "No cholesterol," which is technically true. However, a closer look at the label reveals that Crisco has at least 12 grams of fat per tablespoon, a huge amount, like most other oils or 100 percent fat items. On further inspection, the label informs us that palm oil is used in Crisco (one of the oils highest in saturated fat), and, worse, that these oils are "partially hydrogenated for freshness," meaning that they have been made even more saturated to increase shelf life. In other words, even though Crisco contains no cholesterol, your body will convert most of Crisco into blood cholesterol.

Another example comes from a package of Stouffer's Lean Cuisine Salisbury Steak dinner. Despite its name, this "lean" meal is laden with fat—15 grams, or almost 50 percent fat. It contains only 280 calories because the portion size is so small.

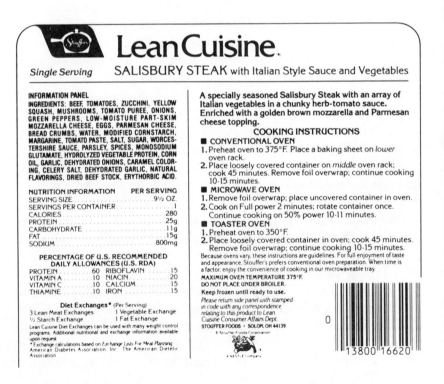

Lean Cuisine.

Single Serving   SALISBURY STEAK with Italian Style Sauce and Vegetables

INFORMATION PANEL

INGREDIENTS: BEEF, TOMATOES, ZUCCHINI, YELLOW SQUASH, MUSHROOMS, TOMATO PUREE, ONIONS, GREEN PEPPERS, LOW-MOISTURE PART-SKIM MOZZARELLA CHEESE, EGGS, PARMESAN CHEESE, BREAD CRUMBS, WATER, MODIFIED CORNSTARCH, MARGARINE, TOMATO PASTE, SALT, SUGAR, WORCESTERSHIRE SAUCE, PARSLEY, SPICES, MONOSODIUM GLUTAMATE, HYDROLYZED VEGETABLE PROTEIN, CORN OIL, GARLIC, DEHYDRATED ONIONS, CARAMEL COLORING, CELERY SALT, DEHYDRATED GARLIC, NATURAL FLAVORINGS, DRIED BEEF STOCK, ERYTHORBIC ACID.

NUTRITION INFORMATION	PER SERVING
SERVING SIZE	9½ OZ.
SERVINGS PER CONTAINER	1
CALORIES	280
PROTEIN	25g
CARBOHYDRATE	11g
FAT	15g
SODIUM	800mg

PERCENTAGE OF U.S. RECOMMENDED DAILY ALLOWANCES (U.S. RDA)

PROTEIN	60	RIBOFLAVIN	15
VITAMIN A	10	NIACIN	20
VITAMIN C	10	CALCIUM	15
THIAMINE	10	IRON	15

Diet Exchanges* (Per Serving)

3 Lean Meat Exchanges   1 Vegetable Exchange
½ Starch Exchange   1 Fat Exchange

Lean Cuisine Diet Exchanges can be used with many weight control programs. Additional nutritional and exchange information available upon request.
* Exchange calculations based on Exchange Lists For Meal Planning, American Diabetes Association, Inc., The American Dietetic Association.

A specially seasoned Salisbury Steak with an array of Italian vegetables in a chunky herb-tomato sauce. Enriched with a golden brown mozzarella and Parmesan cheese topping.

COOKING INSTRUCTIONS

■ **CONVENTIONAL OVEN**
1. Preheat oven to 375°F. Place a baking sheet on *lower* oven rack.
2. Place loosely covered container on *middle* oven rack; cook 45 minutes. Remove foil overwrap; continue cooking 10-15 minutes.

■ **MICROWAVE OVEN**
1. Remove foil overwrap; place uncovered container in oven.
2. Cook on Full power 2 minutes; rotate container once. Continue cooking on 50% power 10-11 minutes.

■ **TOASTER OVEN**
1. Preheat oven to 350°F.
2. Place loosely covered container in oven; cook 45 minutes. Remove foil overwrap; continue cooking 10-15 minutes.

Because ovens vary, these instructions are guidelines. For full enjoyment of taste and appearance, Stouffer's prefers conventional oven preparation. When time is a factor, enjoy the convenience of cooking in our microwaveable tray.

MAXIMUM OVEN TEMPERATURE 375°F.
DO NOT PLACE UNDER BROILER.
Keep frozen until ready to use.

Please return side panel with stamped-in code with any correspondence relating to this product to Lean Cuisine Consumer Affairs Dept.
STOUFFER FOODS · SOLON, OH 44139
© Stouffer Foods Corporation

A NESTLE Company

0   13800 16620

Manufacturers are required to list ingredients in descending order of quantity contained in the package. In this case, beef is the first ingredient, so the package contains more beef than any other ingredient listed. Also, this meal contains whole eggs and two types of cheese. Looking at the Appendix table, we can see that approximately one-half of the fat in beef is saturated, about two-thirds of the fat in the two cheeses is saturated, and about one-third of the fat in an egg is saturated.

So even though the amount of saturated fat is not listed on the label, we can estimate that about one half of the 15 grams of fat are saturated—about an entire day's quota on the Reversal Diet. Thus, this meal has not only a huge amount of total fat but also a large amount of saturated fat. And even though the amount of cholesterol is not listed either, we know that the combination of beef, cheese, and eggs is going to be high in cholesterol as well as in saturated fat. Finally, this meal is high in sodium (800 milligrams) and contains MSG. Not a good choice.

Here's how to determine more precisely your daily quota of total fat or saturated fat:

First, determine your desirable weight using Table 1. Alternatively, decide how much you would like to weigh—the weight at which *you* feel most comfortable.

Second, look at Table 2 and estimate how active you are. *Inactive* means your physical activity is limited—watching television, writing, sewing, a little walking, and so on. *Moderately active* means you spend approximately ten to twenty minutes a day of continuous exercise at least three times per week—such as walking, jogging, swimming, or doubles tennis. *Active* means you spend over twenty minutes exercising continually and vigorously at least three times a week—singles tennis, running, rowing, basketball, and so on. (Exercise is described more fully in chapter 12.)

After you have determined your desirable weight and activity level, then refer to Table 2 for your recommended quota of saturated fat and total fat for each day.

For example, if you are a man with an ideal body weight of 150 pounds and a moderate activity level, then you would eat approximately 25 grams of total fat or about 8 grams of saturated fat per day.

The next step is to determine how much fat you're currently eating. A theme of this book is that increasing awareness is the first step in healing. The stress management techniques, for example, increase our awareness of how stressed we are and help us notice the

Table 1
1983 Metropolitan Height and Weight Tables

MEN					WOMEN				
Height		Small Frame	Medium Frame	Large Frame	Height		Small Frame	Medium Frame	Large Frame
Feet	Inches				Feet	Inches			
5	2	128–134	131–141	138–150	4	10	102–111	109–121	118–131
5	3	130–136	133–143	140–153	4	11	103–113	111–123	120–134
5	4	132–138	135–145	142–156	5	0	104–115	113–126	122–137
5	5	134–140	137–148	144–160	5	1	106–118	115–129	125–140
5	6	136–142	139–151	146–164	5	2	108–121	118–132	128–143
5	7	138–145	142–154	149–168	5	3	111–124	121–135	131–147
5	8	140–148	145–157	152–172	5	4	114–127	124–138	134–151
5	9	142–151	148–160	155–176	5	5	117–130	127–141	137–155
5	10	144–154	151–163	158–180	5	6	120–133	130–144	140–159
5	11	146–157	154–166	161–184	5	7	123–136	133–147	143–163
6	0	149–160	157–170	164–188	5	8	126–139	136–150	146–167
6	1	152–164	160–174	168–192	5	9	129–142	139–153	149–170
6	2	155–168	164–178	172–197	5	10	132–145	142–156	152–173
6	3	158–172	167–182	176–202	5	11	135–148	145–159	155–176
6	4	162–176	171–187	181–207	6	0	138–151	148–162	158–179

Weights at ages 25–59 based on lowest mortality. Weight in pounds according to frame (in indoor clothing weighing 5 lbs., shoes with 1″ heels).

Weights at ages 25–59 based on lowest mortality. Weight in pounds according to frame (in indoor clothing weighing 3 lbs., shoes with 1″ heels).

Source of basic data: *1979 Build Study,* Society of Actuaries and Association of Life Insurance Medical Directors of America, 1980.

early warning signals. Likewise, writing down everything that you consume will dramatically increase your dietary awareness.

The most accurate way to estimate how much fat you're consuming is to write down everything you eat or drink during a three-day period to obtain an average, but even keeping a food log for one day will provide valuable information. Write down everything that you eat or drink, and estimate the amount and quantity as well as you can. (This is only going to be an approximation, so don't get overly concerned about accuracy.)

At the end of the day, consult the Appendix on pages 554–581. These list how much total fat and saturated fat are in a serving of each food item. (If you can't find the food listed, look for one that's similar.) If you eat a prepackaged food, read the label to determine how much fat is in it. Tally up the total fat and, if you have the information, the total saturated fat for that day.

How far are you from your goal? If you already have a diagnosed heart problem, then it will become apparent why, in practical

Table 2
Maximum Total Fat Intake: Men

Ideal Body Weight	Inactive	Moderately Active	Very Active
90	14	15	16
100	16	17	18
110	17	18	20
120	19	20	21
130	20	22	23
140	22	23	25
150	23	25	27
160	25	27	28
170	26	28	30
180	28	30	32
190	30	32	34
200	31	33	36
210	33	35	37
220	34	37	39

Find the figure in the left-hand column that most closely corresponds to the desirable weight you identified in Step 1. Then move across the chart to the vertical column that corresponds to your physical activity level. At the point where your ideal weight and activity level intersect, you will find the maximum amount of total fat (in grams) that you should consume each day.

Maximum Total Fat Intake: Women

Ideal Body Weight	Inactive	Moderately Active	Very Active
90	13	14	14
100	14	15	16
110	15	17	18
120	17	18	19
130	18	20	21
140	20	21	22
150	23	25	27
160	25	27	28
170	26	28	30
180	28	30	32
190	30	32	34
200	31	33	36
210	33	35	37
220	34	37	39

Find the figure in the left-hand column that most closely corresponds to the desirable weight you identified in Step 1. Then move across the chart to the vertical column that corresponds to your physical activity level. At the point where your ideal weight and activity level intersect, you will find the maximum amount of total fat (in grams) that you should consume each day.

Table 2
Saturated Fat Intake: Men

Ideal Body Weight	Inactive	Moderately Active	Very Active
90	5	5	5
100	5	6	6
110	6	6	7
120	6	7	7
130	7	7	8
140	7	8	8
150	8	8	9
160	8	9	9
170	9	9	10
180	9	10	11
190	10	11	11
200	10	11	12
210	11	12	12
220	11	12	13

Find the figure in the left-hand column that most closely corresponds to the desirable weight you identified in Step 1. Then move across the chart to the vertical column that corresponds to your physical activity level. At the point where your ideal weight and activity level intersect, you will find the maximum amount of saturated fat (in grams) that you should consume each day.

Saturated Fat Intake: Women

Ideal Body Weight	Inactive	Moderately Active	Very Active
90	4	5	5
100	5	5	5
110	5	6	6
120	6	6	6
130	6	7	7
140	7	7	7
150	7	8	8
160	7	8	9
170	8	9	9
180	8	9	9
190	9	9	10
200	9	10	11
210	9	11	11
220	10	11	12

Find the figure in the left-hand column that most closely corresponds to the desirable weight you identified in Step 1. Then move across the chart to the vertical column that corresponds to your physical activity level. At the point where your ideal weight and activity level intersect, you will find the maximum amount of saturated fat (in grams) that you should consume each day.

terms, the only way to keep your total fat and cholesterol consumption low enough is to eat a low-fat vegetarian diet such as the Reversal Diet.

For example, let's say your food diary shows that you ate the following foods during a twenty-four-hour period. You would find these foods in the Appendix and write down the number of grams of fat:

FOOD ITEM	GRAMS OF FAT	GRAMS OF SATURATED FAT
Breakfast:		
1 cup of cereal (Quaker Oatmeal)	2.4	0.4
1 cup of skim milk (on the cereal)	0.4	0.3
2 slices of whole wheat bread, toasted	1.6	0.2
2 tablespoons of apple butter (on the toast)	0.2	0.0
1 cup of orange juice	0.0	0.0
Lunch:		
1 cup of canned vegetarian vegetable soup	2.2	0.5
1 cup of spaghetti, egg-free	0.6	0.0
½ cup of tomato sauce (on the spaghetti)	0.0	0.0
1 cup of summer squash	0.2	0.0
1 grapefruit	0.2	0.0
1 club soda	0.0	0.0
Afternoon snack:		
1 apple	0.8	0.0
Dinner:		
1 cup of kidney beans	0.9	0.3
1 cup of brown rice	1.2	0.3
1 cup of lettuce salad	0.1	0.0
1 tablespoon of oil-free salad dressing	0.0	0.0
1 cup of herbal tea	0.0	0.0
1 stalk of broccoli	0.5	0.0
1 slice of angel food cake	0.1	0.1

On that day, your total fat intake was 11.4 grams and your saturated fat intake was 2.1 grams. Since your daily fat quota was 25 grams, you would want to *increase* your fat consumption if this was a typical day's food intake!

To make it easy for you to follow the Reversal Diet, Part 3 of this book provides over 150 recipes. All of these were analyzed by Dr. Shirley Brown, who listed the amount of total fat in each. Also, Part 3 contains 21 days of menus by Dr. Brown and Martha Rose Shulman. Each of these menus fits the guidelines of the Reversal Diet.

You may find that some food items aren't in the Appendix. If you want a more precise analysis of your current diet, contact a registered dietitian.

If you do not wish to keep track of how much fat you consume, then just follow the guidelines for the Reversal Diet outlined on page 256 and avoid eating any commercially prepared foods.

THE PREVENTION DIET

If you already have heart disease, then your body is probably not very efficient at metabolizing dietary cholesterol and saturated fat, so the Reversal Diet is very low in these. If you don't have heart disease, then you may be able to eat a diet higher in fat and cholesterol. But how high?

For many years, doctors have considered a cholesterol level between 240 and 280 as "normal." These values were obtained by taking a sample of everyone's cholesterol level in the United States and finding that the majority of Americans have cholesterol levels between 240 and 280.

But these values are *average*, not *normal*—and the average American gets a heart attack. As I mentioned earlier, no one in the Framingham Study has had a heart attack whose blood cholesterol level has remained consistently under 150. In countries where heart disease is very rare, blood cholesterol levels remain at about this level. Thus, a normal cholesterol level is around 150 or less.

The Prevention Diet is really very simple: If your cholesterol level is less than 150 (and you're not taking cholesterol-lowering drugs), or if your ratio of total cholesterol to HDL is less than 3.0, then whatever you are eating is probably sufficient to prevent heart disease.

Unfortunately, many adults in this country have cholesterol levels higher than this. If your cholesterol level is greater than 150 and you want to prevent heart disease, then gradually begin decreasing the amount of saturated fat and cholesterol in your diet. You may wish to begin by eating no more than double the amount of saturated fat or total fat recommended on the Reversal Diet.

Most people find that a relatively small number of food items account for a disproportionate amount of their daily fat intake: meats, ice cream, butter, eggs, nuts, cheese, and oils are common culprits. If you don't already have coronary heart disease, you may want to eliminate these high-fat foods first and then gradually decrease your fat consumption over a period of time.

After eight weeks, check your cholesterol level again. If it is still above 150, especially if you have other risk factors for heart disease, then you may want to consider reducing the amount of saturated fat and cholesterol in your diet even more. For example, eliminate red meats completely. Take the skin off chicken. Eat more fish. Avoid all fried foods. Have some vegetarian meals each week. Use as little oil as possible when cooking, and avoid using oil-based salad dressings. If you use oil, choose canola (Puritan) oil. Substitute two egg whites for each egg yolk when you bake. Have cereal instead of eggs for breakfast. Switch from whole milk to 2 percent, or even better, to skim milk. After eight weeks, measure your cholesterol level again.

Some people will find that moderate dietary changes are sufficient to bring their cholesterol levels down around 150. Others will find that more comprehensive changes are required in order to accomplish this.

A few people will find that even following the Reversal Diet is not sufficient to bring their cholesterol levels down to 150. Fortunately, the good news is that if you follow the Reversal Diet and the rest of the lifestyle program described in this book, then your risk of coronary heart disease will be low even if your cholesterol level does not come down to 150. As I described earlier, several of the participants in our study followed the program virtually 100 percent and showed some measurable reversal of their coronary atherosclerosis even when their blood cholesterol levels remained above 150.

Since there is a substantial amount of error in measuring cholesterol, be sure to have your cholesterol measured at a reliable laboratory, preferably more than one. For example, one lab may calculate your cholesterol to be 250, another lab might say it's 275, whereas a third laboratory might find it to be only 220. Labs associated with academic medical centers tend to be the most accurate, especially those certified by the Lipid Research Clinics. While there is a lot of variability between laboratories, the relative measures within the same laboratory usually are reliable, so make sure that the same lab does all of your cholesterol analyses.

Be aware that cholesterol levels tend to be about five to seven milligrams higher in the winter months than in the summer months (regardless of the climate where you live). Cholesterol measurements are most accurate when you have been fasting for twelve to fourteen hours before the blood sample is taken. The easiest way to do this is to have your blood drawn in the morning before eating breakfast.

The National Cholesterol Education Project and the American Heart Association recommend that most people reduce their blood level of total cholesterol to 200 and to reduce their LDL to below 130. While this is a step in the right direction, it may not be sufficient to prevent coronary heart disease for many people. How much you are willing to do is a personal choice.

In summary, the most effective way to prevent coronary heart disease is to follow the program outlined in this book and to:

- reduce your consumption of cholesterol and saturated fat sufficiently to keep your blood cholesterol level below 150, or
- follow the Reversal Diet, regardless of your blood cholesterol level

I would like to be able to say, "Just reduce your cholesterol and saturated fat consumption a little, don't worry about your cholesterol level," but it's not true for many people. If your cholesterol level is above 150 and you're not eating the Reversal Diet, then you're taking a chance on developing heart disease. How big a chance is impossible to quantify, since other risk factors are involved such as your age, blood pressure, family history, stress level, and sense of isolation, as well as whether or not you smoke, are overweight, have diabetes, are male or (if you are a woman) whether or not you are post-menopausal.

If your cholesterol level remains elevated and you are unwilling to modify your diet sufficiently, then you may want to consider taking a cholesterol-lowering drug, especially if you have coronary heart disease or several risk factors. While drugs are not the best first choice, it's better than doing nothing. Please discuss this question with your personal physician for more information and guidance.

DINING OUT

In the past, most people used to eat in restaurants only on special occasions. Now, it is the rule rather than the exception for many people. With time at a premium, eating out has become a way of life. Often both heads of a household are working—if there are even two members of a household. And for those whose business requires them to travel frequently, dining in restaurants can become an occupational hazard.

Eating out is also a social activity. Whether as part of a romantic courtship, a business luncheon, or a quiet evening with friends, sharing a meal together is a common way of increasing intimacy and social support. Precisely because of this, we may not want to look "different" when ordering food, especially if our dinner companions are eating a typical American diet.

I have been able to find food that meets the guidelines of both the Reversal Diet and the Prevention Diet in every city and in almost every restaurant, except when traveling in the Soviet Union. Even the large fast food hamburger, pizza, and steakhouse chains are beginning to include salad bars.

On either diet, you can eat at restaurants without much difficulty and without drawing attention to yourself. Staying on the Reversal Diet, though, requires a little more care and preparation, since most restaurants don't believe that a "little" butter or oil would matter.

Here's how:

- If you eat out frequently, get to know the chef and maître d' at two or three favorite restaurants. Most of the time they will be very supportive and flexible, although occasionally not. In general, the better quality the restaurant, the more receptive they will be. Spend a few minutes with them at an off-peak time and explain the guidelines of your dietary preferences. (You might even mention that you will refer other people there who are on the same diet.) This way, when you eat there with friends or business associates, you won't have to spend any time explaining your order to the waiter and drawing attention to yourself. Chances are that no one else will even notice what you're eating.
- When you plan to eat at a new restaurant, call ahead if possible and explain your dietary requests to the chef or maître d'. Is the food made to order or is it a "we heat 'em, you eat 'em" place? Baking, steaming, boiling, and poaching don't require the addition of oil—can the chef prepare something for you

in this way? Will he or she cook something for you without butter and oil? Will they put the sauce on the side? Does the restaurant offer fruit for dessert? Or a fruit sorbet?

- If you're at a new restaurant, and you haven't had time to call ahead, then have a little to eat before you go. When you arrive, look over the entire menu. Vegetable dishes are usually scattered throughout. Avoid foods that are fried, sautéed, au gratin, or creamed. If there are no vegetarian entrées, you may want to order a soup or a salad as your first course and two or three appetizers combined on one plate as an entrée. Avoid *prix fixe* or complete dinners, and order à la carte.
- If you see an interesting item on the menu, ask if the chef could modify it for you. For example, if the restaurant serves mushrooms sautéed in butter, ask if the chef could sauté the mushrooms in wine instead. If they offer a beautiful chef salad, ask if they could leave off the cheese and meat and use vinegar, lemon juice, or pepper instead of an oil-based salad dressing. If the baked potato is usually served with butter and sour cream, ask if it could be served plain, with some salsa, Dijon mustard, or a dollop of nonfat yogurt instead.
- In almost every fine restaurant, the chef will prepare for you a vegetable plate, fruit plate, or a special salad, even if these are not on the menu. If you order a vegetable plate, ask the chef to steam, boil, bake, or grill the vegetables and specify that he or she not use any oil or butter in preparing them.
- When traveling by air, request the dairyless vegetarian plate or the fruit plate. I am working with Continental Airlines to develop in-flight meals that meet the guidelines of the Reversal Diet, and these may soon be available. Carry with you a supply of beverages: herbal tea bags, individual-sized packets of Bambu, Pero, Postum, or whatever you prefer. Or order club soda, seltzer water, or juice during the flight.

Here are a few suggestions for specific types of restaurants:

- *French restaurants* usually have beautiful salads, rice, and vegetable side dishes. And French bread is usually made without oil or butter. Ask for the sauce on the side. Hollandaise/béarnaise and bechamel sauces are loaded with fat and cholesterol, so ask that these be omitted from your dish.

• At an *Italian restaurant,* order egg-free pasta with vegetables and a marinara or similar meatless sauce. In some Italian restaurants, the pizza can be customized: omit the cheese and top the pizza with vegetables and a tomato sauce. Some Italian restaurants serve potato gnocchi (dumplings) made without oil, eggs, or whole milk, and sometimes the minestrone or vegetable soups are vegetarian and made without oil or butter. Ask to be sure.

• *Chinese restaurants* often have a variety of vegetarian side dishes and entrées. Some cities, like San Francisco and New York, have Chinese restaurants with separate vegetarian menus, but almost all Chinese restaurants have at least one vegetarian entrée (usually called the "Buddha's Delight"), and many have more than one. Most Chinese restaurants cook each order separately, so it is easier for them to make the modifications you request. Stir-fried dishes are usually cooked in oil or lard, so ask the chef to stir-fry in water. Some Chinese restaurants use "dry wok cooking," a technique of sautéeing vegetables without using oil. The steamed white rice is fine, but avoid the fried rice, which is cooked with egg yolks and oil. Some Chinese restaurants will serve brown rice. Although Chinese tea may look herbal, it usually has the same amount of caffeine and other stimulants as regular tea.

• In *Mexican restaurants,* finding low-fat food can be challenging. Most Mexican dishes are fried or cooked with lard, meats, or cheeses. Soft "corn tortillas" may be all right since they are usually made only with corn flour, lime, and water, in contrast to "flour tortillas" which are usually made from wheat flour, water, and lard. Pinto beans or red beans are fine when cooked in a clear broth; unfortunately, most Mexican restaurants serve refried beans (frijoles refritos), which are made by frying the cooked beans in oil or lard. If you call ahead, you may be able to persuade the chef to prepare some beans for you in a clear broth and to make Mexican rice without oil. The combination of rice and beans is a complete protein. And you can wrap the beans in the corn tortilla, creating a bean enchilada.

• *Vegetarian, natural foods, or "health food" restaurants* often serve food laden with oils, cheese, avocadoes, nuts, and so on. So be careful. Some of the foods, though, are ideal. Many restaurants will prepare whole grain dishes, whole wheat breads, brown rice, and other healthful foods. Just use the same principles: Ask the chef not to use oil or butter, and search the menu for dishes that fit the guidelines either of the Reversal Diet or the Prevention Diet.

· When *going to a dinner party,* you may want to mention your dietary preferences to your hosts beforehand so that they won't be offended if you don't sample all of their foods. Ask them to prepare a few side dishes without oil or butter, and reassure them that they need not cook a special meal for you. Have a bite to eat before you go so that you're not too hungry when you get there.

QUESTIONS AND ANSWERS:

QUESTION: *Will I get enough calcium on the Reversal Diet? Should I take a calcium supplement?*

In brief, yes, you will get enough calcium on the Reversal Diet, and a calcium supplement is not necessary.

In countries where the majority of people eat a diet similar to the Reversal Diet, the incidence of osteoporosis is quite low, even though average calcium intakes are lower than in this country. Osteoporosis is a disease caused by bone demineralization.

Calcium levels are regulated very carefully by your body, so the amount of calcium in your bloodstream is kept in a very narrow range. Calcium deficiencies usually are caused by two factors: too little calcium in the diet, or too much excretion of calcium in your urine.

If either of these occurs, then your body begins to absorb calcium out of your bones in order to maintain a constant calcium level in your bloodstream. Over time, your bones can become demineralized (depleted of calcium), leading to osteoporosis. If the bones become sufficiently depleted, they'll fracture more easily, even from everyday activities.

Post-menopausal women are especially vulnerable, since high estrogen levels before menopause help to protect them against osteoporosis. When doctors learned of estrogen's protective effects, they began giving it to post-menopausal women to help prevent osteoporosis. Unfortunately, while estrogen does help to prevent osteoporosis, it may also increase the risk of developing breast cancer—not a very good tradeoff. This is another example of the difficulties that occur when we do not go far enough back in the causal chain of events, as described in chapter 2.

The real cause of osteoporosis in this country is not insufficient calcium intake, it's excessive excretion of calcium in the urine. Even calcium supplementation is often not enough to make up for the increased calcium excretion. Vegetarians, in contrast, excrete much less calcium, and this is why they have very low rates of osteoporosis even though their dietary intake of calcium is lower than those on a meat-eating diet.

At the University of Texas Medical School at Dallas, scientists conducted a study reported in the *Journal of Clinical Endocrinology and Metabolism* in 1988. They compared urinary excretion of normal subjects who were given two different diets: one diet contained only vegetable protein while the other diet contained only animal protein. Both diets had the same amount of protein, sodium, potassium, calcium, phosphate, and magnesium.

Urinary calcium excretion was *50 percent greater* on the animal protein diet than on the vegetable protein diet. The authors concluded that the inability of the subjects to compensate for the animal protein-induced loss of calcium in their urine might predispose them to develop osteoporosis as well as kidney stones.

In another report published in the *American Journal of Clinical Nutrition,* 1,600 women in southwestern Michigan were studied using direct photon absorptiometry to measure bone mineral density. Women who had been vegetarians for at least twenty years had only 18 percent less bone mineral by age eighty, whereas closely-paired women who ate a typical American diet had 35 percent less bone mineral.

In the study of 6,500 Chinese by Dr. T. Colin Campbell quoted earlier, he found that although most Chinese consume no dairy products and obtain their calcium from vegetables, osteoperosis is uncommon in China even though the people there consume only half the calcium as Americans. According to Dr. Campbell, "Ironically, osteoperosis tends to occur in countries where calcium intake is highest and most of it comes from protein-rich dairy products," which cause the body to lose more calcium than consumed.

Vegetarians absorb more of their dietary calcium than those eating a typical American diet. Also, exercise helps to prevent osteoporosis.

Eating one cup per day of nonfat milk or yogurt provides some extra calcium to help insure against osteoporosis without increasing protein intake excessively.

QUESTION: *Besides health, what are some of the other reasons that people choose a vegetarian diet?*

Many people are becoming increasingly concerned with our environment. As much as ten pounds of grains and soybeans are needed to produce just one pound of beef. Approximately 20,000 pounds of potatoes can be grown on one acre of land, whereas only 165 pounds of beef can be produced on the same area. Over 80 percent of the corn and 95 percent of the oats grown in the U.S. are eaten by livestock. And part of the reason for the destruction of tropical rain forests is to clear land for grazing to satisfy the demand for beef.

Pesticide residues are much greater in animal products than in plant foods. Also, antibiotics are routinely given to livestock, and there is some concern that these may increase bacterial resistance in animals and humans.

It is less expensive to eat vegetarian foods than meat. Animal products tend to be the most expensive items in the grocery cart. The people who can least afford the high cost of medical care can benefit the most from the low cost of the Reversal Diet.

QUESTION: *What about vitamins?*

Iron deficiency is common in many people in this country, vegetarians and nonvegetarians alike. Dark green leafy vegetables, iron-fortified cereals, and whole grains are good sources of dietary iron. Vitamin C enhances the absorption of dietary iron.

Some evidence indicates that vitamin A and vitamin E help to prevent oxidation of LDL-cholesterol and thus to help prevent coronary atherosclerosis. Vitamin B_6 deficiency may enhance the formation of coronary artery blockages. The requirement for vitamin B_{12} is minute and is contained in nonfat milk or yogurt. Vitamin D is obtained by spending some time in the sun or by eating fortified nonfat milk or yogurt.

Although both the Reversal Diet and the Prevention Diet provide sufficient vitamins, and minerals such as iron, I recommend taking a good multivitamin supplement that contains B_{12}, iron and trace minerals each day.

"Tobacco is a dirty weed. I like it.
It satisfies no normal need. I like it.
It makes you thin, it makes you lean,
It takes the hair right off your bean.
It's the worst darn stuff I've ever seen. I like it."

—Graham Lee Hemminger [1915],
Tobacco

■

"Tobacco is a filthy weed,
That from the devil does proceed;
It drains your purse, it burns your clothes,
And makes a chimney of your nose."

—Dr. Benjamin Waterhouse [1754–1846]

■

"Smoke, smoke, smoke that cigarette
Smoke, smoke, smoke it 'till you puff yourself to death.
Tell St. Peter at the Golden Gate,
That you hate to make him wait,
But you've just gotta have another cigarette."

—Commander Cody and
His Lost Planet Airmen

■

"Smoking is always having to say you're sorry."

—Dr. Tom Ferguson

■

"Smoking is the single most important preventable
cause of death in America."

—U.S. Surgeon General [1989],
The Health Consequences of Smoking

11

How to Quit Smoking

E xcept for the fact that it is addictive, makes you sick, and hastens your death, nicotine is a wonderful drug.

Nicotine calms you down when you feel stressed and wakes you up when you feel tired. It improves memory, decreases anxiety, raises tolerance of pain, lifts depression, increases metabolism (causing weight loss), reduces hunger, and improves performance, concentration, and problem-solving. No wonder people find it so hard to quit smoking!

Smoking cigarettes, in fact, is as physiologically and psychologically addictive as smoking crack cocaine or injecting heroin. Some scientists think it's even more so. A recent report from the Surgeon General stated that nicotine was far more costly and deadly on a national scale than heroin, cocaine, or alcohol. And while it's a crime to buy, sell, or use cocaine or heroin, cigarettes are available at every corner market.

You may have heard that you can become addicted to crack after only a few puffs. What is less well known is that after smoking even a few cigarettes, you can become addicted to nicotine. Up to two thirds of the teenagers who smoke as few as two cigarettes become habitual smokers. The first cigarette—like the first puff of crack cocaine or the first injection of heroin—usually makes you feel apprehensive, dizzy, and nauseous; you may even vomit. But when you ignore those warning signals and continue to smoke, then you quickly become addicted. When that happens, *stopping* smoking makes you feel bad.

It takes less time for the nicotine to reach your brain when you smoke than when you inject nicotine or other drugs intravenously! When you inhale cigarette smoke, it reaches your brain within six seconds, twice as fast as if you injected heroin.

In a recent article in *The New England Journal of Medicine,* Dr. Neal Benowitz wrote: "Many features of nicotine dependence resemble those seen in people dependent on other frequently abused drugs: heroin, alcohol, and cocaine. Cigarette smoking is a convenient and socially acceptable way to administer hundreds of doses of a psychoactive drug to oneself daily (four hundred puffs a day for a two-pack-per-day smoker)."

Dr. Richard Pollin, director of the National Institute on Drug Abuse, says cigarette smoking is now the most serious and most widespread form of addiction in the world—even worse than heroin. He calls smoking "the foremost preventable cause of excess death in the United States."

IT'S HARD TO JUST SAY "NO"

Because nicotine is so addictive, it is very hard to stop smoking. Tobacco has been consumed for many hundreds of years in countries throughout the world, and people have become addicted to nicotine in every one of these.

When smokers try to quit, the relapse rate is high, averaging 70 percent in three months. This relapse rate is similar to that observed in heroin addicts and alcoholics. Surveys indicate that over 90 percent of people who smoke cigarettes would like to quit but find it very hard to do so. The majority have tried to quit one or more times. As is often said, "Quitting smoking is easy—I've done it many times!"

Nicotine withdrawal is not pleasant. About 80 percent of people who stop smoking will experience a withdrawal syndrome and have a strong craving to smoke. Symptoms of withdrawal include restlessness, irritability, anxiety, drowsiness, headache, gastrointestinal disturbances, increasingly frequent wakings from sleep, impatience, confusion, and difficulty concentrating. Some performance measures, such as reaction time, become temporarily impaired. Metabolism slows, so there is a tendency to gain weight even if food intake remains the same.

Physiological withdrawal symptoms are most intense twenty-four to forty-eight hours after the last cigarette and gradually decrease in intensity over a period of two weeks. The psychological addiction, though, can last much longer. The desire to smoke, especially in stressful situations, can persist for months or even years. Some people who have given up cigarettes even have vivid dreams in which they are smoking long after they stopped.

SMOKING AND YOUR BRAIN

One of the remarkable properties of nicotine is that it can affect so many of your brain's hormones. These hormones, also called neuroregulators, include acetylcholine, norepinephrine, adrenaline, dopamine, beta-endorphin, and vasopressin. These brain chemicals make you feel good, and they are powerfully involved in feelings of reward and well being. By altering these chemicals, nicotine helps an individual cope better with stress. The rapid action of nicotine and its diverse neuroregulatory effects make it particularly effective in helping a person cope with the demands of daily living.

Smokers unconsciously learn to adjust their nicotine intake—how much they inhale and how long they wait before having another cigarette—to enhance these effects selectively. Depending on the dose, nicotine can make you calmer or more aroused. In this way, smokers can fine-tune these brain chemicals to make them feel more aroused or more relaxed.

Short, quick puffs (low doses of nicotine) tend to arouse the brain's function, helping a person think and concentrate better.

Long, deep drags (high doses) can help a person relax. In other words, smokers use cigarettes to help control their moods.

WHAT NICOTINE DOES

Sometimes taking risks can be fun. I probably take more chances than the average person. For example, in my personal life I've enjoyed skydiving and scuba diving; in my professional life, conducting this research project was risky. Almost all worthwhile adventures involve taking some chances.

Most smokers know that smoking can be harmful to them, but they often view it as another type of risk-taking behavior, like skydiving. That is, they realize that if something bad happens, it might be catastrophic, but if they're lucky, they might grow old without any harmful effects. Unfortunately, though, it doesn't work that way.

Every cigarette you smoke damages your health. Even if you never get heart disease or cancer later in life, each cigarette you smoke affects your health. And you can feel the difference, *right now.* You may be more motivated to quit by paying attention to these short-term effects rather than whether or not you're going to get cancer some day. What are some of these effects?

Most of nicotine's effects are due to its direct actions on your brain and nervous system. Nicotine, like emotional stress, stimulates your sympathetic nervous system and causes your body to produce more stress hormones such as adrenaline, more thromboxane, and less prostacyclin. As described in chapter 2, these changes cause your heart rate and blood pressure to increase, your blood to clot more easily, and arteries throughout your body to constrict. When you smoke:

- Blood vessels to your skin constrict. Because of this, your skin wrinkles more quickly. (This is one of the reasons why nicotine or stress can make you age faster.)
- Blood vessels to your heart constrict. Chest pain and heart attacks can result.
- Blood vessels to your brain constrict, which can cause strokes.
- Blood vessels to your hands and feet constrict. At a minimum, this causes cold hands and feet. In some cases, especially in people with diabetes, this can lead to gangrene and amputation.

- Blood flow to your sexual organs decreases. Although cigarette ads often suggest that it is macho to smoke, the Marlboro man may be impotent. Studies by Dr. Irving Goldstein of the Boston University Medical School have shown that nearly two thirds of impotent men smoke, almost twice the rate in the general population. He also found that the decrease in blood flow to the penis was directly proportional to the number of cigarettes smoked. Other studies have demonstrated that one in four smokers has poor circulation to the penis, compared to only one in twelve nonsmokers.
- Nicotine clearly decreases your senses of taste, touch, and smell, three of the most important senses of pleasure. Smoking is not a sensual experience.
- Women who smoke are three times more likely to be infertile than nonsmokers. They reach menopause almost two years earlier than nonsmokers. In men, smoking decreases sperm count and motility.
- Over a longer period of time, nicotine damages the lining of the arteries in your heart and throughout your body, causing blockages to form more readily, further decreasing blood flow.
- Nicotine, like chronic stress, causes your body to produce excess cortisol, which suppresses your immune system and increases the formation of arterial blockages.
- Nicotine increases the tendency of your heart to beat irregularly, increasing the risk of sudden cardiac death.
- You inhale a number of toxic gases, including carbon monoxide, formaldehyde, acetone, vinyl chloride, hydrogen cyanide, hydrogen sulfide, ammonia, and many others. Some of these, like polonium, are even radioactive. Besides the long-term risk of cancer, every puff causes a triple-whammy: (1) These gases irritate your lungs, causing more mucus to be produced. (2) Smoking weakens the ability of your immune system to attack harmful bacteria and viruses. (3) Nicotine paralyzes your lungs' natural cleaning mechanisms, so the mucus builds up and makes you more susceptible to bacterial and viral infections. Normally, thousands of small hairs, called cilia, beat back and forth and act as a type of "mucus escalator" to bring mucus in your lungs up to your throat where you can cough it up. Since nicotine paralyzes these cilia, though, the mucus remains deep in your lungs where it makes a home for harmful bacteria and viruses to live and multiply. Only when you are

asleep (and, hopefully, not smoking) do these cilia "wake up" and begin beating again. This is why most smokers cough up mucus when they get up in the morning. But these cilia aren't able to do twenty-four hours of work in only eight hours. Because of this, most smokers have bad breath, a chronic cough and shortness of breath, and they tend to fatigue more easily than nonsmokers.

THE HEALTH EFFECTS OF SMOKING

Over 350,000 people die prematurely in the United States each year from smoking-related deaths, more than the total number of Americans killed in World War I, Korea, and Vietnam combined. It has been estimated that 30 percent of the deaths from coronary heart disease, or 170,000 deaths each year, are attributable to smoking. Those who smoke at least a pack of cigarettes a day have two and a half times the risk of a heart attack as nonsmokers.

Smoking intensifies other health risks. For example, elevated cholesterol levels increase the risk of heart disease much more in smokers than in nonsmokers. Women who take birth control pills— especially those over forty—have a much higher risk of stroke or heart attack if they smoke than if they do not. Women over forty who smoke and take birth control pills have almost ten times the risk of death than nonsmokers who take birth control pills.

Also, 30 percent of the cancer deaths, or 125,000 deaths each year, are due to smoking. Between 80 and 85 percent of deaths from lung cancer are directly attributable to smoking, and lung cancer is one of the most difficult cancers to treat. Chronic bronchitis and emphysema account for another 60,000 smoking-related deaths. Smoking also substantially increases the risks of stroke, peripheral vascular disease, osteoporosis, glaucoma, and cancers of the mouth, esophagus, larynx, bladder, pancreas, stomach, kidney, and cervix.

People who smoke also have twice the amount of peptic ulcer disease. They also have higher rates of asthma, allergies, gum disease, headaches, and cough. Diabetics who smoke are eight times more likely to have complications than nonsmoking diabetics.

Babies of women who smoke have twice the incidence of low birth weights due to direct retardation of fetal growth as well as a higher incidence of birth defects and sudden infant death. Infants and children whose parents smoke have more frequent bouts of bronchitis and pneumonia. Surprisingly, children whose parents smoke have a higher incidence of respiratory illnesses later in life when they become adults, even if they never become smokers. And nonsmoking spouses of smokers face a 25 percent greater risk of contracting lung cancer than nonsmoking spouses of nonsmokers.

Despite this information, and even though the Surgeon General's warning is on every package of cigarettes, about one third of the men and women in this country still smoke. Are you ready to quit?

HOW CAN YOU GET THE BENEFITS OF SMOKING WITHOUT THE RISKS?

Each year 3.3 million Americans stop smoking. You can be one of them. There are many approaches to quitting smoking, and our program can make all of them more effective.

It's hard to quit smoking unless you have something else that can provide the benefits of nicotine. If smoking helps you relax, for example, then you're likely to feel more stressed when you quit smoking unless you have other ways of managing stress that aren't centered around cigarettes.

The Opening Your Heart program provides the beneficial effects of smoking without the harmful ones. This program addresses the underlying causes of why people smoke and offers something better in its place.

Because of this, paradoxically, it's easier to make comprehensive lifestyle changes than to make only a few. At first glance, you might say, "It's hard enough to stop smoking—how can you expect me to stop smoking, practice stress management techniques, begin exercising, change my diet, and give up caffeine, too?" But it's actually easier to make big changes than small ones.

Let's examine some of the benefits of smoking and how you can get these in other ways:

- *Smoking helps me keep my weight down.* Smokers weigh an average of three to five pounds less than nonsmokers because nicotine increases the body's metabolism, so calories are burned faster. Also, nicotine decreases appetite, so smokers tend to eat fewer calories than nonsmokers. Our program can also help you lose weight and keep it off. As explained in chapter 10, the Reversal Diet allows you to eat a larger amount of food yet consume fewer calories, so you can eat whenever you feel hungry. And your metabolism will increase on the Reversal Diet *without* using nicotine.

· *Smoking helps me concentrate better and improves my performance.* So do the meditation and stress management techniques described in chapter 7, and even more effectively. Nicotine does make it easier for people to focus and concentrate on accomplishing the tasks at hand without getting distracted as easily. However, the enhanced ability to concentrate and the "alert relaxation" that comes from meditation is similar to the one produced by nicotine.

· *Smoking helps me control my anger and hostility.* According to a report by British smoking researchers Heather Ashton and Rob Stepney, nicotine can decrease the arousal of the brain's limbic system, the part of the brain associated with anger. Meditation and stress management techniques accomplish something similar. As described earlier, many of the participants in our program who now meditate daily say things like, "I used to have a short fuse and explode easily, but now my fuse is much longer. The situations may not have changed, but *I* have in my reaction to them." More important, though, our program does more than suppress anger pharmacologically; it allows you to begin exploring and changing the roots of the anger.

· *Smoking makes me feel like I'm more in control of my life.* In part, this is due to the fact that people who smoke can regulate their nicotine doses several hundred times a day to fine-tune their mood. But smoking really gives only the illusion of control, since most people find it very difficult to control whether or not they continue smoking. In contrast, our program gives you real control over your health and your life.

· *Smoking helps me control pain, both physical and emotional.* Studies have demonstrated that smoking really does decrease smokers' awareness of both physical pain and emotional distress. As I have described throughout this book, though, becoming aware of pain—whether physical or emotional—can be the first step toward transforming our lives. Meditation, for example, allows you to become more aware of pain yet tolerate it better and to use it as a catalyst for healing.

- *Smoking helps me relax and cope with stress.* This book describes many other ways of relaxing and managing stress without using cigarettes. More important, these approaches can help you address the more fundamental causes of stress without simply using a cigarette to "bypass" them. It's very difficult to change only behaviors like smoking unless you also address emotional and spiritual issues such as loneliness, isolation, and unhappiness. Many people began smoking as teenagers out of a desire to be accepted by their friends.

- *Cigarettes are my friends.* One of the participants in our study described it this way:

When I quit smoking, the physical symptoms of withdrawal weren't as hard as the emotional ones. I've always been able to count on cigarettes to be there for me when I needed them—which hasn't always been true for other people in my life. Cigarettes never let me down. When I smoked a pack a day, I had twenty friends to keep me company throughout the day whenever I felt lonely. I felt like cigarettes loved me!

It was like being an abused woman who stays in the relationship. You know it's bad, but at least a bad relationship is better than being alone and isolated. I'd stopped for months at a time—long enough for the physical addiction to wear off—but when I felt particularly lonely, when I was by myself, I'd find myself reaching for a cigarette.

I can hide behind my cigarettes when people start to get too close. But when I stop smoking and then start again, I feel ashamed and my self-esteem gets even worse. So it's a vicious cycle: my low self-esteem makes me smoke, and smoking makes me feel bad about myself.

When I stopped smoking, at first I felt isolated and very alone. I mourned the loss of my friends. After awhile, I realized that *cigarettes are false friends.* They appeared to be helping me but they were really killing me. True friends are interested in improving my health and well-being, not in destroying it.

Once again, it becomes clear that feeling isolated and alone can lead to self-destructive behaviors like smoking. If we can begin to address the problem at that level, far enough back in the causal chain, then it becomes easier to let go of behaviors that harm us.

Setting up support groups with others who are stopping smoking and using the communication skills described in chapter 8 are some ways to help develop and maintain meaningful relationships and true friendships. These can help us experience the healing power of emotional intimacy rather than the destructive effects of smoking.

Many people report that they smoke as a way of shutting down or walling off their feelings, both from themselves and from others. When they stop smoking, these feelings resurface. While this can be an opportunity for real growth and transformation, as described in chapters 7 and 8, it may seem terrifying at first unless you have some support and guidance.

Sometimes it's a vicious cycle: a person may feel isolated, with low self-esteem and a poor sense of control over one's life. Smoking becomes very beguiling because it helps to block out the bad feelings and provides the illusion of control. Unfortunately, though, when a person decides to quit smoking, he realizes that it is the cigarette that is in control of his life, so the feelings of powerlessness and poor self-worth become magnified. Smoking can help deaden these feelings, and the cycle continues. A friend of mine described it to me in this way:

> Although I didn't realize it at first, I'd been using cigarettes as a way to keep people from getting too close to me. It was literally a smoke-screen—to hide my feelings from others and even from myself. I could conceal myself behind a veil of smoke. I didn't think about it most of the time, but it was very seductive. It was as though the cigarette whispered, "I'm there for you baby, don't worry, it'll be all right." But it wasn't all right.
>
> When I quit smoking, I finally realized how lonely I'd been feeling. For years! It was really hard at first, but allowing myself to experience fully the pain of loneliness helped me to begin overcoming my fears of intimacy.
>
> Now I'm in a real relationship with someone for the first time in several years. I might never have broken out of my shell if I hadn't quit smoking first. I didn't feel such a strong need to reach out when I could just light up another cigarette. But I wasn't very happy then. I'm much happier now, even though it's still really hard at times.

SHORT-TERM BENEFITS OF QUITTING

Efforts to motivate smokers to quit often focus on the long-term health risks of cigarettes—heart disease, cancer, and so on. But let's face it. As an intelligent person, you're probably well aware of the long-term risks, so if you smoke it may be because the perceived short-term gains are more meaningful to you than what seem like distant dangers. You may find it easier to quit if you remind yourself of the short-term gains that come from quitting smoking:

- Food will taste and smell better to you.
- *You* will taste and smell better, instead of tasting and smelling like an ashtray.
- If you're male, your sexual function will often improve. Besides the long-term effects of smoking on impotence described earlier, smoking has an immediate effect on sexual response. In one study, Dr. Mitchell Edson, a urologist in Washington, D.C., studied twenty impotent men who were heavy smokers. Normally, men have frequent erections during sleep, but these men did not, indicating that the problem was physiological and not psychological. Six weeks after they quit smoking, seven of these men had regular nocturnal erections.
- If you already have heart disease, quitting smoking will often decrease the frequency and severity of your chest pain almost immediately. And for everyone, with or without heart disease, quitting smoking will improve your fitness, endurance, and athletic performance.
- It's becoming socially less acceptable to smoke. Recently, smoking has been banned on most U.S. airline flights. More than half of American businesses prohibit smoking in work areas, and the number is increasing rapidly. Some ban smoking altogether. A few, like Turner Broadcasting in Atlanta, won't even hire smokers. Many cities are restricting smoking in public buildings and restaurants. If you quit, you won't have to slink off to the restroom like a junkie in search of a fix.
- You'll save money. A two-and-a-half-pack-a-day habit costs about one thousand dollars over the course of a year—money up in smoke. Cigarette prices have doubled in the past five years, so the costs of smoking are likely to increase even more.
- You'll have fewer colds and infections.
- Your chronic cough may begin to disappear.

LONG-TERM BENEFITS OF QUITTING

In addition to the many short-term benefits of stopping smoking, here are only a few of the long-term benefits:

- Five years after quitting, an ex-smoker has a risk of lung cancer mortality 60 percent lower than a current smoker.
- Fifteen years after quitting, ex-smokers are no more likely to get lung cancer than nonsmokers.
- Only one year after quitting, the risk of dying from a heart attack in male ex-smokers is cut by 50 percent.
- Ten years after quitting, male ex-smokers have the same mortality rate from heart disease as nonsmokers. A recent study by Dr. Lynn Rosenberg found that female ex-smokers have the same mortality rate from heart disease as nonsmokers only two to three years after quitting.

HOW TO QUIT

Most people who give up cigarettes do so on their own, without joining a formal stop-smoking program. The single most important factor for people who successfully quit smoking was the belief and confidence that they could do it. And you *can* do it. But there is no magical quick fix. Don't quit until *you* are ready. Do it in your own way and in your own time.

Quitting smoking is a process, not a one-time event. Alcoholics Anonymous teaches people to abstain from drinking one day at a time, but smokers begin to go through withdrawal several times an hour, so it's especially challenging to quit.

Most people who eventually quit smoking were not able to do so the first time. In a study of 1,000 smokers trying to quit, only 172 succeeded on the first attempt. Another 53 quit after the second try, 48 more quit after three attempts, and so on. In all, 387 of the 1,000 smokers eventually quit, but some required seven or more attempts before they finally stopped smoking. We all fell down many times before we finally learned how to walk or ride a bicycle.

Practicing each part of the Opening Your Heart program on a daily basis is one of the most effective ways of quitting smoking. At first, you may feel ambivalent about quitting. After all, smoking provides a lot of benefits, as described earlier. But if you begin practicing our program on a regular basis, you may find that the desire to smoke begins to decrease on its own.

There are many other resources available to help you stop smoking. One of the best books is *The No-Nag, No-Guilt, Do-It-Your-Own-Way Guide to Quitting Smoking* by Dr. Tom Ferguson. In this book, he reminds the reader that quitting is not simply a matter of willpower; it is a matter of acquiring and practicing a variety of skills. Here are some of the ones that he recommends:

- Buy a package of 3 × 5 index cards and write a reason to quit on each. Carry them with you and review them when you feel the urge to smoke.
- Set a date to quit at a time when you're not likely to be under a lot of stress.
- Visualize yourself as a nonsmoker.
- Write down whenever you smoke and whatever you are feeling at the time.
- Keep plenty of raw fruits and vegetables handy to munch on.
- Avoid caffeine. Some research suggests that caffeine increases the craving for nicotine.
- Avoid alcohol. People often associate drinking and smoking. Also, alcohol diminishes self-control.
- Get your teeth cleaned the day you quit smoking, and brush your teeth several times a day.
- Take lots of warm baths or showers.
- Get a massage.
- Ask your friends to be supportive without being judgmental. Warn them that you're likely to be irritable and grumpy, especially during the first few weeks. Give them specific suggestions on what they can do (and *not* do) that would feel supportive to you. In particular, ask them not to smoke around you, to offer you cigarettes, or to undermine your efforts.
- Find a friend to quit smoking with you. Support one another. Call each other when you feel tempted to start smoking.
- Read everything you can on the effects of smoking and how other people have succeeded in quitting.
- Throw away your ashtrays and smoking paraphernalia.
- Go for a long walk.

- Have your car cleaned. Wash out the ashtray and fill it with toothpicks or flowers.
- Have the inside of your house cleaned, including carpets, drapes, and furniture.
- Have your clothes laundered or dry cleaned.
- Announce that you are quitting to your club, religious group, or friends, and ask them to support you.
- If you find yourself smoking, don't berate yourself for being "weak" or "no good." As Dr. Ferguson writes, "A slip or two on the way to eventual success does not make you a failure. The only real failure would be giving up your efforts to quit."
- Pay attention to the role smoking plays in your life.
- Observe the ways nonsmokers respond to those situations to which you respond by smoking.
- Smoke an entire cigarette while standing in front of a mirror. What feelings do you have while doing this?
- Ask people you know who are former smokers what they found helpful in quitting.
- Sit in the nonsmoking section of airplanes and restaurants.
- Give yourself a reward or special treat each day.
- Notice and write down how your health is improving and how much better you are feeling after the first week of withdrawal is over.
- If possible, schedule frequent vacations or weekend trips.
- After you have been a nonsmoker for at least a few months, offer to help someone else quit.
- Keep your hands busy.
- Put a drop of clove oil on the back of your tongue when you feel the urge to smoke.
- Listen to music.
- During the first few weeks after you stop smoking, avoid social gatherings where there will be drinking and smoking.

CLONIDINE

Clonidine, a medicine used to treat high blood pressure, also has been used to help people withdraw from heroin and other narcotics by reducing the physiological craving for these drugs. More recent studies (including one by my brother Steven Ornish, M.D.) have found that clonidine also helps to reduce the physiological craving for nicotine and the discomfort of nicotine withdrawal.

Clonidine is available in "patches" that are worn for several days while the medication is absorbed slowly through the skin. These patches, manufactured under the brand name Catapres-TTS, are available in different dosages ranging from #1 (0.1 milligram of clonidine per day) to #4 (0.4 milligrams of clonidine per day). Clonidine is available only by prescription and should be used under a doctor's supervision.

One approach is to begin with the #2 strength patch unless you are small or have a blood pressure less than 100/70. (Most people find that the #1 patch is not strong enough to achieve the desired effect.) Since it takes three or four days for the clonidine to reach a therapeutic level, you may wish to quit smoking on the fourth day. Although each patch is supposed to last a week, I find that the dose tends to taper off after five days. Because of this, you'll need to apply a new patch every five days for a total of three or four weeks.

Like all drugs, clonidine has side effects. The most common are drowsiness and a dry mouth. The sedation is mild for some, but for others it can be a problem. Some people report feeling a little "spacy." The sedative effect usually peaks on the third or fourth day and diminishes as the person becomes more used to the clonidine. The dosage can be reduced if side effects remain a problem.

People using clonidine should abstain from alcohol and should not drive or work around machinery if they feel tired. Their blood pressure and heart rate should be monitored at least once a week. If your blood pressure becomes too low, if you become lightheaded, or if you notice an increase in chest pain, then stop using the clonidine. About 10 percent of people develop a contact dermatitis at the site of the patch. If this occurs, a steroid cream can help, or the medication can be discontinued.

While clonidine can help reduce the physiological cravings, it is not a magic treatment and it does not address the more powerful psychological cravings involved in smoking. For some people, though, it can be a useful adjunct to our program in helping them to quit smoking.

WHERE TO GO FOR MORE HELP:

- Your doctor.
- The American Lung Association sponsors stop-smoking groups in most cities. It also publishes *Freedom from Smoking for You and Your Family*, a twenty-day program to help you stop smoking. This book is available from the American Lung Association, 1740 Broadway, New York, NY 10019, or from your local chapter.
- The American Cancer Society's Fresh Start program is also an excellent resource. This program provides four one-hour sessions over a two-week period. The American Cancer Society also publishes a free handbook called the *I Quit Kit*, available from the American Cancer Society, 4 West 35th Street, New York, NY 10001, or from your local chapter.
- The American Heart Association has a number of excellent brochures on the effects of smoking on your heart and suggestions for how to quit. Some local chapters have support groups for people who are stopping smoking and making other lifestyle changes.
- Smokers Anonymous provides information on support groups for people who stop smoking (P.O. Box 25335, West Los Angeles, CA, 90025).
- Other stop-smoking programs are offered at community centers, YMCAs, hospitals, and private companies such as Smokenders or Schick.

Remember, quitting smoking is a process. Even if you don't succeed the first time, don't get disheartened. You *can* do it.

"With an unquiet mind, neither exercise, nor diet, nor physick can be of much use."

—Samuel Johnson (1709–1784)

■

"No less than two hours a day should be devoted to exercise."

—Thomas Jefferson (1743–1826)

■

"If the man who wrote the Declaration of Independence, was Secretary of State, and twice President, could give it two hours, our children can give it ten or fifteen minutes."

—John F. Kennedy (1917–1963)

■

"Do you exercise, Dr. Salk?"
"I exercise restraint."

—conversation with Dr. Jonas Salk

■

"I get my exercise acting as a pallbearer to my friends who exercise."

—Chauncey Depew (1834–1928)

■

"The secret of my abundant health is that whenever the impulse to exercise comes over me, I lie down until it passes away."

—J.P. McEvoy (1938), *American Mercury*

■

"Just do it."

—Nike advertisement

12
How to Exercise

I t took me years before I learned to enjoy exercising. I attended public schools in Dallas, where exercise was often the preferred form of punishment (compounded by the fact that my history teachers were usually football coaches): "Ornish—your homework is late. Run five times around the track!" Or: "You were talking during study hall. Take a lap—now!" I got in good shape from all that running, but I didn't like it.

I still don't enjoy running, but I love tennis, basketball, swimming, cycling, dancing, and other activities. So I do those instead.

Whenever I go to a health club or gym and see people working out with pained expressions on their faces, I find myself thinking, "If they're going to be expending that much energy with so little enjoyment, they might as well be doing something more useful—or at least more fun."

Calvin and Hobbes   **by Bill Watterson**

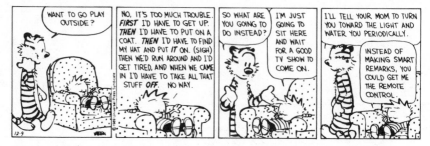

And that is the point: if exercise is fun, then you'll do it. If you do it on a regular basis, then you'll feel better, you'll look better, and you may even live longer. But if it's not fun, or if it's not part of your daily activities, then you probably won't do it for very long.

I mean, let's face it. Exercise is not very complicated, although people sometimes try to make it so. Most people know that exercise is good for them and they know how to do it. Designing a program is relatively easy. *Doing* it on a regular basis, however, is another story.

JUST DO IT

The good news is that you don't really have to exercise very much in order to get most of the health benefits. A recent study by Dr. Steven Blair and his colleagues at the Institute for Aerobics Research, published in the *Journal of the American Medical Association*, indicated that even a little exercise goes a long way. They performed treadmill testing on 10,224 men and 3,120 women who were apparently healthy. Based on their fitness level, these participants were divided into five categories, ranging from least fit (group 1) to most fit (group 5). The researchers followed these people to determine how their level of physical fitness related to their death rates.

After eight years, the least fit (the sedentary group 1) had a death rate more than three times greater than the most fit (the very active group 5). More important, though, was the finding that most of the benefits of physical fitness came between group 1 and group 2, particularly in men (see figure 12.1).

The Reward of Fitness: Longevity

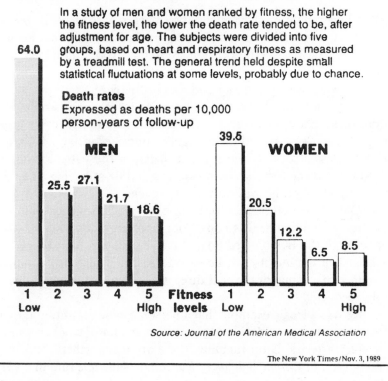

In a study of men and women ranked by fitness, the higher
the fitness level, the lower the death rate tended to be, after
adjustment for age. The subjects were divided into five
groups, based on heart and respiratory fitness as measured
by a treadmill test. The general trend held despite small
statistical fluctuations at some levels, probably due to chance.

Death rates
Expressed as deaths per 10,000
person-years of follow-up

64.0

MEN

25.5 27.1

21.7

18.6

39.5

WOMEN

20.5

12.2

6.5   8.5

| 1 Low | 2 | 3 | 4 | 5 High | Fitness levels | 1 Low | 2 | 3 | 4 | 5 High |

Source: Journal of the American Medical Association

The New York Times/Nov. 3, 1989

Figure 12.1

In other words, walking 30 minutes a day (the activity level of group
2) reduced premature death almost as much as running 30 to 40
miles a week (the activity level of group 5). Further, in groups 2
through 5, deaths were lower from *all* causes, including heart disease
and cancer, when compared with the sedentary people in group 1.

Similar results were found in 12,138 middle-aged men who
participated in the Multiple Risk Factor Intervention Trial. The
investigators, directed by Dr. Arthur S. Leon, divided these men into
three groups based on level of exercise. During seven years of follow-
up, those who exercised moderately had one-third fewer deaths from
all causes (including heart disease) than those who were sedentary.
Moderate exercise was defined as at least 30 minutes a day of light
or moderate intensity activities such as walking, gardening, or home
repairs. Mortality rates of those with high levels of exercise were not
significantly different from those with moderate levels of exercise.

FITNESS AND HEALTH ARE NOT THE SAME

When I was an intern, working in the emergency room at the Massachusetts General Hospital in Boston on January 9, 1982, a nurse announced on the overhead paging system, "Room three, five minutes away." Room three was the cardiac arrest room, so all of us stopped what we were doing and ran in there.

A few minutes later, the paramedics wheeled a stretcher into room three. On it lay an unconscious man with no pulse. We began pumping his chest, inserting intravenous lines, recording EKGs, and so on. I was struck by the contrast between the patient's athletic physique and the fact that he was in the middle of having a massive heart attack. And he was only thirty-seven.

Then I noticed he was wearing a World Series ring. Someone else recognized that he was Tony Conigliaro, formerly a star baseball player with the Boston Red Sox. Because his heart had stopped for at least five minutes before he arrived in the emergency room, he remained in a coma for the next three weeks. Unfortunately, he never fully recovered.

He was a tragic example that a person can be very fit, muscular, even a world-class athlete, and yet still have a lot of blockages in his coronary arteries. Unfortunately, there are many others. Jim Fixx, who wrote *The Complete Book of Running*, died while running. Peter Maravich, the former basketball star, died while playing basketball with some friends. French athlete Jacques Bussereau died while running in the 1984 New York Marathon.

Exercise will make you fit, but fitness and health are not synonymous. Exercise alone is not enough to make you healthy. To achieve good health, exercise is an essential part of a comprehensive lifestyle program, such as the Opening Your Heart program.

"Fitness" refers to your level of conditioning, also referred to as the "training effect." The simplest measurement of fitness is how long it takes for your heart rate to return to normal after vigorous exercise. The sooner your pulse returns to its usual resting rate, the more fit you are. Another measurement of fitness is your resting pulse rate—the slower it is, the more fit you are (assuming you are not taking cardiac medications). A third measurement of fitness is how far and long you can exercise.

"Health" refers to your overall state, defined by the *American Heritage Dictionary* as "the overall condition of an organism at a given time; optimal functioning with freedom from disease or abnormality." The World Health Organization defined health as "a state of complete physical, mental, and social well-being, not merely the absence of disease or infirmity." With respect to your heart, "health" refers to how much blockage is present in your coronary arteries and how much blood flow your heart receives.

SHOULD YOU EXERCISE TO LIVE LONGER?

Moderate exercise seems to be enough to make you *healthy*—only 30 minutes of walking or similar activities once a day or an hour of walking three times per week. If you want to become more *fit*, in contrast, you'll need to expend a minimum of 2,000 calories a week on some form of continuous, sustained (also called "aerobic") exercise.

Approximately 100 calories are burned off per mile, whether the mile is covered by walking briskly or jogging. For example, approximately 2,000 calories are consumed in:

- running three miles in 30 minutes, six days a week;
- swimming for 30 minutes, six days a week;
- playing singles tennis for 1 hour, five days a week;
- walking four miles in 1 hour, five days a week;
- cross-country skiing for 30 minutes, six days a week;
- aerobic dancing for 40 minutes, five days a week.

Dr. Ralph Paffenbarger of Stanford University sent questionnaires to 16,936 Harvard alumni, aged thirty-five to seventy-four, to determine the influence of exercise on longevity. (His study is considered less precise than the Blair study, since he used self-reported questionnaires rather than actually measuring fitness levels.) Dr. Paffenbarger found that men who expended 2,000 calories per week exercising lived one to two years longer than sedentary individuals.

The problem is that over the course of your adult life, you would need to spend about one and a half years running to live one to two years longer. To run off 2,000 calories per week, you need to run three miles in 30 minutes six days a week. Since it takes another 30 minutes to go to and from the track and to get dressed, shower, and undressed, then it will require at least 1 hour six days a week, or 6 hours per week, or over 300 hours per year. If you begin exercising when you are thirty, then by the time you are seventy-five you will have spent $45 \times 300 = 13,500$ hours running. If you calculate that the average person spends 16 hours awake every day, then $365 \times 16 = 7,940$ hours per year awake. In other words, you may spend one and a half years of your waking hours running—about as much time as you lengthen your life by running.

For this reason, it may be a mistake to exercise more than walking 30 minutes a day just to live longer. If you choose to do more, then do it because you *enjoy* it, not just to live longer. If you enjoy running, for example, then run. Even if you don't enjoy running but you like the way it makes you look or feel afterwards, then do it for those reasons.

Fortunately, according to the studies of Dr. Blair and Dr. Leon, people who walk 30 minutes a day live longer anyway, without having to do more vigorous exercise.

NO PAIN, NO PAIN

At a national meeting of the American College of Sports Medicine (ACSM), University of Pittsburgh epidemiologist Dr. Ron LaPorte noted the lack of data to support what he termed the "myth" that the reason people who exercise have lower rates of heart disease is because they are more fit. He said:

> I think the ACSM guidelines are probably wrong. Our belief system and the ACSM guidelines predict that you have to do aerobic exercise three times a week at 80 percent of maximum heart rate to reap the benefits of physical activity—that you have to be at the upper end of the fitness dimension to reduce risk. But in fact the primary reduction of heart disease is in moving from extremely low levels of fitness to the next higher level.

Recent ACSM president Peter Raven agreed that it's time to "back off on the Mr. Macho concept. The idea that if you can't run a marathon, you're not fit, is ridiculous. We've been bombarded with going for the burn, and it's probably totally incorrect." He also pointed out that that kind of attitude may have turned off many individuals who could benefit from moderate exercise.

Some of the early exercise enthusiasts, ranging from Jane Fonda to Dr. Kenneth Cooper, wrote about the importance of regular, vigorous exercise. Jane Fonda preached, "Go for the burn—no pain, no gain." People began discussing their resting pulse rates at dinner parties. A person's level of fitness became still another way to set himself apart from other people.

But you don't have to suffer to feel good. You can make exercise a "playout" instead of a workout. I play tennis whenever I can because I enjoy the game and I like the way it makes me feel afterwards. And I walk daily. I have more energy and endurance when I exercise regularly.

In summary, then, moderate exercise is enough to provide you with almost all of the health and longevity benefits without most of the risks of more intense exercise. If you want to do more, the rest of this chapter will explain how to do it more safely. But do more only if you *want* to, not because you think you *have* to.

This is especially reassuring since the risks of sudden cardiac death during exercise increase in direct proportion to the intensity of exercise. The association of exercise with sudden death is rare but more than coincidental. In a study of sudden death while jogging in Rhode Island from 1975 through 1980, Dr. Paul Thompson found that only one death per year occurred for every 7,620 joggers. Nevertheless, the death rate during jogging was estimated to be seven times more than during sedentary activities. The risk of sudden death during exercise was particularly high for men who were unaccustomed to physical activity. As Dr. Thompson wrote, "Vigorous exercise both protects against and provokes sudden cardiac death. Similar findings were reported in a different study by Dr. David Siscovick when he was at the University of Washington in Seattle. He found that while vigorous exercise was protective overall, it increased the risk of death during exercise.

But moderate exercise, like walking, helps protect against sudden cardiac death (and other diseases, even cancer) without substantially increasing the risk of sudden cardiac death. This is particularly important for people who already have diagnosed heart disease, for whom the risks of exercising are even greater.

In our research, we chose walking as the preferred form of exercise, since *walking provides most of the health benefits along with the lowest risk of injury or sudden cardiac death.* We asked our study participants to walk for only thirty minutes a day or for an hour every other day.

Walking thirty minutes a day or for an hour three times a week is the minimum amount of exercise recommended in the Opening Your Heart program. This amount of exercise is enough to receive most of the health benefits with the least risk of injury or death. Doing this on a regular basis will make you feel better, and you may live longer, too.

Almost anyone can find enough time to walk this amount—consider going for a walk on your lunch hour. You won't even have to change clothes or shower afterwards. Instead of settling in for a drink and the evening paper when you get home, try first going out for a walk before dinner. Bring your spouse or a friend and talk about your day; use the time to unwind and build friendship and intimacy. Or try getting up a half hour earlier and taking a refreshing morning walk to start your day.

More exercise than this will make you more fit—but not necessarily healthier. Consistency is more important than intensity.

USE IT OR LOSE IT

If you'd like to become more fit as well as healthier, you'll receive additional benefits. Your muscles, like your capacity to love, only increase with use. If you want to do more than walk thirty minutes a day, you'll primarily benefit your skeletal muscles used during exercise rather than your heart.

Fitness, also called the training effect, refers to how efficiently your body can extract oxygen from the blood and transport it to your muscles during exercise. Regular exercise increases the number of small blood vessels to your muscles, thereby supplying them with more blood and oxygen, and also increases the number of mitochondria that supply energy inside muscle cells. In other words, a fit person can exercise longer before getting tired—more work with less effort.

Regular exercise can also help you reduce your percentage of body fat. As you age, your weight may remain constant but your percentage of body fat may increase. Over time, your total body weight may begin to increase as well. Exercise can help to reverse this process.

Also, exercise can increase your bone density, reduce your blood pressure, decrease the formation of blood clots, raise the level of

HDL ("good") cholesterol, and lower your triglycerides. Exercise allows diabetics to burn off fat instead of carbohydrate more efficiently.

HOW TO EXERCISE SAFELY

If you decide you want to do more than walking, and if you are over thirty, then consult your physician first. This is especially true if you have diagnosed heart disease, hypertension, or other special conditions. Your doctor, knowing your specific medical history, may be able to tailor a program to better fit your condition. He or she may suggest that you take an exercise stress test (in which you run on a treadmill while your blood pressure and electrocardiogram are monitored) before you begin a vigorous exercise program to screen for any underlying heart disease and to identify the appropriate intensity of exercise for you.

Health clubs and gyms are one way to exercise, but many people can't afford to join these. Other people don't have time to go on a regular basis. Some think it's a little absurd to get in a car and drive to a health club where they pay to walk on a treadmill—instead of just walking around the block a few times. It's all a question of what motivates you and what you find fun and relaxing.

The most efficient way to exercise is to make it part of your daily activities and routine.

- Instead of driving, walk or bicycle to work or to the store. If that's not practical, park a little farther away (where the parking places are usually easier to find, thereby also reducing your stress level).
- Take the stairs instead of an elevator, especially if you're going only one or two floors.
- If you use the moving sidewalks at airports, don't just stand there—walk!
- Set aside some time after work to go for a walk with a friend, a loved one, or a family member. Going for a walk with a loved one is a way to increase intimacy as well as exercise.
- If you play golf, walk instead of using an electric cart.
- Exercise with family or friends to provide social support for more motivation and a double benefit.

- Dance.
- Take little adventures—walk in new environments.
- On a vacation, walk rather than drive to see and experience the sights.
- Write time for exercise in your appointment book—in ink.

To achieve a training effect, exercise must be of a particular type, frequency, intensity, and duration.

Type of Exercise

Your body produces energy in two ways: the *anaerobic* system (which doesn't require oxygen) and the *aerobic* system (which does).

The anaerobic system is designed for short, quick, intense bursts of energy, the kind you use sprinting or dashing for a train. The anaerobic system provides you with instant energy, but it is relatively inefficient. Because of this, it generates large amounts of waste products such as lactic acid, which causes muscle cramps, soreness, and pain.

The aerobic system is much more efficient, and it provides most of the energy you use when you exercise for more than a few minutes. When you first begin to exercise, or during short bursts of high-intensity exercise, your body draws on anaerobic metabolic sources. After the first minute or so, an increased amount of oxygen-rich blood reaches your muscles. At that point, the aerobic energy system is turned on.

Understanding the differences between these two systems explains why it's so important to warm up before exercising. If you begin exercising too quickly, without warming up, you'll draw too heavily on your anaerobic system. As a result, you'll fatigue quickly and build up a lot of lactic acid. Likewise, cooling down for a few minutes after exercising allows your body time to return to normal.

Regular activation of the aerobic energy system causes it to become more efficient. In order to get a training effect, the type of exercise you choose must use large muscle groups (such as your arms and legs), be rhythmical, and be continuous. Examples of aerobic exercise are brisk walking, biking, jogging, rowing, swimming, cross-country skiing, and aerobic dance. Activities in which you move only intermittently, such as golf, baseball, or bowling, tend to activate the anaerobic system and thus do not help to achieve as much of a training effect.

Frequency of Exercise

If you exercise at least three times per week, you will show a conditioning response. However, there is a proportional increase in orthopedic or overuse injuries in people who exercise at high intensities more than five days per week. This is an area where you will need to personalize your program to fit your schedule and how your body reacts to exercise. Respect your body's limits and avoid exercising to the point of pain or injury.

Intensity of Exercise

If you regularly exercise between 45 and 80 percent of your functional capacity (also called your maximum heart rate), you will exhibit a training effect and improve your fitness level. But how do you know what your functional capacity is?

If you have had an exercise treadmill test, then your functional capacity is simply the maximum heart rate, measured in beats per minute, reached during your test. If you have not had an exercise test, you can estimate your maximum heart rate by subtracting your age from 220.

For example, let's say you are forty-two years old and you reached a maximum heart rate of 170 on your treadmill test. To exercise between 45 and 80 percent of your functional capacity, simply:

      (a) take 45 percent of 170 = 77.1;
      (b) take 80 percent of 170 = 136.

Thus, to achieve a training effect, you should keep your pulse rate between 77 and 136 beats per minute. This range is called the "target heart rate."

Let's say you are thirty years old and you've never had a treadmill test. Your estimated maximum heart rate is 220 − 30 = 190. To exercise between 45 and 80 percent of your functional capacity, simply:

      (a) take 45 percent of 190 = 85.5;
      (b) take 80 percent of 190 = 152.

Thus, to achieve a training effect, you need to keep your pulse rate between 85 and 152 beats per minute. Clearly, this is a wide spectrum, so begin exercising at the low end of this range and *gradually* begin to increase it over time. Most of our research participants began exercising at 45 percent of their functional capacity and gradually increased over the first three months of the study to 60 percent and, in a few cases, as high as 80 percent. Use common sense and avoid overdoing it.

Another method is called the Karvonen Equation, which takes into account your resting heart rate:

Training heart rate$_1$ = [(maximum heart rate − resting heart rate) × (0.45)] + resting heart rate

Training heart rate$_2$ = [(maximum heart rate − resting heart rate) × (0.80)] + resting heart rate

The Karvonen Equation is more complicated but is currently the one recommended by the American College of Sports Medicine.

If you have known heart disease or are on any heart medications, then these formulae may not be appropriate for you. If so, then please consult your physician for your proper target heart rates. In general, your physician will ask you to keep your maximum heart rate approximately ten beats per minute slower than the heart rate at which abnormalities begin to appear on your exercise electrocardiogram.

The average target heart rate for asymptomatic adults should be between 60 and 75 percent of maximum heart rate. People with low functional capacities, including some cardiac patients or those who have never exercised, should begin at 45 to 50 percent.

HOW TO TAKE YOUR PULSE

· Using the pads (not fingertips) of the first two fingers, find your pulse at either the carotid artery (at the neck), as shown in figure 12.2, or at the radial artery (at the wrist), as shown in figure 12.3. Do not press hard, especially at the carotid pulse, as pressure on this artery can sometimes slow the heart.

· Begin counting when the second hand of a clock or watch is at a point where a ten-second interval will be easily distinguished.

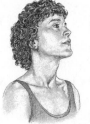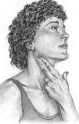

Figure 12.2

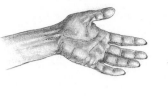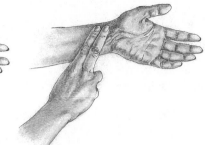

Figure 12.3

- Starting with the number 0 as a baseline, begin counting the number of heart beats felt for a ten-second interval.
- Multiply this number by six to get your pulse rate for one minute.
- Take your pulse before, during, and after exercise to properly monitor your exercise.

There are two other ways to monitor the intensity of your exercise: the Talk Test and the Rate of Perceived Exertion.

THE TALK TEST   If you're not exerting yourself too much, then you should be able to carry on a conversation while you exercise—that is, to "talk while you walk." If you can't talk while you exercise, then you may soon experience the "talk while you drop" phenomenon because you probably don't have enough oxygen available for your working muscles.

The talk test is particularly good for those who have difficulty in taking their pulse. The limitation of this method is that it will only indicate if you are exercising too hard or at too high an intensity, but it will not identify if you are at the minimum intensity level for proper exercise training.

THE RATE OF PERCEIVED EXERTION TEST   The other measure of intensity is purely subjective, based on your perceived exertion—in other words, how hard you *feel* like you are exercising. The Borg Scale for Rate of Perceived Exertion (RPE), developed by Gunnar Borg, is based on the premise that people are very capable of identifying their exertion levels. It also reminds us to listen to our bodies and to modify our exercise levels based on how we feel day to day and even moment to moment.

Rate of Perceived Exertion (RPE)		
6		
7	Very, very light	
8		
9	Very light	
10		
11	Fairly light	
12		Ideal Aerobic Exercise Levels
13	Somewhat hard	of Perceived Exertion
14		
15	Hard	
16		
17	Very hard	
18		
19	Very, very hard	
20		

The Borg Scale for Rate of Perceived Exertion (adapted from: G.V. Borg, *Medical Science Sports Exercise*, 14:377–87, 1982).

To use the RPE scale, simply identify which number (6 to 20) best identifies how you are feeling while you exercise. The number six is equivalent to lying down, doing nothing at all. The number twenty is equivalent to your maximal effort, the hardest you've ever exercised. Ideally, when you exercise aerobically, your RPE should be between 11 and 15.

Duration of Exercise

For an optimal training effect, exercise continuously for thirty to sixty minutes at your target heart rate, not including warm-up or cool-down periods. Although they were required to walk only thirty minutes, the participants in our study averaged forty minutes of aerobic exercise a day, five to seven times per week.

You will likely experience the most significant training effect during the first four to eight weeks of the Opening Your Heart Program. Younger, healthier, and more fit people may experience changes a little faster than older, symptomatic, or sedentary individuals.

Ideally, I suggest that you increase the duration of exercise before increasing its intensity. Your first goal should be to exercise a minimum of thirty minutes a day in whatever blocks of time you can sustain (for example, one thirty-minute walk, two fifteen-minute walks, five six-minute walks, and so on). Once you can do thirty minutes of sustained exercise, you only need to exercise once a day. After reaching the thirty-minute goal, you may want to gradually increase the time by five-minute increments every one or two weeks. In our study, the people who demonstrated the most reversal of their coronary artery blockages exercised five to seven hours per week. Those people also tended to follow the Reversal Diet better and to do the stress management techniques more regularly, so it's hard to determine how much of their improvement was due to the exercise alone.

You will notice that along with your increased ability to exercise longer, you'll be able to exercise more intensively. To decrease your risk for injury, which might cause you to stop exercising altogether, begin your program at 50 to 70 percent of your maximal heart rate and an RPE = 10 to 13, and as soon as you can tolerate forty-five minutes of continuous exercise, *gradually* increase to 60 to 80 percent of your maximal heart rate or an RPE = 11 to 15.

Twelve-Week Walking Program for the Low Fit and Beginning Exerciser.

> Week 1—Walk fifteen minutes, two times per day at a target heart rate (THR) of 50–60 percent maximum intensity, six to seven days per week. RPE = 10–12
>
> Week 2—Walk twenty minutes, two times per day at THR of 50–60 percent maximum intensity, six to seven days per week. RPE = 10–12
>
> Weeks 3–5—Walk thirty minutes per day at a THR of 50–70 percent maximum intensity, six to seven days per week. Add 5 minutes each week. RPE = 10–13
>
> Weeks 6–8—Walk forty to fifty minutes per day at a THR of 60–75 percent maximum intensity, six to seven days per week. RPE = 11–14
>
> Weeks 9–12—Walk forty to sixty minutes per day at a THR of 60–80 percent maximum intensity, six to seven days per week. RPE = 11–15

The elements of training for fitness can be summarized using the FITT Principle of Frequency, Intensity, Time/Duration, and Type:

The FITT Principle

*F*requency—three to seven times per week

*I*ntensity—Target Heart Rate (THR) of 45
          to 80 percent of maximum
         —Rate of Perceived Exertion (RPE)
         of 11 to 15
         —"Talk While You Walk"

*T*ime/Duration—thirty to sixty minutes *not*
               including warm up/cool
               down. Minimum of three
               hours per week.

*T*ype—Exercise that uses large muscles, is
         continuous and aerobic.

THE EXERCISE SESSION

Your exercise session contains three phases:

Warm-up phase (five to ten minutes): This helps to make the transition from anaerobic to aerobic metabolism. During this time, you gradually increase your cardiovascular system workload (heart rate and blood pressure) and body temperature to help avoid injuries and muscle soreness. Start your warm-up with gentle stretching of the muscles you plan to use. (For example, stretching the leg muscles if you are going to walk.) The stretches described in chapter 7 are ideal; some others are included here. Follow this brief stretching with three to five minutes of low-intensity aerobic exercise.

Exercise phase (twenty to sixty minutes): Do the aerobic exercise of your choice at an appropriate intensity.

Cool-down phase (Ten to fifteen minutes): Ease into three to five minutes of low-intensity aerobic exercise followed by a few minutes of stretching. The cool-down phase is at least as important as the warm-up phase. During aerobic exercise, your blood vessels begin to dilate in order to supply more blood (and oxygen) to your muscles.

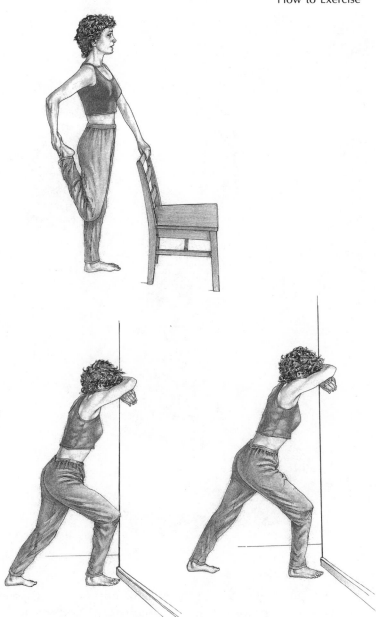

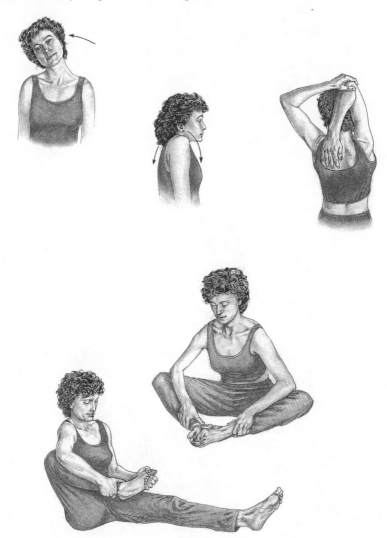

The cool-down phase allows time for your blood vessels and your heart to resume their normal state. Otherwise, blood pools in your legs if you stop suddenly, so you may not get enough blood to your brain. This is the reason some people feel lightheaded if they stop exercising too quickly without cooling down first. It's a good idea to continue to cool down until your heart rate is within ten beats per minute of your pre-exercise heart rate.

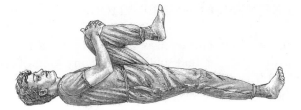

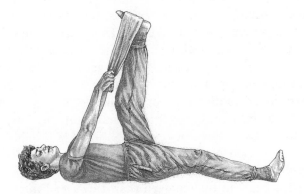

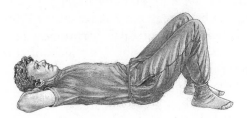

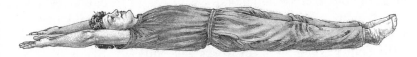

SPECIAL EXERCISE CONSIDERATIONS

After eating. Your mother was right—it's not a good idea to swim after eating. Or, for that matter, to do any kind of strenuous exercise on a full stomach.

Your body is continually making decisions regarding where to send blood. Some organs, like your brain, always have priority and are assured of getting enough blood flow except in the most dire circumstances. Blood flow to other organs, such as your muscles or your digestive system, can vary considerably during the day.

When you eat a big meal, your digestive system tells the brain, "Hey, send more blood down here—we've got a lot of work to do!" When you run, your legs tell your brain the same thing. There isn't enough extra blood to do both jobs adequately, so if you run on a full stomach, you may find that your legs will cramp or your stomach will begin to hurt.

This is one reason why people who have heart disease sometimes experience chest pain following a big meal. Enough blood is shunted away from the heart to the stomach that it can lead to chest pain.

After smoking. Smoking at any time is not a very good idea, as I described in chapter 11, but it's a particularly bad idea to smoke within two hours of beginning to exercise. Smoking limits your blood's oxygen-carrying capacity and constricts your coronary arteries, so there may not be enough oxygen available to your muscles and your heart. This can lead to chest pain (or worse, a heart attack).

After drinking alcohol. Exercising after alcohol consumption may precipitate heart arrhythmias.

Hot weather. Because it puts an extra burden on your cardiovascular system, hot weather can greatly decrease your tolerance for exercise. It can cause potentially serious problems such as heat cramps, dehydration, and heat stroke. This is particularly true when it's humid, since humidity makes it more difficult for your body to cool itself (sweat evaporates less readily).

When exercising in heat or humidity, decrease the duration and intensity of your exercise and monitor your heart rate closely. Allow your body more time to warm up and cool down. Also, drink plenty of fluids, preferably water, before, during, and after exercise to ensure the body's cooling system works efficiently.

Cold weather. Like excessive heat, cold weather also makes your cardiovascular system work harder and can cause your arteries to constrict. Both of these factors can lead to chest pain in people with heart disease who exercise in cold weather. Cold weather also can cause frostbite and hypothermia. When the wind chill factor is less than 15° Fahrenheit, the risk of problems increases greatly.

Avoid heat loss. Dress in layers, and remove extra clothing as you warm up. Keep your skin dry. Wear a hat and gloves to protect your extremities. Decrease your exercise intensity and pace yourself. If it's cold and windy, begin your session by walking into the wind and end by walking with the wind, you'll tire less easily.

Altitude. The higher you go, the less oxygen is available to breathe. Because of this, it takes more effort to run the same distance in Denver, the "Mile-High City," as it does in Houston. (Because of the high altitude, not many world records were set by runners at the Olympics when it was held in Mexico City.) Those with heart disease may experience increased angina when exercising at high altitudes.

Therefore, decrease both the intensity and duration of your exercise at high altitudes. If you plan to hike or exercise above 8,000 feet, consult your doctor first. To avoid high altitude sickness, acclimatize yourself by ascending only 1,000 to 2,000 feet per day.

Medications. Many prescription drugs can affect your body's response to exercise and your exercise tolerance. Below is a chart of commonly prescribed medications and their effects on the body during exercise.

These effects are dose-related—the higher the dose, the greater the effect. For some medications (especially heart medications) it is important to exercise when the drug levels are constant and at their peak level. It is probably a good idea for those taking cardiac drugs to exercise two to four hours after taking their medications. On the other hand, it's important to limit your exercise if you've missed a dose of medication or right before taking a scheduled dose because your blood levels of the drug may be low.

Illness. Avoid exercising when you're ill, especially when you have a fever. Exercise may exacerbate the illness. Rest, take it easy, and let your body heal itself. Then resume your exercise program at a lower intensity and duration and gradually increase to previous levels.

Injuries and other warning signs. Exercise with awareness. Listen to your body before, during, and after you exercise.

Overexertion. When you've overdone it, you will feel fatigued long after your usual recovery time. Your heart rate may not

Commonly Prescribed Medications and Their Effect on the Body During Exercise

MEDICATION	EFFECT ON CARDIOVASCULAR SYSTEM WITH EXERCISE
Cardiovascular	
1. Beta blockers (Inderal, Lopressor, Visken, Corgard, Tenormin, Blocadren)	Decreases heart rate, decreases blood pressure, sometimes increases exercise tolerance
2. Diuretics (Hydrochlorothiazide, Lasix, Diuril)	Potential for decreasing potassium, which can increase arrhythmias
3. Nitrates (Isordil, Nitro-Bid, Persantine, Nitro-Dur, Peritrate, Cardilate)	Increases heart rate, decreases blood pressure
4. Calcium channel blockers (Procardia, Calan, Isoptin, Cardizem)	Decreases blood pressure, may increase or decrease heart rate
Non-Cardiovascular	
1. Bronchodilators (aminophylline, theophylline, albuterol, isoproterenol)	Increases heart rate, may increase or decrease blood pressure. May cause arrhythmias and ischemia
2. Thyroid medications (levothyroxine)	Increases heart rate and blood pressure
Other	
1. Nicotine	Increases heart rate and blood pressure. May provoke ischemia and arrhythmias
2. Alcohol	May provoke arrhythmias

return to its pre-exercise level as quickly as normal. Review why this may have happened. Did you get enough sleep the previous night? Did you push yourself too much in the workout?

Orthopedic injury. Orthopedic injuries can occur not only from direct injury, as when you twist your ankle or knee, but also from overuse or from improper or worn-out workout shoes or equipment. If you get hurt, use the RICE Principle below to decrease the pain and inflammation. If you suspect any serious injury, then consult your physician.

The RICE Principle

*R*est

*I*ce the injured area twenty minutes at a time each hour the first day and then twice a day for the next two days. (Those with peripheral circulatory problems should not use ice.)

*C*ompression—use an elastic bandage to hold ice pack on injured area.

*E*levate the injured area to a level above the heart.

Other warning signs. If you experience any of the following during or after exercise, see your doctor promptly:

· Dizziness
· Recurrent and excessive fatigue
· Unusually heavy sweating
· Rapid or irregular heartbeats
· Unusual shortness of breath
· Poor recovery
· New or increased chest, jaw, back or arm pain, or anginal pain that does not go away with rest or after taking two nitroglycerin pills

SPECIAL CONDITIONS

Diagnosed medical problems may affect your exercise performance, so it is important to modify and adapt your exercise program to allow for safe, optimal cardiovascular conditioning. The following are guidelines to modify the FITT Principle on page 338 for those in special circumstances. Consult a physician before starting an exercise program if you have a medical illness.

Diabetes Mellitus

Exercise can be beneficial for both Type I (childhood-onset) and Type II (adult-onset) diabetics. In general, an exercise program is not recommended for diabetics whose blood sugar is out of control.

If you have insulin-dependent Type I diabetes, you need to monitor your blood sugar carefully, especially when beginning an exercise program. Physical activity has an insulinlike effect on the body, so you may need to decrease your usual amount of insulin. Especially during exercise and immediately afterwards, be aware of hypoglycemic symptoms (dizziness, hunger, weakness). To avoid hypoglycemia:

- Monitor your blood glucose before and after activity and modify your insulin dosage accordingly.
- Keep easily digested carbohydrates such as fruit juices easily accessible.
- Avoid exercise at times of peak insulin response.
- To keep absorption of insulin more constant, inject the insulin in a non-exercising muscle (e.g., your abdomen).
- You may need to decrease insulin by one to two units or increase your consumption of carbohydrates by ten to fifteen grams for each thirty minutes of exercise. Keep track of your blood glucose levels and show these to your physician for more precise advice on how to titrate your insulin level when you exercise.

Diabetics have an increased incidence of peripheral circulatory problems. If you have diabetes, wear clean cotton socks and shoes that cushion and support your feet well. Shower afterward to avoid athlete's foot.

If you have diabetic retinopathy, avoid any jumping or jarring activities that increase pressure around the eyes (for example, toe-touches, sit-ups, or any exercise where the head is in a dangling position).

Diabetics can modify the FITT Principle as follows:

Frequency—seven days per week for Type I diabetics with stable insulin and diet patterns; five to seven days per week for Type II diabetics with stable insulin and diet patterns.

Intensity—Target Heart Rate (THR) of 50 to 70 percent of maximum due to high exercise frequency. Those with neuropathy who often have difficulty taking pulses should use an RPE of 10 to 13.

Time/Duration—thirty to forty minutes for Type I; forty to sixty minutes for Type II.

Type—Any aerobic exercise; although overweight Type II diabetics and those with retinopathy should choose nonweight bearing exercise (cycling, swimming) to decrease risk for orthopedic injury.

Hypertension

Although exercise raises your blood pressure while you exercise, regular exercise tends to lower it the rest of the time. Even without weight loss, regular exercise helps prevent high blood pressure. In Dr. Paffenbarger's study of Harvard alumni described earlier, those who did not engage in sports were 35 percent more likely to develop high blood pressure than those who did play sports.

Sometimes exercise and dietary changes help normalize blood pressure so that medications are no longer needed, as many of our study participants found out. Blood pressure medications can sometimes alter a person's response to exercise, so if you are taking medication for your blood pressure, be aware of possible side effects. People with hypertension can follow the FITT Principle as described on page 338.

Peripheral Vascular Disease

People who have peripheral vascular disease often must limit their daily activities because they develop leg pains (claudication) during exercise. Regular aerobic exercise will often help to increase the time they can exercise before getting claudication.

Exercise physiologists generally recommend that even if exercise causes some mild leg pain when you begin, you may be able to work through it. You should consult with your physician to be sure. Use a pain scale to help judge the pain: 0 = no pain; 1 = light, barely noticeable pain; 2 = moderate pain; 3 = intense pain; 4 = excruciating, unbearable pain. Modifying the intensity of exercise according to the pain scale and your target heart rate, as indicated below:

Frequency—five to seven days per week.

Intensity—THR of 50 to 80 percent of maximum capacity, RPE of 11 to 15, up to a 2 on the 0 to 4 pain scale.

Time/Duration—Thirty to sixty minutes, with intermittent rests if claudication pains exceed 2 on the pain scale.

Type—Limit weight-bearing activity which increases leg pain. Try cycling or swimming or exercising in a warm pool.

Pulmonary Disease (Emphysema)

People with chronic obstructive pulmonary disease (COPD) should be screened by a pulmonary specialist before beginning an exercise program. They should develop an exercise program with their physician, one that will probably follow the following FITT Principle.

Frequency—Seven days per week.

Intensity—50 to 75 percent of maximum exercise ventilation (determined by a pulmonary exercise test).

Time/Duration—Four 5-minute sessions, two 10-minute sessions, or whatever is tolerated, then gradually increase time to 40 minutes per day.

Type—Anything aerobic, except for upper body exercise (rowing) due to the increased ventilatory effort it requires.

Arthritis

If you have osteoarthritis, avoid any exercise that produces excessive stress on your affected joints. Exercise is important to increase and maintain flexibility, strength, and range of motion, but it should not provoke excessive pain. The following FITT Principles apply:

Frequency—Seven days per week.

Intensity—THR of 50 to 80 percent of maximal capacity or as joints tolerate

Time/Duration—Thirty to sixty minutes per day. Break your exercise sessions down into smaller segments with multiple sessions per day, if necessary.

Type—Aerobic exercise, but no weight-bearing exercise during inflammatory periods. Try swimming or exercising in a warm pool.

In summary, if your goal is a healthier heart and a longer life, then walking thirty minutes a day, or one hour three times a week, is enough to provide you with most of the benefits of exercise with few of the risks. Other than a pair of comfortable shoes, you don't need any special equipment or training. It's easy, it's not complicated, and it can be fun. So get moving!

PART THREE

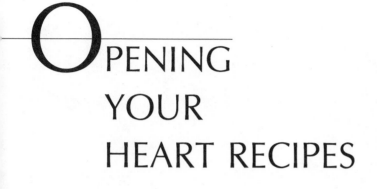

OPENING YOUR HEART RECIPES

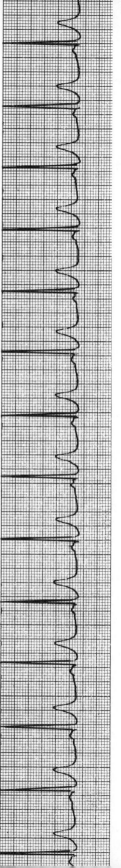

Introduction to the Recipes

by Shirley Elizabeth Brown, M.D.,
and Martha Rose Shulman

One look at the recipes in this book and you will let go of any preconceived ideas you may have had about the incompatibility of healthy, meatless, low-fat eating and gastronomic pleasure. This is not a diet of deprivation; it is, on the contrary, a diet vibrant with color and rich with the flavors and textures of many different foods—fresh vegetables, tangy herbs and pungent spices, chewy, wholesome grains, savory beans, elegant pastas, and sweet, enticing fruit dishes. There are enough delicious and beautiful dishes here for you to cook something different every day for months. And you will quickly appreciate how light and satisfied these meals leave you feeling.

Vegetables, grains, and dried beans are the backbone of the diet. If you have been used to a meat-and-potatoes diet up until now, some of the grains and beans might be new to you, but none are exotic; they are all easy to find in most supermarkets and natural foods stores, and getting to know them will be an adventure. All of the recipes and menus have been conceived with great attention to color and vivid taste, so that when you begin to work with the grains and beans you won't be disappointed by the drab characteristics you may have associated with vegetarian cuisines in the past. The ingredients will quickly become familiar and indispensable as you begin to use them in salads, main dishes, side dishes, soups, and even desserts, flavoring them with various herbs and spices and combining them with sparkling, crunchy vegetables and sweet, juicy fruits.

Over the last few years in the United States a new awareness and demand for good, fresh, seasonal produce has evolved, so that the fruits, vegetables, and herbs you will come across in these recipes will be easily available in supermarkets and farmers' markets. Walk through these markets and let the beauty of the produce inspire you; you will find recipes here for practically any vegetable that catches your eye.

You will also discover that many of your favorite dishes are easily adapted to the new dietary guidelines. Thumb through the recipes here and you'll find appetizers like the Red Pepper Coulis (page 400), chili recipes that can be used in sumptuous offerings like the Black Bean Burritos (page 443), hearty stews, lasagna and manicotti. And there are many other luscious pasta dishes such as Pasta with Asparagus and Asparagus Cream (page 461) or Linguini with Roasted Red Pepper and Herbed Tomato Sauce (page 463). You'll find enchiladas, burritos, and many familiar soups and curries. Those who like Chinese and Japanese food will have plenty of marvelous stir-fries to choose from ("fried" without oil), pungent combinations of vegetables, tofu, noodles, and grains. And if you have a sweet tooth you needn't despair: It's easy to make melt-in-your-mouth desserts without pounds of butter and sugar, fruit desserts such as Pear Cobbler (page 537) or Glazed Fruit Tart (page 539), warm compotes, baked and poached apples and pears, elegant combinations of fresh fruits and sweet wines, and comforting puddings.

Salads will take on a whole new meaning to you as you discover combinations such as Cauliflower with Lime and Hot Pepper Vinaigrette (page 404), Watercress, Fennel, and Orange Salad (page 416), Potato Salad with Tomatillo Sauce (page 412), and Baby Lima Bean

Salad (page 424), to name just a few. Hearty soups such as Lentil-Hominy Soup with Lime and Chili (page 487), White Bean and Tomato Soup with Fresh Herbs (page 486), Spanish Chick-Pea and Garlic Soup (page 485) and lighter soups such as Gazpacho (page 477) and Carrot Soup with Ginger, Orange, and Cilantro (page 477) will surprise and delight the palate. You'll find an international array of main dishes. Asceticism just doesn't have a place here.

On each recipe page you will find information to help you with menu planning.

The *yield* will tell you the quantity or volume that the recipe as written will produce. The *number of servings* will help you plan how many people you'd like to feed with a certain dish. Although a specific serving size will be used for the nutrient analysis (see below), you can of course vary it.

At the bottom of each recipe there is information regarding the calories, fat, cholesterol, and sometimes salt content for each recipe. If you have any concern over portion size, it will probably center around the amount of total fat and saturated fat in the recipes given here. Most of the *nutrient analysis* is based on some reasonable serving size, often a 1-cup portion. Use this as a reference and not as a guide to how much you can or should eat.

For explanatory purposes, let's assume that you are on a 10 percent fat diet and that you are limiting yourself to a total of 15 grams of fat for each day. If you eat three meals a day, the average total fat content for each meal should be approximately 5 grams of fat.

Look at the Spanish Chick-Pea and Garlic Soup (page 485). One cup of this soup contains a total of 2.9 grams of fat per cup (most of the other soups contain less fat). One and a half cups of this soup will contain 4.4 grams of fat, and two cups will have 5.8 grams of fat. What you have had for breakfast or plan to have for supper will determine how much of the soup you will have, and what you plan to eat with it. This is how to use the nutritional information.

The number of calories are provided for those watching their weight, although calorie count isn't really necessary because you will probably lose excess weight naturally while eating as much as you want. For those with high blood pressure or congestive heart failure problems, the amount of sodium is given wherever it may be an issue for that recipe.

BEGINNING THE TRANSITION

Although you may find these recipes and menus so tempting that you want to plunge right into the new diet, it may make sense to some of you to make a gradual transition. If this way of eating is completely new to you, small progressive changes will be easiest. Start by reducing your consumption of red meat by having lean cuts no more than once or twice a week, then once every two weeks, and so on until you've cut it out altogether. Do the same with poultry and fish. Gradually eliminate cheese and other high-fat dairy products. Replace full fat or partially skimmed milk and yogurt with their nonfat counterparts. You can use Butter Buds and similar products as a substitute for butter and margarine. You'll also find egg substitutes such as Egg Beaters, but read the labels carefully; some of these products are high in fat.

Take it one step at a time. As you begin to switch the focus of your diet, begin to experiment with grains, legumes, vegetables, and tofu. Try a new grain, bean, or vegetable dish every week. You will discover a new world of textures and flavors as you explore these new dishes.

ADAPTING RECIPES

There is no need for you to throw out all of your old cookbooks. You can learn to adapt dishes you already enjoy. Certain familiar meals, such as lasagna, pizza, and chili and soups such as split pea soup and minestrone can be adapted to meatless versions without sacrificing their character (see, for example, the recipes on pages 464, 516, 445, and 488). Recipes that contain oil can be easily adapted by changing a few simple techniques. In many cases, you'll find you can omit the oil altogether without changing the character of the dish; other times, as in the salad dressings and purees in this book, you can substitute another ingredient, such as yogurt, tofu, or tomato juice, for oil, with good results.

Begin by leafing through your cookbooks. Turn first to the vegetables section, then look at pasta and rice dishes, salads, soups, and whole-grain baked goods and grains. Some contain meat, and almost all will contain oil or butter and salt. Many will contain milk, eggs, cream, or cheese. If you want to convert a recipe to a low-fat, vegetarian version, try making it first without the oil and/or animal products. If the recipe contains meat (such as stews, stir-fries, pastas, casseroles, and soups), simply eliminate the meat. If you want to substitute something for texture or bulk, try equivalent measures of one of the following:

- cooked grains such as rice, bulgur, millet, couscous, or wheat berries (perfect for many casseroles)
- cooked beans, texturized vegetable protein, dehydrated bean flakes (in casseroles)
- finely chopped steamed vegetables, such as carrots, onions, squash, or mushrooms (in pasta sauces or stews)
- grated carrots (in pasta sauces, chili, and stews)
- diced or crumbled tofu (as a cheese or ground beef substitute in sauces; as a meat substitute in stews and soups)

If a recipe calls for sautéing vegetables in oil or butter, cook them until tender in a small amount of water, vegetable stock, or wine. This can be done with or without covering the pan and is called braising. The longer the cooking time, the softer the vegetables will become, and if they cook too long they will lose some of their color. After braising the vegetables, you can add the remaining ingredients. Many vegetable dish recipes call for sautéing, but they will taste just as good if the vegetables are steamed, braised, baked, or microwaved before being mixed with other ingredients. Experiment with these cooking methods.

Here are some examples of how to modify recipes using these guidelines:

UNMODIFIED WHITE BEAN AND FRESH TOMATO SOUP
WITH PARSLEY SAUCE
FROM *The Greens Cookbook*

BY DEBORAH MADISON

The Stock

Use the broth from the beans alone or in combination with the Summer Vegetable Soup Stock (page 472).

The Soup

3/4 cup dry navy beans
10 cups water
10 fresh sage leaves or 1 teaspoon
  dried sage
4 cloves garlic
3 bay leaves
6 thyme branches or 1/4 teaspoon
  dried thyme
3 tablespoons virgin olive oil
Salt
1 medium red or yellow onion,
  finely chopped
1 pound ripe tomatoes, peeled,
  seeded, and chopped

Freshly ground black pepper
Parsley Sauce

Parsley Sauce

1 cup Italian parsley leaves,
  loosely packed
2 cloves garlic
1/4 teaspoon salt, preferably coarse
  sea salt
3 tablespoons virgin olive oil
3 tablespoons freshly grated
  Parmesan
Red wine vinegar

Sort through the beans and remove any small stones and chaff. Rinse the beans well, cover them generously with water, and set them aside to soak overnight.

Next day, pour off the soaking water and cover the beans with 10 cups fresh water. Add half the sage, 3 garlic cloves (peeled and left whole), 2 bay leaves, the thyme, and 1 tablespoon olive oil. Bring to a boil, add 1 teaspoon salt, lower the heat, and cook the beans at a simmer or slow boil until they are tender but not mushy, about 1 hour. Remove them from the heat and strain, reserving the broth.

Slowly warm the rest of the oil in a soup pot with the remaining sage, garlic (roughly chopped), and bay leaf for 1 or 2 minutes; then add the onion and cook until it is soft, about 8 to 10 minutes. Stir in the tomatoes; then add 6 to 7 cups of the bean broth or vegetable stock and 1/2 teaspoon salt. Bring to a boil and simmer for 20 minutes. Add the beans and cook another 10 minutes.

Season to taste with salt and freshly ground black pepper. The soup may be served immediately or set aside for later. Just before serving, prepare the Parsley Sauce. Reheat the soup and garnish each bowl with a generous spoonful of sauce.

To make the parsley sauce, finely chop the parsley. Pound the garlic with the salt in a mortar until it is a smooth paste. Add a tablespoon or so of the parsley and work it vigorously into the garlic; then stir in the olive oil, cheese, and remaining parsley. Add red wine vinegar to taste, and season with salt if necessary.

The above recipe contains 6 tablespoons of olive oil and 3 table-spoons of cheese. The easiest way to modify the recipe and lower its fat content is simply to delete the oil and cheese without changing the other ingredients. The rich flavor of this soup will not be lost.

The parsley sauce calls for olive oil and the required cheese. These add flavor, and the olive oil gives the ground herbs and garlic a smoother, more saucelike consistency.

If the oil is omitted, there are several options available to provide the appropriate texture. Lemon juice, wine, vegetable stock, herbed or wine vinegars will all add flavor to the sauce and the right consistency. Just plain water could also be used, but it would take away from the flavor of the herbs.

If you don't need to eliminate salt, you could add it here for further flavor enhancement.

MODIFIED VERSION OF WHITE BEAN AND TOMATO SOUP WITH PARSLEY SAUCE

The Stock

Use the broth from the beans alone or in combination with the Summer Vegetable Soup Stock (page 472).

The Soup

¾ cup dry navy beans
10 cups water or vegetable stock
10 fresh sage leaves or 1 teaspoon
    dried sage
4 cloves garlic
3 bay leaves
6 thyme branches or ¼ teaspoon
    dried thyme
Salt
1 medium red or yellow onion,
    finely chopped
1 pound ripe tomatoes, peeled,
    seeded, and chopped

Freshly ground black pepper
Parsley Sauce

Parsley Sauce

1 cup Italian parsley leaves,
    loosely packed
2 cloves garlic
Salt to taste
3 tablespoons vegetable stock
Red wine vinegar
Freshly ground black pepper
    (optional)

Follow the original recipe as written except for those instructions that pertain to the olive oil. After the beans have been soaked and drained, add half of the sage, 3 cloves garlic, 2 bay leaves and the thyme. Omit the olive oil from this step.

Use a small amount (about 2 to 4 tablespoons) of the reserved bean broth or vegetable stock to braise the onions to which have been added the remaining sage, garlic, and bay leaf. When the onions have softened, add the tomatoes with the bean broth and salt and pepper as per the instructions above.

Finely chop the parsley. Pound the garlic and salt in a mortar until it is a smooth paste. Add 1 to 2 tablespoons of the parsley to the garlic paste and mix well. Gradually add the remaining parsley, alternating with the vegetable stock in small amounts. For a smoother and more uniform sauce, you may want to process a portion of the herb-garlic mix in your food processor or blender. Add red wine vinegar to taste, and season with black pepper if desired.

Deborah Madison has another version of this soup on page 486. Instead of sautéing the vegetables in oil, note that she cooks them with the beans so they infuse their savory flavor into the bean broth. Prolonged cooking weakens the flavor of some herbs; by adding them toward the end of the cooking you can retain their fullest flavors. The herbs are so tasty in themselves that it's really not necessary to make an oil-based paste. Deborah Madison chose lemon juice and its peel to add to the herb-garlic paste for added flavor and smoothness of texture.

Another good example of a modified recipe is Stuffed Manicotti (page 514). Manicotti are usually filled with a rich cheese filling and often topped with a bechamel sauce as well as a tomato sauce. Here the manicotti noodles are filled with an herbed tofu mixture and topped with a blended tomato sauce containing no oil. It's baked in the oven and comes out as bubbly and savory as a traditional manicotti.

Salad dressings are also easy to modify. The ideal dressing is a mixture that will coat and season the salad, and oil is not the only solution.

UNMODIFIED VINAIGRETTE DRESSING

1 tablespoon lemon juice
3 tablespoons vinegar
1 clove garlic, minced or put
* through a press*

1 teaspoon Dijon mustard
Salt and freshly ground pepper to
* taste*
¾ cup olive oil

Mix together the lemon juice, vinegar, garlic, mustard, salt and pepper.
Whisk in the oil.

Modified Low-Fat Versions:

NONFAT YOGURT VINAIGRETTE

1 tablespoon lemon juice
3 tablespoons vinegar
1 clove garlic, minced or put
* through a press*

1 teaspoon Dijon mustard
Salt and freshly ground pepper to
* taste*
¾ cup plain nonfat yogurt

Mix together the lemon juice, vinegar, garlic, mustard, salt, and pepper.
Whisk in the yogurt.

TOMATO VINAIGRETTE

1 tablespoon lemon juice
3 tablespoons vinegar
1 clove garlic, minced or put
* through a press*

1 teaspoon Dijon mustard
Salt and freshly ground pepper to
* taste*
¾ cup tomato juice

Mix together the lemon juice, vinegar, garlic, mustard, salt, and pepper.
Whisk in the tomato juice.

TOFU VINAIGRETTE

1 tablespoon lemon juice
3 tablespoons vinegar
1 clove garlic, minced or put
* through a press*

1 teaspoon Dijon mustard
Salt and freshly ground pepper to
* taste*
¾ cup soft tofu

Process all the ingredients in a blender or food processor until the mixture is smooth. If this is too thick, gradually add more juice or vinegar.

You'll see by the many recipes here that heaps of sugar aren't necessary for sweet, satisfying desserts. Fruits have so much inherent sweetness, and flavors can be enhanced by marinating fruits in sweet wines, lemon or lime juice, and in other fruit juices or fruit juice concentrates (which also serve to sweeten many puddings and baked goods). Sherbets really don't require the vast amounts of sugar that traditional recipes call for (see the Apple and Apple Cider Sherbet on page 530 and the Berry Sorbet on page 534). Fruit juice can almost always replace a sugar syrup.

Here is a traditional recipe for Bananas Poached in Wine, followed by a modified one.

UNMODIFIED BANANAS POACHED IN WINE

2 cups dry or semidry white wine
³/₄ cup sugar
2 teaspoons vanilla extract
3-inch stick cinnamon
¹/₂ cup raisins or currants

3 to 4 firm, ripe bananas
Freshly grated nutmeg to taste
1 cup heavy whipping cream, whipped and flavored with vanilla

Combine the white wine, sugar, vanilla, cinnamon, and raisins or currants in a saucepan, and bring to a simmer. Stir to dissolve the sugar, cover, and simmer 5 minutes. Peel and slice the bananas, and add to the poaching liquid. Cover and simmer 10 minutes. Add nutmeg and serve topped with whipped cream.

MODIFIED VERSION: BANANAS POACHED IN APPLE JUICE

2 cups apple juice
1 tablespoon vanilla extract
3-inch stick cinnamon
3 tablespoons raisins or currants
3 to 4 firm, ripe bananas

Freshly grated nutmeg to taste
4 to 6 tablespoons plain nonfat yogurt, flavored with vanilla or Whipped "Cream" (page 542) (optional)

Combine the apple juice, vanilla, cinnamon, and raisins or currants in a saucepan, bring to a simmer, and cook for 5 minutes. Peel and slice the bananas, and add to the poaching liquid. Cover and simmer for 10 minutes. Add nutmeg and serve topped with yogurt flavored with vanilla or the Whipped "Cream," if desired.

While the wine may be just fine for some, here the apple juice replaces the wine and sugar and produces just as heady a compote. The quantity of raisins or currants has been reduced but you still have them to bite into, and the yogurt or Whipped "Cream" gives you a nice creamy topping.

For sweetening and moistening breakfast cereals, use nonfat milk with fresh or a little dried fruit. You may also want to add some fruit juice or fruit juice concentrate as a sweetener (the concentrate will be very sweet, so try small amounts at first).

Once you become familiar with the recipes here, it won't be difficult for you to see how to modify some of your old favorites.

EQUIPMENT

Pots and Pans
If you want to invest in some helpful items, begin with some good nonstick cookware. Some of the heavier Silverstone pots and pans are especially useful. With these you can sauté with virtually no oil, yet food will not stick. Whatever kind of cookware you choose, equip yourself with two or three *saucepans* (1-, 2- and 4-quart) *with lids, a large, heavy-bottomed soup pot or casserole with a lid,* and *a 10- or 12-inch skillet. A large lidded skillet* will also come in handy. I also recommend the following:

NONSTICK CRÊPE PAN   A 7-inch crêpe pan will be useful for some of the recipes here.

STEAMER   This inexpensive item is indispensable for low-fat cooking. Use either a stainless steel fold-up type that you can fit into a saucepan or a tiered Chinese steamer, either bamboo or aluminum.

WOK   A very useful item for stir-fry and also for steaming if you have a tiered Chinese steamer. Get a wok with a lid, preferably a nonstick one.

A LARGE POT FOR PASTA   This can be an inexpensive enameled pot, such as the kind used for canning. Since you fill it with water, a light vessel might be easier to handle than a heavy one.

PRESSURE COOKER   This isn't required, but if you're pressed for time, it's useful for cooking beans, since it reduces the cooking time by half. But don't cook split peas or lentils in a pressure cooker; the cooking liquid may froth and bubble and may clog the pressure gauge.

Baking Dishes

> *A 3- or 4-quart lidded baking dish or casserole*
> *A 1- or 2-quart baking dish or soufflé dish*
> *One or two 10-inch pie pans*
> *Two or three nonstick baking sheets or jelly-roll pans*
> *Two nonstick bread pans*
> *Two 10- or 12-inch nonstick pizza pans*

Utensils

KNIVES   Good kitchen knives are the most important utensils to have. You should also have a sharpening stone and a steel for keeping the sharp edge on the blades. Dull knives make chopping vegetables time-consuming and dangerous.

You should have a 10-inch stainless or carbon steel knife, a couple of paring knives, and a serrated bread knife. Carbon steel keeps a sharper blade, but will rust if you don't keep it dry and will color when you cut acidy fruits. So I would recommend stainless as the most practical. You should also have:

> *Two or three wooden spoons*
> *Whisk*
> *Metal spatula*
> *Plastic or rubber spatula*
> *Four-sided grater or Mouli grater*
> *Nutmeg grater, for fresh nutmeg*
> *Garlic press*
> *Pepper mill*
> *Citrus juicer*
> *Bread board for kneading and rolling out dough*
> *A heavy rolling pin*

Colander
Strainer
Lettuce dryer
Kitchen timer
Potato peeler
At least three mixing bowls (stainless are the most useful)
A large bread bowl either ceramic or stainless
Mortar and pestle (marble ones are the most effective)
Mouli food mill for pureeing soups and sauces

Measures

2-cup Pyrex measuring cup
4-cup Pyrex measuring cup
Set of individual measuring cups
One or two sets of measuring spoons
Kitchen scale

Electrical Appliances

BLENDER

FOOD PROCESSOR   Not essential, but very handy for making purees and some sauces (although these can also be done in a blender with a little more effort). It's especially useful for grating vegetables.

ELECTRIC MIXER   Not essential, but if you have one with a dough hook it can save time with breadmaking.

SORBETTIER OR ELECTRIC ICE CREAM MAKER   Although these appliances can be expensive and are not essential, either an electric ice cream freezer or a sorbettier that fits into your freezer will allow you to make all kinds of fruit ices with very little effort.

SPICE MILL   Spices are much more vibrant when stored whole and ground just before using. You can also grind spices in an electric coffee grinder, although you should be careful to break whole cinnamon sticks into small pieces before grinding them, or you could jam the blade and burn out the motor.

The Glossary and General Cooking Instructions are meant to familiarize you with ingredients that may not be part of your cooking repertoire.

An attempt has been made to include most of the grains and legumes mentioned within the recipe section, as well as information about some of the more unusual vegetables, wine vinegars, sauce thickeners, and soy products. It is by no means a complete listing.

Most of these ingredients are relatively easy to find. Many are available in your local supermarkets, whereas others may be found in specialty shops, ethnic markets, or health food stores. While some of these ingredients are familiar, others may be new to you. You do not need to try any new ingredients to follow the Reversal Diet or the Prevention Diet, although you may enjoy experimenting with some new ones.

A GLOSSARY OF INGREDIENTS

Grains
When you ask people how they would typify the American diet, the answer is frequently "meat and potatoes." There is little understanding of how prominent a role grains play in our diets. Completely overlooked is the fact that one fifth of our diet is from wheat in the form of bread, hamburger buns, cakes, cookies, pies, and rolls. It is understandable that this grain is overlooked since these wheat products don't look like wheat kernels and are in their least nutritious form. They are also usually heavily laden with fats and simple sugars.

Grains (wheat, corn, rice, oats, millet, rye, barley) are the seeds of grasses. The nutrients within each kernel are not distributed evenly. Each grain contains a seed (germ), food for the seed (endosperm) and a covering to protect the seed and its food sources (hull and bran). The goal of milling and refining in this century has been to remove the germ and the bran layers to shorten the grain's cooking time and allow it to be processed into flours. These layers contain 28 percent of the grain's protein, all of its fiber, and the vast majority of the B vitamins. The germ layer in particular contains fats that are essential to our diet and health. The refining process may include bleaching to whiten the flour; this process removes even more vitamins. "Enriched" breads have had some of the B vitamins returned to the flour that were removed in the milling and refinement process, but these breads still lack protein and fiber.

Recently the American public has moved away from white bread in favor of whole wheat bread with its higher fiber and nutrient content. The same interest should be taken in other grains.

The following is by no means a complete list of grains. Some of the items listed are not truly even grains (amaranth, buckwheat, quinoa, wild rice) but are seeds from various sources or other parts of plants that are used similarly to grains. The list includes only those items that are called for in the recipes in this book. Have fun experimenting with these and other grains that you find in your grocery or health food outlet. Hopefully you will develop a taste for "whole grain" products, which contain more fiber, protein, B vitamins and essential fats than their refined counterparts.

Store grains in tightly covered jars in a cool, dark place.

AMARANTH   This is not actually a grain but it can be considered as one. It is a complete protein and contains more iron and fiber than wheat (the most frequently eaten grain in this country). It is widely available as a flaked cereal or granola mix. It can be prepared as you would do with other grains in pilafs, stews, and soups. The flour is available for baking and commercial pastas.

ARBORIO RICE   This is a polished short-grain white rice. It is grown in northern Italy and is round with a chewy, hearty texture and a very rich flavor. It is the traditional rice for risotto and can be used in salads, and pilafs.

BARLEY   A hearty grain with a chewy texture and nutty taste. It looks a little like rice and puffs up when cooked. It is especially good in soups.

BROWN RICE   This is mostly the whole, unpolished rice grain and has a very nutty, wholesome flavor. Both long- and short-grain brown rice is available, and it is easy to find in supermarkets as well as health food stores. It takes longer to cook than white rice, but is worth the wait. Brown rice is high in B vitamins, essential fatty acids, complex carbohydrates, and an excellent source of fiber. It is a high-quality protein when eaten in combination with dried beans.

BUCKWHEAT   This is actually the pyramid-shaped seed of a fruit rather than being a true grain. It has a rich and earthy flavor. It is used in all of the ways that the true grains are used, such as in cereals, pilafs, and salads. It is also ground into flours for use in baked goods, pancakes and noodles.

BULGUR   As cracked wheat that has been precooked and dried, bulgur has a nutty taste and fluffy texture, with the same nutritional characteristics as brown rice. The smaller-sized varieties are traditionally used for tabbouleh. Coarser varieties are used for pilafs and salads. Stir a little cooked bulgur into chili to give it more texture.

CORN, CORNMEAL, MASA HARINA AND HOMINY   Corn is not

usually thought of as a grain but it is. The kernels do not have the husk that some of the other grains have, but nutritionally they are not much different, although they do contain a little less protein and fat.

Who doesn't love the sweet taste of corn on the cob in season? The kernels can be scraped from the cob and eaten as is or pureed to use as a soup base. The whole kernels can be added to stews, ground into grits or more finely ground into flour. Corn is also available as flakes. Cornmeal can be used to make cereals, polenta, muffins, and tortillas. The silken-textured corn flours are used to make pasta.

Masa harina is a type of flour made from corn kernels that have been soaked in lye or lime (hominy). The soaking process allows easier removal of the germ and the hull from each kernel and bleaches the corn to a near white color. Masa harina is used in the making of tortillas.

COUSCOUS   This is another precooked cracked wheat product. It is made from white durum wheat from which the bran and germ has been removed. It is therefore a refined wheat product. Once cooked it has a very light, airy quality and a silky texture. It's fabulous with bean and vegetable stews, and makes a delicious, quick breakfast grain. It is available in imported food sections in stores and many whole food stores.

CRACKED WHEAT   A cracked wheat product that differs from bulgur only in that it hasn't been precooked. It makes a great breakfast cereal and is good in breads.

FLAKED WHEAT, RYE, BARLEY, AND TRITICALE   All of these resemble oat flakes, but they are a little stiffer in texture. Triticale is a hybrid grain made from wheat and rye. All of these flakes are made by pressing the whole wheat, rye, or triticale berries. Mix them together with oat flakes for granolas and mixed grain cereals.

MILLET   A delicate, nutty-tasting grain that looks like tiny yellow beads. The millet that is sold as bird feed has not been hulled and is not suitable for consumption. It has been a dietary staple in Africa for centuries and is eaten in the form of cereals, stews, and flat breads. Substitute it for brown rice whenever you want a change. It also makes a nice breakfast grain.

MIRIN   A sweet Japanese cooking wine made from fermented rice.

NUTRITIONAL YEAST   Unlike the more active yeast forms, this has no activity to raise bread. It is occasionally added to food for its sharply fermented, almost salty flavor.

OATS Oats and oat products have captured increasing amounts of interest because of their beneficial effect on lowering cholesterol. Oat bran has the greatest amount of lipid-lowering fiber of the oat products and can be used as a cereal, sprinkled on other cereals, and added to baked goods such as cookies, muffins, and breads. Oat flakes have a little less fiber than oat bran. Rolled oats can be used similarly and in granola mixes.

QUINOA This Peruvian Indian staple is like a grain, except, unlike a grain, it is said to contain all of the essential amino acids. This makes its high protein content readily usable by the body to build muscle and repair tissues. It is a little higher in fat than most grains and therefore is higher in calories.

Quinoa can be used like rice, couscous, bulgur, or millet. Think of it when you are planning stuffings, pilafs, desserts, or puddings. It is also commercially available as a cereal.

SEITAN Seitan is a firm, usually wheat-based food that because of its texture and versatility is frequently used a meat or poultry substitute. It is essentially wheat flour that is kneaded to develop the gluten fibers, then rinsed of the bran and starch. The resulting gluten-rich dough is high in protein but does not have much flavor on its own. It must be cooked and simmered in a well-seasoned sauce to allow the flavors of the sauce to become infused. It can then be sliced and used in various ways. You will see it disguised as chicken, beef or pork in many Asian vegetarian restaurants (e.g sweet and sour pork, almond chicken ding, Mongolian beef). You can also find it canned in food stores catering to Seventh Day Adventists who do not eat meat. It is becoming more widely available and can be found precooked in a soy, vegetable or herb broth in health food stores in airtight containers.

Here are instructions to make your own seitan: Gradually add 6 cups of water to a mixing bowl with 7½ cups of whole wheat flour. Mix well until a ball is formed. Knead for 5 to 10 minutes. Remove the dough from the bowl and hold it under cold running water. Stretch and work the dough under the water to rinse away the bran and starch. Do this for 10 minutes. You will observe that the dough ball will become more sticky and will stretch quite easily. Shape the dough into a loaf. Wrap it in cheesecloth and tie the ends of the cheesecloth together to keep the loaf from slipping out. Drop the loaf into boiling vegetable stock or mushroom broth and simmer for an hour. Make sure that the loaf remains covered by the stock while it is cooking. It can then be sliced or cubed for use. This will make 1 loaf weighing 1½ to 2 pounds.

SOBA NOODLES   These dried buckwheat noodles were introduced from Japan and are widely available in large supermarket chains as well as health food stores. They are traditionally used in soups but can also be used as you would any pasta. For a light lunch, add some cooked soba noodles to a vegetable stock that has simmered for 5 to 10 minutes with some sliced ginger, green onions, bean curd, and bok choy (Chinese cabbage) or spinach. You could even add some dried sea vegetables such as nori or hijiki.

WHOLE WHEAT BERRIES   Each berry is one whole wheat kernel. The grain is very hard and when cooked has a hearty, chewy texture and sweet flavor. It looks like dark brown rice. Whole wheat berries can be sprouted, cracked, left whole to be eaten as is, or added to other grains.

WILD RICE   This is not a true grain but is actually the seed of an aquatic grass from the northern United States. The hull may be loosened but the grain is never refined. Wild rice is naturally higher in protein, iron, fiber and B vitamins than brown rice. It is also very low in total fat, much lower than brown rice. It has not been widely cultivated and is quite expensive, so it is usually reserved for special occasions, or used sparingly in combination with other grains. The individual grains are long and dark brown to black and have a nutty flavor. They are chewy in texture and are also used in salad and stuffings.

Legumes or Dried Beans

Dried beans and peas are generally underrated as a food source by most Americans. Compared to ground beef chuck, dried kidney beans, for example, have much greater protein and other nutrients except for a few B vitamins. Remember, legumes must sometimes be eaten with grains to get the most benefit from their protein. They are also effective in reducing your LDL (the harmful fraction) cholesterol.

They can do more than be used as the basis for soups and stews, or sprinkled into salads. Mash them to form dips, stuffings for pastas, or sandwich spreads. Use them along with the vegetables of your choice as a filling for corn tacos and flour tortillas (enchiladas and burritos).

Store dried beans in tightly covered jars in a cool, dark place. Once cooked, they freeze well and will keep for several months.

BLACK BEANS   Black, medium-sized beans with a rich, satisfying flavor. Great for tacos, soups and salads.

BLACK-EYED PEAS   Medium-sized, oval, creamy white beans with a black spot on one side. They have a savory flavor.

CHICK-PEAS   Large round beige beans with a nutty, distinctive taste. Great in salads, in soups, and blended as a spread.

GREEN SPLIT PEAS   These have a familiar earthy flavor and slightly mealy texture. Traditional split pea soups usually contain ham hocks, but meatless versions are delicious.

LENTILS   Various colored small beans with a distinctive, satisfying flavor. Delicious in soups or salads. They are also good when combined with tomatoes as a sauce for pasta (page 469). There are many varieties with differing tastes, textures, and cooking times. The green and brown varieties take longer to cook than the red ones. French lentils are a variety of tiny green lentils. They're available in imported food stores and health food stores.

MUNG BEANS   The only form of this small olive-colored bean that would be familiar to most Americans would be the bean sprouts that appear in some very popular Chinese dishes. The cooked whole bean can be eaten as well. The starch of the mung bean is used to make *cellophane noodles.* Also called bean thread noodles, they are translucent and have very little taste on their own. Use the noodles in soups and, as demonstrated within this book, as a salad.

PINTO BEANS AND BORLOTTI BEANS   Medium-sized, speckled light brown beans. Pintos are standard in Mexican food, borlottis in Italian food. They have a rich, succulent texture and a less pronounced flavor than either kidney beans or black beans.

RED KIDNEY BEANS   Red kidney-shaped beans, good in salads, stews, chili, and soups.

SOYBEANS   These are a very attractive addition to your diet since they contain more protein than any other vegetable source. Whole soybeans are not particularly flavorful and when compared to other beans they are relatively high in fat, although compared to other food sources with comparable amounts of protein (meats, fish, and fowl), the fat content of most soy products is very low. The major problem with this bean is that it is extremely difficult to digest and causes considerable bloating in most people. For these reasons, whole soybeans (roasted or stewed), soy grits (ground soybeans), and soy flakes are *not* recommended.

There are other ways to benefit from soybeans that are easier to digest.

Soybean Products

SOY FLOUR   This is sometimes added to grain-based flours to increase their protein content. It contains no gluten and therefore yeasted breads will not rise without the addition of a gluten-containing flour. Look for the defatted varieties.

SOY MILK   This is made from soaked, ground, and strained soybeans. It is frequently used for bottle-fed infants who are allergic to cow's milk. It is much higher in fat, lower in vitamin B_{12} and lower in calcium than nonfat cow's milk.

SOY SAUCE, TAMARI, AND MISO   All are made from fermented soybeans, wheat and considerable amounts of salt. Soy sauce has a little alcohol and corn syrup added; miso may have other grains mixed in. One tablespoon of soy sauce is nearly equivalent to ½ teaspoon of salt. Consider this when you use it. The "Low Salt" varieties of both soy sauce and tamari are misleading, since they retain approximately 75 percent of the original salt content. Miso contains about half as much salt as regular soy sauce and there are even varieties that have reduced amounts of salt such as sweet white shiro miso. There is also a salt-free variety called muen.

SOY CHEESES   These are generally not recommended for those with heart disease and are discussed for the sake of education. Widely found in the dairy cases of health food stores, these nonmilk-based cheeses are made from soybeans, milk proteins, and various oils. They do "melt." There is some controversy about whether or not the milk proteins they contain (specifically one called casein) promote cholesterol plaques in arteries. Soy cheeses contain about 5 to 7 grams of fat per ounce. That's equivalent to a piece the size of a slice of American cheese and contains more than half the amount of fat in the American cheese slice.

TEMPEH   Made from partially mashed, fermented soybeans, tempeh is easier to digest than soybeans. Vitamin B_{12} is produced in the fermentation process, some of which can be absorbed by consumers of this vegetable product. It has a distinctive taste and is frequently marinated or cooked in sauces. It is very firm and can be eaten with lettuce, tomatoes, onions, and mustard or ketchup as a "burger" or cubed for kabobs or stews.

TEXTURIZED VEGETABLE PROTEIN   This is also known as isolated soy protein and is the basis for products such as Tuna or Hamburger Helper. It is also used as a meat substitute in foods like soy sausage or bacon. It can be found in some health food stores and added to stews or vegetables and gives the appearance, texture, and, if done right, the taste of ground beef. The products vary widely in sodium content and may contain added oils. Read the packaging carefully or ask your grocer about the sodium and fat if it is sold in bulk.

TOFU   Bean curd is another name for tofu. It is the equivalent of soy cheese. Tofu is a miracle food; it is very easy to digest, very high in protein, low in calories and fat, economical, and extremely versatile. By itself it is bland, with a spongy texture. Like a sponge it will absorb the flavors of whatever it is mixed with. As it cooks its texture firms up. It can be mixed with herbs, blended into sauces or a low-fat mayonnaise-like vinaigrette, or baked as a quiche. It can be used in bread spreads, vegetable dips, pizza toppings, and stir-frys, and substituted for cheese in some recipes. It doesn't behave like cheese in that it doesn't melt.

In the supermarket or natural food store, tofu is found refrigerated sitting in water in bins, or in vacuum-packed containers of water. Be sure to keep it sitting in water in your own refrigerator or it will dry out.

YELLOW SPLIT PEAS   Yellow split peas are popular in Greek and Indian cuisines. Their flavor is more subtle than that of green split peas, with a more agreeable texture.

WHITE BEANS (GREAT NORTHERNS OR SMALL WHITE BEANS) These white beans have a subtle, elegant flavor and are terrific in soups, in salads, and with pasta.

Seasonings, Flavorings, Condiments, and Miscellaneous

AGAR-AGAR   This product is derived from seaweed and is used to make gelatin-based molded salads, desserts or aspic. It can also be used to thicken sauces. It is sold in bars, sheets, granules or flakes. For savory or dessert aspics, soak the agar flakes or granules in ¼ cup cold liquid for a few minutes until the agar has softened. Then add ¾ cup hot liquid (sauce, stock or juice) to dissolve it. Use 1 teaspoon of agar per cup of cooking liquid.

ARROWROOT POWDER   A thickening agent like cornstarch. It is used in some of the sauces in this collection. Store it with spices.

Dissolve arrowroot in cold liquid before adding it to sauces or they will be lumpy.

BALSAMIC VINEGAR   This is a thick, strong, slightly sweet vinegar imported from Italy. It has a marvelous, distinctive flavor. Use it more sparingly than regular red wine vinegar. Store in a cool, dry place.

CAPERS   These large, round green seeds of the caper plant, pickled in a vinegary brine, add a pungent flavor to dishes. Keep them on hand for salads, pasta, and vegetable dishes. Rinse them before adding them to dishes, because the brine is very salty. Store in the refrigerator.

DRY WHITE AND RED WINE FOR COOKING   Always have a bottle of both dry white wine and red wine on hand. Recommended for the whites are a not too expensive Loire Valley wine, such as a Sauvignon or a Muscadet, or a California Chenin Blanc; for a red, a Cotes du Rhone, Cabernet or a Chianti. Store in a cool, dry place, and once opened, in the refrigerator.

CURRANTS   These tiny raisins, originally from Corinth (thus the name), add an intensely sweet flavor to desserts, and are also excellent in salads and grain dishes. Store in a tightly covered jar in a cool, dry place or in the refrigerator.

DIJON MUSTARD   Easy to find in supermarkets, this strong French mustard is a must for a good vinaigrette. Store in the refrigerator. Avoid the varieties with added oils and the English varieties of mustards with eggs.

GARLIC   There are two varieties, white-skinned and pink-skinned. The white-skinned bulbs have a stronger flavor, the pink-skinned variety is slightly sweeter and some think a more refined flavor. Look for bulbs with large cloves; a head of garlic with large cloves usually contains about thirteen. "Giant" or "elephant" garlic are large bulbs containing huge cloves, sometimes only a few per head. They are milder than the normal-sized varieties, with a sweet, nutty taste. New or fresh garlic, harvested in the spring in France, Italy, and Spain, has green stems like onion stems, and soft, thick skins. Once you get through the skins to the cloves, you will find this garlic to be a great delicacy, juicy, tender, and sweet. If you have trouble digesting garlic, it may help to cut the cloves in half and pull out the green stem that runs down the middle.

Garlic becomes quite mild when slowly cooked or simmered, so don't let recipes like the Garlic-Herb Soup (page 481) or the Spanish

Chick-Pea and Garlic Soup (page 485) intimidate you. Store in a cool, dry place.

HIJIKI   One of the many sea vegetables (kombu, nori, dulse, wakame) available in this country. Hijiki has a very salty flavor and is sold dried in packages or bulk. It must be soaked 10 to 20 minutes in hot water before using.

LEMONS AND LIMES   These deserve to be listed as a condiment because fresh lemon juice and fresh lime juice are so often used to season dishes in this diet. Many salads require nothing more than lemon juice and herbs and/or spices for seasoning. Store in the refrigerator, or if using within a few days, in a fruit bowl.

ORANGE PEEL   A strip of orange zest, with the bitter white part cut away from an orange peel, often adds an alluring perfume to soups and vegetable dishes.

ORANGE FLOWER WATER   Orange flower water, extracted from the blossoms of the bitter orange tree, is used to perfume many Moroccan and Provençal dishes. It has a sweet aroma and slightly bitter taste. You can find it in imported food stores and in some pharmacies. Store in a cool, dry place.

RED WINE, WHITE WINE AND CIDER VINEGARS   Quality vinegars are important seasonings in this cuisine. Many are available commercially, but consider buying an imported French wine vinegar, such as Dessaux, or making your own. It's easy: take a half-empty bottle of decent red wine, cover it loosely and wait until a cloud appears in the wine (you can also use vinegar in which a cloud has appeared). This is called a *mere,* or mother, and will generate more vinegar when you add wine to it. Taste the vinegar before you use it, as homemade vinegars are sometimes very strong, and you may need less than a given recipe calls for. Store in a cool, dry place.

SALT SUBSTITUTES   The sodium in table salt is associated with hypertension in many people. Most of the commercial salt substitutes use potassium chloride, which is bitter tasting, so many people have difficulty using them. Instead, you might want to try using the various spice blends that are commercially available, making your own, or learning how to use wines and vinegars. The simplest method is to reduce your salt intake. Give your palate time to adjust, and to discover the naturally sweet and savory natures of all that we eat. The salt substitutes containing potassium may be a problem for some people with kidney diseases.

TOMATILLOS   These are a variety of green Mexican tomatoes

with a papery husk that must be removed. They can be eaten raw, crushed or pureed for salsa, but many find that cooking improves the flavor. Tomatillos are excellent in sauces and soups.

UNSWEETENED PRESERVES, JAMS AND FRUIT SPREADS Found in most health food stores and supermarkets, these are more and more common. Some of the easiest to find are unsweetened apple butter and apricot butter. Spread on toast for breakfast. Once opened, store in the refrigerator.

Herbs

Store dried herbs in tightly covered jars in a cool, dark, dry place. To keep fresh herbs for a few days in the refrigerator, cut the stems off about half an inch from the end. Wrap the cut end of the bunch in a moistened double thickness of paper towels. Wrap this, in turn, in foil so that the paper towels stay wrapped around the stems, and seal the herbs in a dry plastic bag.

BASIL   Known as "the royal herb" in France, basil and tomatoes were made for each other. The herb is sweet and slightly pungent, sometimes a little peppery. Dried basil hardly resembles fresh and is usually not an acceptable substitute (the exceptions are certain soups and sauces). If you're using dried basil, you may want to add it in the last few minutes of the cooking process. If it is cooked for more than 15 minutes, it will tend to lose most of its flavor.

BAY LEAF   Used to flavor soups, stews, beans, and vegetables, these leaves have an earthy, somewhat musty flavor. Fresh bay leaves are shiny, pliable, and dark green, unlike the faded dry leaves we get in our supermarkets. If you can find fresh leaves, buy them, but the dry ones still pack a lot of flavor.

CHERVIL   These pretty, delicate stems with their bright green, featherlike leaves have a distinctive sweet, slightly anise-like flavor. Chervil looks a little bit like flat-leaf parsley, although it is a lighter green and more fernlike. Chervil is marvelous in salads, and makes a beautiful garnish.

CHIVES   These look like tiny stems of green onions and have a sweet, mild oniony taste. Add to salads, soups, and potato dishes.

CILANTRO (FRESH CORIANDER)   This herb, with its strong, pungent flavor is a favorite in Mexican, Indian, Middle Eastern, Chinese, and North African dishes. It tastes nothing like the seeds from which it grows (see spices, below). Cilantro resembles flat-leaf parsley, although its color is lighter and its leaves more delicate.

DILL   Fresh dill, with its refreshing, feathery green leaves, goes beautifully with cucumbers, potatoes, and yogurt. Like basil, chervil, and cilantro, it loses its flavor when dried. Dill looks like wild fennel, but the flavor is not at all similar.

MINT   There are many variations of mint. The herb adds a wonderful touch to many salads and soups (it goes especially well with cucumbers and fresh peas). It is a brilliant seasoning for fruit desserts. The simple addition of a few leaves of fresh mint to a bowl of peaches, melon, or strawberries transforms a simple dessert into an unforgettable one.

MARJORAM AND OREGANO   These herbs come from the same family and are a common ingredient in Greek and Italian cuisines. Marjoram has a minty, somewhat thyme-like flavor and is great in salads and soups. Oregano is more rustic than marjoram, with a slightly peppery fragrance, and more widely used.

PARSLEY (FLAT AND CURLY LEAF)   A widely used herb in all manner of dishes. The flat-leafed variety, often referred to as Italian parsley, has a richer, more satisfying flavor than the curly leafed herb.

ROSEMARY   Rosemary imparts a pungent, savory flavor to veg-etable dishes, salads, breads, and soups. Dried rosemary has a less acrid taste than fresh, and is sometimes preferable.

SAGE   The gray-green, knobbly textured leaves of this herb have a stunningly earthy, slightly bitter flavor. It goes beautifully with beans, potatoes, and all manner of vegetables. Rubbed dried sage has a much stronger, more bitter flavor than fresh and cannot be substituted in recipes that call for fresh.

TARRAGON   The long, elegant leaves of French tarragon have a luxurious, sweet flavor, somewhat resembling basil but more tangy and slightly like anise. A few tablespoons of freshly chopped tarra-gon added to a soup or salad will transform an ordinary dish into a truly elegant one. Dried tarragon has the sweetness but not the punch of its fresh counterpart.

THYME   Thyme, either fresh or dried, is an important ingredi-ent in many soups, sauces, and vegetable dishes. It has a strong, savory, slightly bitter flavor, and a little goes a long way.

WILD FENNEL   This stalky, feathery-leafed herb, with the fla-vor of anise, is great in salads and vegetable dishes. The leaves of wild fennel should be fresh, but you can use the dried stalks for *bouquet garni* in soups.

Spices

Store spices in tightly covered jars in a cool, dark, dry place. They will lose their freshness and pungency after 6 months. You might want to buy them whole and grind in a mortar, spice mill, or coffee grinder as needed; the spices will retain more of their pungency that way.

ALLSPICE   Whole allspice berries, slightly larger than peppercorns, are picked green and dried in the sun, whereupon they take on their rusty-brown color. As for all spices, it's best to purchase allspice berries whole and grind them as you use them.

The name allspice derives from the flavor of this sweet spice, which is reminiscent of several other sweet spices, most notably cinnamon and cloves, with a hint of nutmeg.

ANISE SEEDS   Anise seeds have a sweet licorice flavor, like fennel but a bit stronger, and can be used in vegetable dishes and salads, as well as some desserts.

CARAWAY SEEDS   These seeds have a distinctive flavor that is associated with Jewish rye bread. Caraway is ground and used in North African dishes and many salads.

CARDAMOM SEEDS   These are small, black fragrant seeds which come in white or green pods. The pods are easy to open to extract the seeds, and the spice should always be bought in this whole form, because it will quickly lose its perfume once ground. Cardamom has a distinctive earthy perfume and flavor.

CINNAMON   A familiar spice with a sweet, pungent flavor.

CORIANDER SEEDS   These light brown round seeds, slightly larger than peppercorns, have a completely different flavor than the fresh leaves of the plant. The flavor is mild and musky-sweet, with a subtle hint of orange peel.

CUMIN SEEDS   Cumin seeds in their whole and ground state are an essential ingredient in many Mexican, Middle Eastern, Indian, and North African dishes. The spice has a very special, unmistakable nutty-earthy taste.

FENNEL SEEDS   The seeds of the fennel herb plant. They have a licorice flavor like anise, and can be used interchangeably.

FENUGREEK SEEDS   The seeds of fenugreek, an annual herb which is a member of the bean family. Native to Asia Minor and India, the small, hard, vaguely triangular seeds have a very strong aroma and bitter taste. Recipes call for a very few, and they impart a distinctive curry flavor. They are known to be a digestive, and for this reason are often cooked with legumes.

GINGER   Ginger has a strong, pungent flavor that lends itself to many soup stocks, salads, and fruit and vegetable dishes. Fresh ginger is associated with Oriental and Indian cuisines; dried ginger appears in many Mediterranean recipes.

HOT PEPPERS   Hot peppers, both dried and fresh, are a staple in many recipes. Mexican chilis such as *ancho, chipotle* and *serrano,* and small dried chilis such as cayenne and *peperoncini,* add fire and deep, complex flavor to various dishes and are rich in vitamin C.

MUSTARD SEEDS   These are the seeds that are ground to make dry mustard powder and all prepared mustards. They can be used in some of the marinated vegetable dishes. They are widely used in pickling.

NUTMEG   The inner part of the fruit of the nutmeg tree, this spice has a delicious sweet and pungent, nutty flavor. It is used to sweeten baked goods and sweets, also to season soups, vegetables (especially spinach), sauces, and many pasta dishes. It should always be freshly grated, as it will quickly lose its zesty aroma in powdered form. The spice should be used with discretion, as the flavor can overpower a dish.

PAPRIKA   Also known as Hungarian pepper and Spanish pepper, this is the national spice of Hungary, but has also found its way into many Spanish, Turkish, North African, and Middle Eastern dishes. Paprika is the dried powder of a mild, sweet, bright red pepper. It should have a mild, sweet flavor. It must be very fresh or it will be bitter; if the color has gone from bright red to rust brown, it has deteriorated. Look for Hungarian paprika, which is the best (look for the word "Hungarian" or "Magyar" on the label). The next best is Spanish. Store it in the refrigerator in an airtight container.

SAFFRON   This is the most luxurious and expensive spice. It is made from the dried stamens of the saffron plant's flowers, a member of the crocus family. The reason it is so costly is that it takes about 250,000 dried stamens, collected by hand from about 75,000 flowers, to make a pound of saffron. It is usually sold by the twentieth of an ounce or by the gram, in thread and powdered form. Saffron's magic lies in the gorgeous yellow hue it imparts to its dishes and its strong, sweet aroma. A little of this spice goes a long way, luckily. It only takes ¼ teaspoon to color and flavor a cup of rice. To achieve even coloring and flavoring, powder the saffron threads with your fingers or the back of a spoon in a small bowl and soak in a little hot water for 15 minutes. Add this solution, with the threads, to whatever you are cooking.

TURMERIC   Native to India, turmeric belongs to the ginger family. It imparts a lovely yellow color to dishes and has a woody, slightly bitter flavor.

Sweeteners

APPLE CONCENTRATE   A very concentrated apple juice that can be used to sweeten some dishes. The recipes in the book call for undiluted concentrate. And very little is generally used. You can of course add water if you wish.

BLACK CHERRY CONCENTRATE   A sweet concentrate made from black cherries. Excellent as a syrup for some fruits. It can be found in the large grocery chain stores and health food stores.

MILD-FLAVORED HONEYS   Choose light-colored varieties for the mildest flavors—clover, acacia, and lavender honeys are the mildest.

MAPLE SYRUP   With its distinctive taste, this makes a special sweetening for certain dishes. Look for pure maple syrup.

GENERAL TECHNIQUES
AND COOKING INSTRUCTIONS

Preparing Fruits and Vegetables

APPLES AND PEARS   To *dice* or *chop,* cut into quarters lengthwise through the core, pare away the core, then slice each piece in one direction, turn a quarter turn and cut again.

BROCCOLI AND CAULIFLOWER   To break into florets, cut cauliflower in half, cut away the stem and break off the flowers. Cut the tops off the broccoli stems to break into smaller flowers. The stems are also edible.

CABBAGE   To shred cabbage, cut in quarters and cut away the thick stem. Then cut in thin strips, using a long, sharp knife.

CORN ON THE COB   To remove corn kernels from the cob, stand the cob upright on a plate and run the knife down between the kernels and the cob. This can be done before or after cooking.

GARLIC   First pull off the number of cloves you need from the head. To peel, place the clove on a cutting board and pound it once with the bottom of a jar, or place the flat side of a wide cutting knife over it and lean on the knife. The clove will burst and the skin will pop off. Either put the clove through a garlic press or chop, holding down the tip of your knife with one hand while you rock the knife up and down with your other. Continue with this motion until the garlic is as finely chopped as you desire. Some recipes call for roasting whole heads of garlic. You'll find the directions for roasting garlic in the recipe for the Pizza Provençal (page 524).

HERBS   To chop herbs such as parsley and basil, pick the leaves off the stems, place on a cutting board, and, using a large knife, chop with quick, rapid strokes, holding the tip of the knife down with your spare hand. The herbs will spread out as you chop, but just keep pushing them back to the center. Or pick the leaves off the stems, place in a wide-mouth jar, and cut with a scissors. Herbs can also be chopped very efficiently in a food processor, but be careful to process in very short bursts to avoid pureeing them.

LETTUCE AND SPINACH   Washing leafy vegetables can be very tedious, but there's nothing worse than chomping down on sandy lettuce. If you wash a large quantity at a time you won't have to deal with the task every time you want a salad. Separate the leaves and fill the sink or a bowl with cold water. Place in the water, and take each individual leaf and run under cold water, rubbing with your thumbs if necessary to make sure all the grit is washed off. Drain on towels and pat dry, or dry in a salad spinner (one of the greatest inventions of the modern kitchen). To store, wrap in towels and place, towel and all, in plastic bags (or cheesecloth salad bags). Seal well and keep in the crisper of your refrigerator.

MUSHROOMS   If the mushrooms aren't at all sandy, simply cut off the very end of the stem and wipe with a damp cloth or use a mushroom brush. If they are sandy, cut away the stem end, run briefly under cold water, and rub the sand off with your thumbs. Wipe dry with a paper towel or cloth and trim off the end of the stems. Slice thin.

ONIONS   First cut in half lengthwise, that is, from the stem end to the other, along one of the lines. Cut the very ends off and remove the skin. Do this near the sink with the cold water running, or put the onions in the freezer for an hour before chopping, and you won't cry as much. To *chop,* lay one half flat-side down on your cutting board and cut across the onion in thin strips, starting at one end, working toward the center and holding the onion down at the opposite end with your other hand. As the knife nears your fingers, turn the onion around, and holding onto the side you have already cut to steady the onion, cut again toward the center. Now turn the onion a quarter turn and cut across the slices at a right angle to dice. Repeat for the other half.

If a recipe instructs you to cut an onion in *strips,* place the cut onion on your work surface and cut along the lines of the onion, in the same manner as above, but don't repeat the cut at a right angle.

For cutting *rings* do not cut the onion in half first. Remove the skin by cutting a lengthwise slit through the skin one layer deep, all the way around, then removing the skin. Cut the onion crosswise (across the lines) into rings.

ORANGES AND GRAPEFRUIT   To peel and cut away the white pith at the same time, use a very sharp knife to cut the skin off in a spiral, starting at the stem end and tilting the knife in slightly. Hold the fruit over a bowl, as it will drip. If you are just peeling to eat or to divide into sections and you don't need to get rid of the pith, quarter the fruit just through the skin with a sharp knife, then peel off the skin.

SWEET PEPPERS   To chop or dice, cut in half lengthwise (from the stem down) and gently remove the stem, seeds, and membranes. Proceed as for onions, cutting into lengthwise strips, then crosswise into dice. For rings, cut the top off, remove the seeds and membranes, and cut crosswise. Information on roasting peppers can be found in the recipe for Asparagus with Roasted Red Peppers (page 406).

TOMATOES   To *peel,* bring a pot of water to a rolling boil and gently drop in the tomatoes. Count to twenty, remove from the boiling water, and run under cold water for several seconds. The skin will come away easily. To *seed,* cut in half crosswise (halfway between the stem end and the bottom) and squeeze over a bin or bowl. Don't worry about crushing the tomato, because you are going to cook it anyway. To *chop,* cut several strips in one direction, then turn the tomatoes a quarter turn and cut strips in the other direction. You can make satisfying tomato sauces by baking tomatoes in a hot oven until they're soft, removing the skins, and pureeing or mashing them with garlic and herbs.

SLICING SEVERAL VEGETABLES AT ONCE   Long vegetables such as carrots, cucumbers, and zucchini can be lined up on a cutting board and simultaneously cut into crosswise slices using a long sharp knife. Work carefully to avoid cutting yourself.

GENERAL COOKING DIRECTIONS FOR VEGETABLES

BAKING   Potatoes, yams, onions, eggplant, beets, pumpkin, and winter squash lend themselves to baking. The slow cooking brings out the natural sugars in the vegetables and gives much more satisfactory results than a microwave.

BRAISING   This is cooking in a covered pan in a small amount of liquid. Check the vegetables frequently to make sure the liquid has not evaporated.

MICROWAVING   The amount of water used, the length of time cooked, how the vegetables are sliced, and the amount to be cooked will all determine how well cooked or soft the vegetables will turn out to be. The vegetables will need to be cooked in a small amount of water and covered with a vented plastic wrap designated for use in microwaves, or a cover also specifically made for microwave cooking.

Fresh vegetables will vary widely in the amount of time needed for cooking. As you would expect, the green and leafy vegetables will take less time than the coarser and more fibrous root vegetables.

For example, at the high or 100 percent output setting, cabbage, endive, spinach and kale will require 5 to 7 minutes, while root vegetables such as potatoes, parsnips, rutabagas, and carrots will need approximately 15 minutes. Trimmed artichokes should take 12 to 15 minutes.

The microwave instructions for frozen vegetables are frequently listed on the package. Because they, like canned vegetables, are already cooked and only need thawing or reheating, they will require less time than fresh vegetables in the microwave.

"SAUTÉING" IN LIQUID   Instead of sautéing vegetables in oil, cook over high heat in a small amount of water, vegetable stock, or wine, until the vegetables begin to soften. Stir constantly to keep the vegetables from sticking, and add liquid as necessary.

STEAMING   Steaming vegetables allows them to retain their color, texture, and many of their water-soluble vitamins. Place the vegetables (on a plate if your steamer is large enough) in a stainless steel or bamboo steamer above 1 or 2 inches of water in a saucepan. (Putting the vegetables on a plate or bowl allows you to save the liquid that escapes as they cook. You can then use this liquid in a sauce, soup, or dressing.) Bring the water to a boil, cover the pot, and reduce the heat.

Vegetables vary in their steaming times. Steam green vegetables, squash, and cauliflower for 5 to 10 minutes, then refresh them under cold water to stop the cooking, or serve them right away, piping hot.

Artichokes and root vegetables take longer. Artichokes take 45 minutes to an hour. Carrots cut in sticks and small turnips, quartered, take about 10 to 15 minutes. Large turnips, sliced, take 15 to 20 minutes. Beets and potatoes can take anywhere from 15 to 40 minutes, depending on their size. To hasten the cooking time you can cut them into smaller pieces.

Most eggplant recipes require salting the eggplant and then sautéing it in a great deal of oil. Instead, "steam" eggplant in a hot oven. This method not only draws out the liquid but also brings out the eggplant's marvelous aroma.

To "steam" eggplant, preheat the oven to 450°F. Cut the eggplant in half lengthwise. Pierce each half in several places with a sharp knife, or make one or two slashes down the middle, cutting almost down to the skin but not through it. Brush a baking sheet with a tiny amount of oil (or use a nonstick baking sheet or cooking spray) and place the eggplant on it, cut-side down. Place in the oven for 20 minutes, or until the skins begin to shrivel. If you are going to puree the eggplant, bake until thoroughly soft, approximately 45 minutes to an hour. Remove from the oven and allow to cool. The eggplant will be soft and fragrant. When cool enough to handle, proceed with your recipe.

GENERAL COOKING DIRECTIONS FOR DRIED BEANS

With the exception of lentils and split peas, dried beans must be soaked for at least 4 hours, and preferably overnight, before you cook them. Wash the beans and pick over them to remove any small pebbles. Generally you can use three parts water per one part beans to soak, and if your water is very hard, use bottled water. Drain the water before you cook, and cook in fresh water. For a very tasty pot of beans, cook with a chopped onion and a few cloves of garlic. Make sure the volume of the pot is at least one-third greater than the beans and water, as they will bubble up fairly dramatically. Bring the beans to a boil, reduce heat, cover, and simmer 1 hour (45 minutes for lentils and split peas). Add additional garlic and herbs to taste and continue to simmer, covered, until soft but not mushy.

When do you add the salt? If you plan to use it, you may add the salt at the beginning of cooking, but be prepared to increase the length of time it will take for the beans to become tender enough to eat. Adding salt at this stage will make it more difficult to adjust the other seasonings at the end of cooking. If you learn how to season the beans with herbs and spices, you will find that you won't need as much salt to give the beans a wonderful flavor. If you must use salt, it is best to add it toward the end of cooking, after you have added your other seasonings.

By changing the water several times during the soaking process you can minimize the gassy effect that beans may have on your digestive system. This will rid the beans of the sugars that your body is not used to handling. The problem with this is that with every rinse you end up washing away some of the vitamins and minerals that make legumes an especially important food source.

Other tricks can help combat any stomach problems you might have with beans. None of these suggestions have been scientifically proven but have come anecdotally from different sources. Try adding a large pinch of baking soda to the soaking water or a piece of dried kombu seaweed to the cooking water. Kombu is a sea vegetable that can be found in health food stores or Asian markets. Adding a slice of ginger root to the cooking pot is also said to help.

If bloating remains a problem, be reassured that with time, your digestive tract should eventually develop the enzymes needed to break down these discomforting sugars.

GENERAL COOKING INSTRUCTIONS FOR GRAINS

Generally, one cup of raw grains feeds four people.

BROWN RICE AND BARLEY   Use one part brown rice to two parts water. Barley requires one part grain to three parts water. Combine the grain and water in a saucepan and bring to a boil. Add ¼ teaspoon salt (optional), reduce heat, cover, and simmer for 35–45 minutes, until most of the liquid is absorbed. Remove the lid and if any liquid remains, continue to cook, uncovered, for 5 to 10 more minutes, or until all the liquid has evaporated.

BULGUR   Use one part bulgur to two parts water. Place the bulgur in a bowl. Bring the water to a boil and pour over the bulgur. Add ¼ teaspoon salt (optional). Let sit until most of the water is

GENERAL INSTRUCTIONS FOR PREPARING DRIED
UNSOAKED LEGUMES

Legume (1 Cup Dry)	Water	Cooking Time	Yield
Aduki beans	3 cups	2 hours	2 cups
Baby lima beans	2 cups	1½ hours	1¾ cups
Black beans	4 cups	1½ hours	2 cups
Black-eyed peas	3 cups	1 hour	2 cups
Chick-peas (Garbanzo beans)	4 cups	3 hours	2½ cups
Cranberry beans	3 cups	1½ hours	2½ cups
Fava beans	3 cups	3 hours	2 cups
Great northern beans	3½ cups	2 hours	2 cups
Kidney beans	3 cups	1½ hours	2 cups
Lentils	3 cups	45 minutes	2¼ cups
Lima beans	2 cups	1½ minutes	1¼ cups
Mung beans	2½ cups	1½ hours	2 cups
Navy beans	3 cups	2½ hours	2 cups
Pigeon peas	3 cups	30 minutes	2¼ cups
Pinto beans	3 cups	2½ hours	2 cups
Red beans	3 cups	3 hours	2 cups
Split peas	3 cups	45 minutes	2¼ cups

absorbed and the bulgur becomes soft (about 20 minutes). Pour off the excess water and fluff with a fork.

COUSCOUS   Use one part couscous to two parts water or vegetable stock (tepid or hot, but not boiling). Place the couscous in a bowl, pour the water over it, cover, and let sit 10 to 15 minutes. Fluff with a fork.

The more traditional method of preparing couscous involves steaming and produces a lighter, more separate "grain." After soaking couscous as above, if it is wetter and not as tender as you would like, drain it and then steam the couscous for 20–25 minutes. You can use a simple vegetable steamer by placing a double layer of cheesecloth over the steamer to prevent the couscous from falling through the venting holes.

If you want to add couscous to a vegetable stew, add the uncooked couscous at the end of cooking. Simmer for 2 to 3 minutes, and then let stand for 5–10 minutes before adding the seasonings to taste.

KASHA (BUCKWHEAT GROATS)   Use one part kasha to two parts water or stock. Have the stock simmering. Roast the kasha over

GENERAL INSTRUCTIONS FOR PREPARING GRAINS

Grain (1 Cup Dry)	Water	Cooking Time	Yield
Amaranth	1½ cups	20 minutes	2 cups
Arborio rice	2 cups	25 minutes	2½ cups
Barley (whole)	3 cups	45 minutes	3½ cups
Basmati rice	2½ cups	20 minutes	3 cups
Brown rice	2 cups	45 minutes	3 cups
Buckwheat (kasha)	2 cups	15 minutes	2½ cups
Bulgur wheat	2 cups	15–20 minutes	2½ cups
Couscous (precooked)	1 cup	15 minutes soaking	2¾ cups
Cracked wheat	2 cups	25 minutes	2⅓ cups
Millet	2½ to 3 cups	35–45 minutes	3½ cups
Oats (whole grain)	2 cups	1 hour	2½ cups
Polenta	4 cups	25 minutes	3 cups
Rye berries	2½ to 3 cups	1 hour	2 cups
Quinoa	2 cups	15 minutes	2½ cups
White rice	2 cups	20 minutes	3 cups
Wild rice	3 cups	1 hour or more	3½ cups
Whole grain wheat berries	2½ to 3 cups	2 hours	2¾ cups

medium heat in a dry heavy-bottomed saucepan or frying pan with a lid, stirring until the grains begin to smell toasty, about 2 minutes. Add the simmering stock, cover, and simmer 20 to 30 minutes, until the kasha is tender but not mushy. Pour off any remaining stock.

MILLET   Roast the millet in a dry saucepan until it begins to smell toasty—about 2 minutes. Use one part millet to two and one half parts water. Add the water and bring to a boil. Add ¼ teaspoon salt (optional), reduce heat, cover, and simmer for 35 minutes. Remove the lid and continue to simmer until the liquid is evaporated (up to 10 minutes).

QUINOA   This grainlike food needs to be rinsed well prior to cooking. For its preparation, use one part quinoa to two parts water. Combine quinoa and water in a saucepan and bring to a boil. Reduce heat, cover, and simmer for 15 minutes, until most of the liquid is absorbed. Remove the lid and if any liquid remains, continue to cook, uncovered, for 5 to 10 minutes more or until all the liquid has evaporated.

WHEAT BERRIES, WHOLE RYE, AND TRITICALE   Use one part

grain to three parts water. Combine the grains and water and bring to a boil. Add ¼ teaspoon salt (optional), reduce heat, cover, and simmer for 50 minutes. Wheat berries and triticale require 2 hours. Remove from the heat and pour off any excess liquid.

GENERAL COOKING INSTRUCTIONS FOR PASTA AND NOODLES

Bring a large pot of water to a rolling boil. Add salt (optional) and drop in the pasta. With a long-handled spoon, give the pasta a stir so that it doesn't stick together. You only want to cook the pasta until it is cooked through but still firm to the bite—*al dente*—and this will take anywhere from 4 to 10 minutes, depending on the kind of pasta. Test after 4 minutes and keep testing every minute until done. Drain and proceed with your recipe.

Since no oil is being added to the cooking water, and we are not using oil-based pasta sauces, there may be a problem with the cooked pasta clumping together. Consider rinsing the pasta in cold water after draining, particularly if you are not planning to serve it immediately after tossing it with your sauce or vegetables.

Cellophane Noodles

These noodles are found commercially in Asian food markets or the Oriental foods sections in the larger supermarket chains. They are sold as large bundles of dried noodles. Soak them for 20 minutes in warm water and then cook for no more than 3 minutes in boiling water or vegetable stock.

Soba Noodles

Use 2 to 3 quarts of water for 8 ounces of noodles. Put the water into a very large pot and bring to a rolling boil. Add the soba noodles and continue boiling. When the water starts to foam, add 1 cup of cold water and reduce the heat to medium. When the water comes to a boil again, add another cup of cold water. Repeat this 3 more times. Check the noodles for texture after the third time. If they are not al dente, continue cooking. After cooking, drain and rinse under cold water.

TWENTY-ONE DAYS OF MENUS

Day 1

Breakfast

Waffles
Nonfat yogurt
Fresh strawberries
Orange juice
Brewed tea

Lunch

Hummus
Tabbouleh

Tossed green salad
Pita bread
Fresh fruit

Dinner

Black Bean Burritos
Quinoa Mexican Style
Salsa Cruda
Orange-Jicama Salad with
    Pickled Onions
Berry Sorbet

Day 2

Breakfast

Oatmeal with Raisins and
    Cinnamon
Nonfat milk
Grapefruit half
Brewed tea or warm beverage

Lunch

Black Bean Chili
Toasted corn tortillas
Green Pea "Guacamole"

Tossed green salad
Salsa Cruda
Fresh fruit

Dinner

White Bean and Tomato Soup
    with Fresh Herbs
Vegetable Cakes with Red
    Pepper Coulis
Corn Salad with Lime-Cilantro
    Dressing on lettuce greens
Garlic Bread
Peach Bread Pudding

Day 3

Breakfast

Dry cereal
Nonfat milk or yogurt
Grapefruit half
Brewed tea or beverage
Peach Bread Pudding

Lunch

Pizza Provençal
Tossed green salad
Sorbet with fresh fruit

Dinner

Tomato and Lentil Soup
Wild Mushroom Flan
Roasted Potatoes

Julienned Vegetables with
    Lemon-Mustard Vinaigrette
Pears with Black Cherry Sauce
French Bread

Day 4

Breakfast

Buckwheat Pancakes
Nonfat yogurt
Sliced bananas
Sliced kiwi
Fresh berries
Orange juice

Lunch

Tomato and Lentil Soup

Zucchini Salad
Bread
Fresh fruit

Dinner

Sweet and Sour Wok-Cooked
    Vegetables with Tofu
Broccoli with Teriyaki Sauce
Golden Rice Pilaf
Tossed green salad
Orange sections

Day 5

Breakfast

Apple-Cinnamon Oat Bran
    Muffins
Nonfat yogurt
Fresh berries
Orange juice

Lunch

Pasta with Asparagus and
    Asparagus Cream
Baby Lima Bean Salad

Tossed green salad
Fresh fruit

Dinner

Spanish Chick-Pea and Garlic
    Soup
Linguini with Roasted Red
    Pepper and Herbed Tomato
    Sauce
Onion Confit with Croutons
Watercress, Fennel, and Orange
    Salad
Poached Pears

Day 6

Breakfast

Toasted Carrot Cake
Dry cereal
Nonfat milk
Fresh berries
Brewed tea or beverage

Lunch

Southwestern Vegetable Stew
Tofu Cheese with Herbs
Garlic Bread
Tossed green salad
Sorbet

Dinner

White Bean and Tomato Soup
  with Fresh Herbs
Mushroom and Leek Crêpes

Wild and Arborio Rice
Broccoli with Honey and
  Mustard Sauce
Apple Strudel

Day 7

Breakfast

Apple Strudel
Dry cereal
Nonfat yogurt
Grapefruit half
Brewed tea or beverage

Lunch

White Bean Salad
Pasta Primavera with Dijon
  Vinaigrette

Tossed green salad
Fresh fruit

Dinner

Minestrone Soup
Stuffed Zucchini with Tomato
  Sauce and Fennel Seeds
Red Onion and Cucumber
  Vinaigrette
Risotto
Apple and Apple Cider Sherbet

Day 8

Breakfast

Waffles
Nonfat yogurt
Sliced kiwi
Raisins
Mango juice
Brewed tea or beverage

Lunch

Minestrone Soup
Bread

Tossed green salad
Fresh fruit

Dinner

Kappa Maki
Marinated Tofu
Eggplant Puree
Marinated Cucumber and Red
  Bell Pepper Salad with
  Cellophane Noodles
Rice
Melon with Ginger Lemon Syrup

Day 9

Breakfast

Oatmeal with Raisins and
  Cinnamon
Nonfat yogurt and fruit

Orange juice
Brewed tea or beverage

Lunch

Gazpacho
Tamale Pie

Garlic Bread
Jicama-Cucumber Salad with
    Lime and Chili
Fresh fruit

Dinner

Ratatouille
Polenta with Tomato Sauce

French Lentil Salad
Tossed green salad
Banana Bread

Day 10

Breakfast

Banana Bread
Nonfat yogurt and fruit
Orange juice
Brewed tea or beverage

Lunch

Chick-Pea and Vegetable Stew
    with Couscous

Tossed green salad
Fresh fruit

Dinner

Stuffed Red Pepper with Spanish
    Rice and Tomatillo Sauce
Tossed green salad
Red Bean Chili
Corn tortillas
Balsamic Strawberries

Day 11

Breakfast

Corn Bread
Jam
Nonfat yogurt with fruit
Brewed tea or beverage

Lunch

Pasta with Eggplant-Red Pepper
    Sauce
Tofu Cheese with Fresh Herbs

Bread
Tossed green salad
Fresh fruit

Dinner

Green Split Pea Soup with
    Carrots and Celery
Eggplant Lasagna
Mushrooms Braised with Herbs
Broccoli with Lemon Sauce
Bread
Poached Pears

Day 12

Breakfast

Millet Cereal with Raisins
Nonfat yogurt

Toast
Jam
Fresh berries
Brewed tea or beverage

Lunch

Black Bean Salad on lettuce
    greens
Zucchini Pancakes
Salsa Cruda
Potatoes Cooked in Wine with
    Basil
Bread
Fresh fruit

Dinner

Chinese Eggplant and Tofu
Asparagus with Roasted Red
    Peppers
Rice Salad with Apricots and
    Currants
Semolina Lemon Pudding

Day 13

Breakfast

Fresh raspberries
Dry cereal
Nonfat milk or yogurt
Toast
Brewed tea or beverage

Lunch

Red Bean Chili
Scalloped Potatoes

Coleslaw
Corn Bread or tortillas
Fresh fruit or sorbet

Dinner

Carrot Soup with Ginger,
    Orange, and Cilantro
Indian Vegetable Stew
Couscous
Apple Chutney
Tossed green salad
Peach Bread Pudding

Day 14

Breakfast

Peach Bread Pudding
Dry cereal
Nonfat milk or yogurt
Orange juice
Brewed tea or beverage

Lunch

Gazpacho
Green Pea "Guacamole"

Corn tortilla chips
Tossed green salad
Fresh fruit

Dinner

Garlic-Herb Soup
Stuffed Manicotti
Brussel Sprouts with Maple
    Syrup
Tossed green salad
Mango Compote

Day 15

Breakfast

Apple-Cinnamon Oat Bran
    Muffins
Nonfat yogurt
Sliced bananas
Brewed tea or beverage

Lunch

Stuffed Manicotti

Tossed green salad
Garlic Bread
Fresh fruit

Dinner

Enchiladas with Tomatillo Sauce
Rice Pilaf with Saffron Peppers
Black Bean Salad on tossed
    lettuce greens
Baked Bananas

Day 16

Breakfast

Buckwheat Pancakes
Nonfat yogurt
Fresh berries
Sliced kiwi
Orange juice

Lunch

Spicy Carrot and Tomato Soup
Mushroom and Artichoke
    Frittata

Quinoa Salad on tossed lettuce
    greens
Melon slices with sorbet

Dinner

Pasta with Red Pepper and
    Lentil Sauce
Tossed green salad
Garlic Bread
Broccoli with Honey and
    Mustard Sauce
Pear Cobbler

Day 17

Breakfast

Pear Cobbler
Dry cereal
Nonfat milk or yogurt
Orange juice

Lunch

Tofu Stew with Miso
Saffron rice

Steamed Spinach with
    Honey-Mustard Sauce
Fresh fruit

Dinner

Lentil-Hominy Soup with Lime
    and Chili
Potato Pancakes
Applesauce
Tossed green salad
Carrot Cake

Day 18

Breakfast

Buckwheat Pancakes
Baked Bananas
Raisins
Nonfat yogurt
Orange juice
Brewed tea or beverage

Lunch

Lentil-Hominy Soup with Lime
   and Chili

Garlic Bread
Celery Root with
   Lemon-Mustard Vinaigrette
Fresh fruit

Dinner

Garlic-Herb Soup
Lydia's Mexican Casserole
Tossed green salad
Berry Sorbet

Day 19

Breakfast

Waffles
Nonfat yogurt
Sliced peaches
Strawberries
Brewed tea or beverage

Lunch

Scrambled Tofu and Vegetables
Garlic Bread

Salsa Picante
Tossed green salad
Fresh fruit

Dinner

Eggplant Lasagna
Zucchini "Pasta" with Yogurt
   Sauce
Pickled Red Onions
Tossed green salad
Rice Pudding

Day 20

Breakfast

Plantain Pancakes (without Red
   Pepper-Jalapeño Sauce)
Salsa
Nonfat yogurt with fruit
Jam
Orange juice
Brewed tea or beverage

Lunch

Hearty Bean and Vegetable Stew
Waldorf Salad
Bread
Fresh fruit

Dinner

Tomatillo Soup with Corn and
   Cilantro

Black Bean Burritos
Zucchini and Mushrooms with
  Ancho Chili Sauce

Apple and Apple Cider Sherbet

Day 21

Breakfast

Oatmeal with Raisins and
  Cinnamon
Nonfat yogurt
Fresh berries
Orange juice

Lunch

Tomatillo Soup with Corn and
  Cilantro
Baby Lima Bean Salad on tossed
  greens

Roasted Potatoes
Bread
Fresh fruit

Dinner

Steamed Fresh Vegetables and
  Tofu with Soba Noodles
Misoyaki Sauce
Yams with Ginger and Dried
  Apricots
Banana Bread

SALADS, DRESSINGS, CONDIMENTS, AND STARTERS

You will see from the number of recipes in this section that you can practically live on salads. They're perfect for all the beautiful fresh vegetables in the market, as well as for many leftovers, especially grains and beans. There are plenty of substantial salads to choose from here: bean salads like the French Lentil Salad (page 423), or the White Bean Salad (page 422); salads made from grains, like the Rice Salad with Apricots and Currants (page 419) or the Tabbouleh (page 419). Potato salad is also filling and delicious, and there are plenty to choose from here. These substantial salads can easily serve as main dishes. The chutneys make nice accompaniments for these and for curries.

More delicate combinations that would make nice starters, light lunches, or side dishes, are also plentiful here. They are colorful and bursting with the fresh, vibrant flavors of herbs and fresh produce. All of the recipes should make your mouth water.

The pureed bean and vegetable spreads—Hummus (page 411), Eggplant Puree (page 411), and Green Pea "Guacamole" (page 444)—are delicious spread on bread and accompany these salads beautifully. They also make nice hors d'oeuvres as dips or served with bread or crackers.

You will see here that oil is not essential for a good salad. The dressings are lively ones based on tasty vinegars, lemon juice, lime juice, tomato juice, and orange juice. They combine brilliantly with the ingredients in the salads to bring out their flavors in the most delicious ways.

ITALIAN DRESSING

YIELD: 2 CUPS (16 SERVINGS)   BY CHRISTIAN JANSELME

If this dressing is too thick, reduce the amount of recommended cornstarch the next time that you make it.

2 cups water
2 tablespoons cornstarch
1 teaspoon salt substitute
1/8 teaspoon freshly ground black pepper
2 shallots, minced

1/4 red bell pepper, minced
2 tablespoons Dijon mustard
2 cloves garlic, minced
1/2 teaspoon freshly minced Italian parsley
1/2 teaspoon paprika

7 tablespoons plus 2 teaspoons   *1 tablespoon honey*
   white wine vinegar

Bring the water to a boil and stir in the cornstarch. Let cool. If the mixture is lumpy, you may want to pass it through a blender. Mix the remaining ingredients together, then add to the water and cornstarch mixture. Mix well and keep refrigerated.

Serving size = 2 tablespoons
11 calories
0.1 grams total fat
trace saturated fat
0 milligrams cholesterol

CHINESE DRESSING

YIELD: 2 CUPS (16 SERVINGS)   BY CHRISTIAN JANSELME

This works well as a salad dressing or dipping sauce. Please note that with the soy sauce and pickles this has a fair amount of sodium and should probably not be used by those with hypertension or congestive heart failure.

6½ tablespoons finely chopped   *6 tablespoons plus 2 teaspoons soy*
   sweet gherkins   *sauce*
1 teaspoon freshly minced garlic   *3 tablespoons plus 1 teaspoon*
½ cup or ½ bunch freshly   *honey*
   minced cilantro   *6 tablespoons plus 2 teaspoons*
2 teaspoons finely minced onion   *balsamic vinegar*
4 teaspoons Dijon mustard   *2 cups water*

Mix the gherkins, garlic, cilantro, onion, mustard, soy sauce, honey, and vinegar together. Set aside. Bring the water to a boil and then add the mixed ingredients. Either mix this well or process it in a blender or food processor for a smoother dressing.

Serving size = 2 tablespoons
13 calories
trace total fat
trace saturated fat
0 milligrams cholesterol
461 milligrams sodium

LEMON AND MUSTARD VINAIGRETTE WITH GARLIC

YIELD: 1/4 CUP (2 SERVINGS)   BY MARK HALL

Use this for any of your favorite steamed vegetables such as broccoli, spinach, zucchini or other varieties of squash. It is also good on cold salads.

3 tablespoons fresh lemon juice
1 tablespoon Dijon mustard
1/4 teaspoon balsamic vinegar
1/4 teaspoon freshly minced garlic

1 teaspoon dried tarragon leaf
Salt
Freshly ground black pepper

Mix the first five ingredients. Add salt and pepper to taste.

Serving size = 2 tablespoons
2 calories
0.1 grams total fat
trace saturated fat
0 milligrams cholesterol

TOMATO VINAIGRETTE

YIELD: 2/3 CUP (5 TO 6 SERVINGS)   BY MARK HALL

This can be used on a crisp green salad or mixed blanched vegetables on a bed of lettuce.

1/2 cup tomato juice
1/4 teaspoon freshly minced garlic
1 tablespoon balsamic vinegar
1/2 tablespoon Dijon mustard
2 teaspoons dried chopped basil

1/4 teaspoon freshly ground black
 pepper
2 tablespoons fresh basil
Salt

Very briefly blend or puree all ingredients except for the salt in a food processor or blender. Add salt to taste.

Serving size = 2 tablespoons
8 calories
0.1 grams total fat
trace saturated fat
0 milligrams cholesterol

RED PEPPER COULIS

YIELD: 1½ CUPS (10 SERVINGS)   BY WOLFGANG PUCK

The vibrant color and flavor make this an excellent accompaniment to many dishes, such as the Vegetable Cakes recipe on page 490.

½ pound (2 small) cored, seeded and diced red peppers
1 medium (about 6 oz.) peeled, seeded and diced tomato
½ large (about 6 oz.) onion, diced

1¾ cups Vegetable Stock (page 475)
¼ cup chopped basil
Pinch of thyme

In a medium skillet, combine the red pepper, tomato, onion and vegetable stock and cook until the vegetables are tender, 10 to 15 minutes. Stir in the basil and thyme.

Puree in a blender and pour back into a clean skillet. Reduce until about 1½ cups remain. Use as needed.

Serving size = ¼ cup
32 calories
0.3 grams total fat
trace saturated fat
0 milligrams cholesterol

RED ONION AND CUCUMBER VINAIGRETTE

YIELD: 6 CUPS (6 SERVINGS)   BY ALICE WATERS

3 medium-sized red onions
1 cucumber (preferably Japanese, 6 to 7 inches long)

About ½ cup rice wine vinegar

Peel and thinly slice 3 medium red onions and 1 cucumber. Toss the vegetables with ½ cup rice wine vinegar and arrange on a serving platter.

Serving size = 1 cup
32 calories
0.3 grams total fat
0.1 grams saturated fat
0 milligrams cholesterol

PICKLED RED ONIONS

YIELD: 2 CUPS (4 SERVINGS)   BY DEBORAH MADISON

This recipe is quick to make and may well become a standard preparation to have on hand in your refrigerator. The onions become completely infused with pink and make a beautiful and lively tasting garnish for all kinds of salads. Keep the rings whole or finely dice the onion. They'll keep a week or so refrigerated, though they may loose their crispness as they sit.

1 pound firm, smooth red onions
boiling water
1 cup white wine, champagne,
    tarragon, or rice vinegar or
    other mild vinegar
1 cup cold water
1 tablespoon pickling spice or

½ teaspoon peppercorns,
½ teaspoon coriander seeds,
2 bay leaves, and ¼ teaspoon
    red peppercorns
1 teaspoon sugar
1 clove garlic, sliced (optional)

Peel the onion and slice into thin rounds. Separate the rounds and put them in a colander large enough to hold them comfortably. Place the colander in the sink.

Bring about a quart of water to a boil and pour it over the onions, letting it drip right through the colander. Transfer the onions to a bowl and add the vinegar, cold water, spices, sugar, and garlic, if using. If the onions aren't covered by the liquid, add more as necessary, using equal parts water and vinegar. Cover with plastic wrap and refrigerate until cool and the color is diffused, about 30 minutes. Keep in the liquid, refrigerated, and use as needed.

Serving size = ½ cup
52 calories
0.4 grams total fat
0.05 grams saturated fat
0 mg cholesterol

COMPOSED SALAD OF MANGOES AND BEETS WITH MANGO VINAIGRETTE

YIELD: 8 CUPS (4 TO 6 SERVINGS)   BY PAM MORGAN

Although the combination of mangoes and beets may seem strange, they taste wonderful together. The green of the lettuces, the dark pink of the beets, and the orange of the mango makes a spectacular presentation. The beets and the vinaigrette can be prepared and refrigerated up to two days in advance.

4 medium-sized fresh beets, leaves
   and stems removed
1/2 cup chopped red onion
1 bunch watercress, large stems
   removed
1 small bunch Frisee or American
   chicory
2 small heads Bibb lettuce
2 peeled and sliced (strips) ripe
   mangoes

Mango Vinaigrette:
1/4 cup cider vinegar
1 tablespoon honey mustard
1/2 teaspoon curry powder
1 tablespoon fresh lime juice
1 peeled, seeded, and chunked
   ripe mango
Pinch salt
Freshly ground black pepper to
   taste

All of the ingredients for the vinaigrette can be added to a food processor or blender. Process with a steel blade, or blend until smooth.

Cook the beets in boiling water for thirty minutes and drain. When they have cooled enough to permit handling, peel and chop into small cubes. Toss the beets with the red onions and three tablespoons of the vinaigrette. Set aside.

On a medium-sized serving platter, arrange the lettuces on the outside of the plate. Place the watercress in the center of the platter and spoon the beets and onions over it. The mango strips can be arranged around the beets. Transfer the remaining dressing to a serving bowl and serve on the side with the salad.

Serving size = 2 cups
110 calories
0.7 grams total fat
0.1 grams saturated fat
0 milligrams cholesterol

Mango Vinaigrette
Serving size = 2 tablespoons
39 calories
0.4 grams total fat
trace saturated fat
0 milligrams cholesterol

JULIENNED VEGETABLES WITH LEMON-MUSTARD VINAIGRETTE

YIELD: 2½ CUPS VEGETABLES (2 TO 3 SERVINGS)   BY MARK HALL

For the fresh herbs in the dressing use Italian parsley in combination with others. If you like the taste of tarragon and plan to use it, do so without other herbs because the flavor is quite distinctive. This colorful salad can be served warm or chilled.

½ cup julienned red onions
½ cup julienned carrots
½ cup julienned celery
½ cup julienned red or yellow
   bell peppers
½ cup bean sprouts

2½ tablespoons fresh lemon juice
1 tablespoon Dijon mustard
Salt
Freshly ground black pepper
1 tablespoon chopped fresh herbs

Briefly blanch together the red onions, carrots, celery, peppers, and bean sprouts. This should take no more than 45 seconds. Mix together the lemon juice, mustard, and salt and pepper to taste. Toss this with the vegetables and fresh herbs.

Serving size = 1 cup
44 calories
0.6 grams total fat
trace saturated fat
0 milligrams cholesterol

MARINATED CUCUMBER AND RED BELL PEPPER SALAD WITH CELLOPHANE NOODLES

YIELD: 4½ CUPS (4 TO 5 SERVINGS)   BY CAROL CONNELL

This is a particularly refreshing, crunchy summer salad.

2 ounces dry cellophane or bean
   thread noodles
Vegetable broth (optional)
2 cups peeled, seeded, and sliced
   cucumbers
2 cups thinly sliced red bell
   peppers

1 cup no-oil Italian dressing or
   vinaigrette
1 tablespoon freshly minced basil
1 tablespoon freshly minced
   cilantro
⅛ teaspoon red hot chili flakes
Lettuce

Drop the noodles into boiling water or vegetable broth for 5 to 10 minutes or until done. Toss all ingredients together and marinate for at least 1 hour. Serve on a bed of lettuce.

Serving size = 1 cup
84 calories
0.5 grams total fat
trace saturated fat
0 milligrams cholesterol

CAULIFLOWER WITH LIME AND HOT PEPPER VINAIGRETTE

YIELD: 4½ CUPS (4½ SERVINGS)   BY MARK HALL

This dressing has just a hint of fire. You should not find it overwhelming.

5 cups cauliflower florets
2 tablespoons lime juice
1½ teaspoons rice wine vinegar
⅜ teaspoon red hot chili flakes

½ teaspoon freshly minced garlic
½ teaspoon ground cumin
1½ tablespoons finely minced cilantro

Blanch the cauliflower and plunge into ice cold water to stop the cooking. Heat the lime juice, vinegar, and chili flakes in a saucepan over medium heat until the flakes have softened. Pour over the cauliflower. Add the garlic, cumin, and cilantro. Let marinate for at least 1 hour.

Serving size = 1 cup
44 calories
0.5 grams total fat
trace saturated fat
0 milligrams cholesterol

ZUCCHINI SALAD

YIELD: 2½ CUPS (2 TO 3 SERVINGS)   BY MARK HALL

This can be served warm or cold.

1 cup sliced red onion
½ teaspoon freshly minced garlic
4 teaspoons rice wine vinegar
2 cups julienned zucchini
    (approximately 1 medium-sized
    zucchini)

1 cup halved cherry tomatoes
2 teaspoons freshly minced Italian
    parsley
Salt
Freshly ground black pepper

Put the onions and garlic in a large pan with 2 teaspoons rice wine vinegar. Cover the pan and let braise over medium heat. When the onion is translucent but not soft, remove the pan from the heat, add the zucchini, and toss. The goal is to let the heat from the onions just wilt the zucchini. Toss with the remaining 2 teaspoons rice wine vinegar, the cherry tomatoes, and parsley. Season with salt and pepper to taste and serve.

Serving size = 1 cup
54 calories
0.5 grams total fat
0.1 grams saturated fat
0 milligrams cholesterol

CELERY ROOT WITH LEMON AND MUSTARD VINAIGRETTE WITH GARLIC

YIELD: 2 CUPS (4 SERVINGS)   BY MARK HALL

The Lemon and Mustard Vinaigrette dressing gives this traditional salad a spicy and piquant quality. It can be served at room temperature or chilled.

2 cups celery root
¼ cup Lemon and Mustard
    Vinaigrette with Garlic (page
    399)

Remove coarse husk from the celery root. The root turns brown quickly, so put it in some water with lemon juice while you are slicing it to keep it from turning. Cut it into matchstick shapes and blanch in boiling water, being careful not to overcook it. This should take about 2 minutes, depending on how large the "matchsticks" are. Then plunge the celery root into ice cold water to stop the cooking.

Toss the dressing with the celery root. Let it marinate for at least 1 hour.

VARIATION: Use 1 cup celery root and 1 cup julienned carrots. Blanch each vegetable separately and plunge into ice cold water to stop the cooking. Toss with the dressing, marinate, and serve.

Serving size = ½ cup
23 calories
0.3 grams total fat
trace saturated fat
0 milligrams cholesterol

ASPARAGUS WITH ROASTED RED PEPPERS

YIELD: 2 CUPS (4 SERVINGS)   BY MARK HALL

1½ cups asparagus   1 teaspoon balsamic vinegar
1 medium red pepper   Salt
1 teaspoon freshly minced garlic   Pepper

Remove the hard bottom stem of the asparagus and slice the rest of the stalk into approximately 1-inch pieces. Blanch the asparagus and put into ice-cold water to stop it from cooking further. Drain and set aside.

Roast the red pepper in a 500 degree oven for 20 to 30 minutes, turning occasionally. When the skin has darkened and blistered, remove the pepper from the oven. Transfer it to a bowl and cover with aluminum foil. Let it cool for 30 minutes, then peel off the skin and seed the pepper. Slice into julienne strips and toss ½ cup roasted pepper with the garlic and vinegar. Let marinate for a few minutes then toss the peppers with the asparagus. Add salt and pepper to taste and serve.

Serving size = ½ cup
16 calories
0.2 grams total fat
trace saturated fat
0 mg cholesterol

ROASTED PEPPERS WITH SAFFRON

YIELD: 1 CUP (4 SERVINGS)   BY DEBORAH MADISON

You can eat these tender roasted peppers by themselves for an appetizer, combine them with other elements to make a larger salad, toss them with pasta, or add to cooked rice and millet. They'll keep for several days if well covered and refrigerated.

For the best results and easiest handling, choose thick-fleshed red or yellow peppers whose sides are as flat and even as possible. For a really pretty salad, use both red and yellow peppers.

Appetizer for four

2 medium to large peppers
1 small garlic clove, slivered
Pinch of saffron threads
1 tablespoon boiling water
Balsamic vinegar, to taste

Fresh herbs, such as basil or
   marjoram, chopped
Chopped nasturtium flowers or
   slivered opal basil (optional)

Grill the peppers directly over an open flame. (If you don't have a gas-burning stove, place the peppers under the electric element in the oven and turn them every few minutes.) Set them right on the burner, turn the flame on high, and every few minutes, rotate, using a pair of tongs. Continue doing this until the pepper is completely charred, then immediately drop in plastic bag and twist shut, or set in a bowl and cover with a plate. Allow the peppers to steam for at least 15 minutes to soften the flesh and make the peels easier to remove.

After the pepper has steamed, you'll notice an amber-colored juice in the bottom of the bowl. Carefully reserve it. If it is full of ash, pour it through a sieve. This sweet, syrupy juice will become part of the dressing. If you hold the pepper up and pierce it at the bottom, more juice will run out, which you can add to the syrup. Set aside in a bowl.

Using a paper towel, wipe off the charred skin. Remove the top, open up the pepper, scrape out the seeds and slice into pieces as wide as you like. Add them to the juices along with the slivered garlic. Cover the saffron threads with the boiling water, allow to stand several minutes, then pour over the peppers. Toss, season with vinegar to taste, and just before serving, toss with the herbs.

For a pretty garnish, you could toss the peppers with chopped nasturtium flowers or the slivered leaves of opal basil.

---

1 serving = ¼ cup
9 calories
0.1 gram total fat
trace saturated fat
0 milligrams cholesterol

CORN SALAD WITH LIME-CILANTRO DRESSING

YIELD: 4 CUPS (4 TO 8 SERVINGS)   BY MARK HALL

You can use canned corn for this salad but sweet corn, at the height of the season, makes this very colorful salad something special.

2 cups fresh corn kernels (from 2
    to 4 ears)
½ teaspoon freshly minced garlic
¼ cup white wine
¾ cup finely diced red bell
    pepper
¾ cup finely diced green bell
    pepper
½ cup finely diced red onion

2 tablespoons freshly chopped
    cilantro
1 tablespoon freshly chopped
    parsley
⅛ teaspoon cayenne
¼ teaspoon freshly ground black
    pepper
½ teaspoon salt

Lime-Cilantro Dressing:

2 tablespoons rice wine vinegar
2 teaspoons lime juice

Braise the corn with the garlic in the white wine for about 5 minutes. When the corn is cooked, toss with the diced peppers and onion. Mix the dressing and toss with the vegetables. Serve at room temperature.

Serving size = 1 cup
91 calories
1.1 grams total fat
0.1 grams saturated fat
0 milligrams cholesterol

COLESLAW

YIELD: 4 CUPS (8 SERVINGS)   BY MARK HALL

This can be prepared in one of two methods. The salad can be dressed immediately after tossing the vegetables or it can be "wilted" before dressing and serving. Wilting changes the texture and taste. It requires a fair amount of salt which can be rinsed off at the end of this procedure. Keep in mind that there will still be some residual salt. Therefore, if hypertension or heart failure is a problem, this step should be omitted.

*3 cups thinly sliced cabbage
1 cup thinly sliced carrots
1/2 to 1 teaspoon kosher salt*

*2 tablespoons Dijon mustard
1 teaspoon caraway seeds
1/4 teaspoon freshly ground black
    pepper*

Dressing:

*1 tablespoon rice wine vinegar
1 tablespoon red vine vinegar*

In a large bowl toss the cabbage and carrots together. If you plan to wilt the vegetables, sprinkle some salt onto the cabbage-carrot mixture and distribute it well. Cover it with a heavy plate or pot cover that will weight down on the mixture. The salt will pull the water out of the vegetables. Let this sit for about 1 hour. Drain and rinse.

To prepare the dressing, mix the rice and red wine vinegars with the mustard, caraway seeds, and pepper. When the slaw has been rinsed, toss it with the dressing.

CITA PINNOCK'S VARIATION: For a creamy dressing, blend or process the following ingredients and toss with the cabbage and carrots:

*1/2 cup nonfat yogurt
1/4 cup Italian Dressing (page 397)
1 tablespoon freshly minced onion
1/4 teaspoon celery seed*

*1/2 teaspoon honey
1/4 teaspoon white pepper
1 tablespoon minced Italian
    parsley*

Serving size = 1/2 cup
19 calories
0.2 grams total fat
trace saturated fat
0 milligrams cholesterol

Variation with creamy dressing:
Serving size = 1/2 cup
24 caloires
trace total fat
trace saturated fat
trace cholesterol

CRANBERRY ASPIC

YIELD: 1 CUP (4 SERVINGS)   BY MARY CARROLL

The bright red color and texture of this aspic bring a warm holiday feeling to your most special fall and winter occasions.

½ cup fresh cranberries
¼ cup chopped, seeded, and
  peeled oranges
¼ cup cored and peeled ripe
  persimmons or apples
⅓ teaspoon freshly grated nutmeg

1 tablespoon agar-agar gelatin
  flakes
Lettuce, parsley, or other greenery
  for garnish

Pulse all the ingredients except the garnish in a food processor or blender until chunky. Place in a saucepan and heat to boiling, stirring constantly, until agar-agar flakes are completely dissolved. Pour into a nonstick or lightly oil-sprayed gelatin mold or decorative glass bowl and chill until firm. To unmold, run the bottom of the bowl under hot water for a few seconds, then turn the aspic onto a platter. Decorate with lettuce, parsley, or other greenery.

Serving size = ¼ cup
17 calories
0.2 grams total fat
0.1 grams saturated fat
0 milligrams cholesterol

HUMMUS

YIELD: 2 CUPS (4 SERVINGS)   BY DONNA NICOLETTI

This Middle Eastern dip is perfect with pita bread, crackers, or a salad.

1 cup dry chick-peas (garbanzos)
5 cups water
6 to 7 bay leaves
¾ cup chopped onion
1 clove garlic
⅔ cup tomato puree
2 tablespoons lemon juice
¾ teaspoon ground cumin

¼ teaspoon paprika
⅛ teaspoon cayenne
¼ teaspoon freshly ground black
  pepper
¾ teaspoon salt
Chopped fresh Italian parsley,
  mint, or cilantro for garnish
  (optional)

Sort and rinse the chick-peas, then soak overnight in water. Drain them, then add 5 cups water and bay leaves. Bring to a boil, then reduce the heat to medium and cook for approximately 1½ hours, or until the beans are completely soft. When cooked, drain the beans and puree until completely smooth in a food processor with the rest of the ingredients except the garnish.

Garnish with parsley, mint, or cilantro.

Serving size = ½ cup
204 calories
2.9 grams total fat
0.3 grams saturated fat
0 milligrams cholesterol

EGGPLANT PUREE

YIELD: 1½ CUPS (3 SERVINGS)   BY MARK HALL

This puree works as a side dish to Asian-inspired dishes. It can also be used as a spread for pita bread or as a dip with fresh vegetables.

*1 pound coarsely chopped
   American eggplant
½ cup water
2 teaspoons freshly grated or
   minced ginger
1 teaspoon freshly minced garlic
½ tablespoon molasses*

*3½ tablespoons freshly chopped
   cilantro
⅛ teaspoon hot red pepper flakes
½ tablespoon soy sauce
1 tablespoon rice wine vinegar
Salt (optional)*

Peel and chop the eggplant. Place in a pot with ½ cup water. Bring to a boil, cover, and let steam about 7 minutes, until thoroughly cooked, stirring frequently. Puree in a food processor until smooth. Season with the ginger, garlic, molasses, cilantro, hot pepper flakes, soy sauce, and rice wine vinegar. Taste and add salt, if desired.

Serving size = ½ cup
55 calories
0.3 grams total fat
trace saturated fat
0 milligrams cholesterol
183 milligrams sodium

POTATO SALAD

YIELD: 6 CUPS (6 SERVINGS)   BY CAROL CONNELL

This has all the creaminess, crunch and flavor that you would expect from potato salad.

¼ cup freshly minced dill
¼ cup nonfat yogurt
½ cup Dijon mustard
¼ cup no-oil Italian dressing
5 cups boiled, cooled, and cubed
* new potatoes*

½ cup diced celery
½ tablespoon minced red onion
Salt
Freshly ground white pepper

Mix together the dill, yogurt, mustard, and oil-free dressing. Toss with the potatoes, celery, and onion. Add salt and freshly ground white pepper to taste. Serve chilled or at room temperature.

Serving size = 1 cup
148 calories
1.1 grams total fat
trace saturated fat
trace cholesterol

POTATO SALAD WITH TOMATILLO SAUCE

YIELD: 6 CUPS (6 SERVINGS)   BY DEBORAH MADISON

This tomatillo sauce brings a lot of sparkle to potatoes. It is naturally good without oil and salt. Cooking the ingredients first softens the effect of the

garlic and chilies, but if you want a sauce with more punch, stir in some fresh garlic and chile just before serving.

There may be more sauce than you wish to use on the potatoes, but leftovers will keep, refrigerated, for 3 or 4 days. It makes an excellent flavoring when stirred into soups, beans, rice, or pasta.

THE SAUCE

10 tomatillos
½ yellow onion, cut in large pieces
2 jalapeño peppers, seeds and veins removed

4 cloves garlic, peeled
1 large bunch cilantro, trimmed and washed
Ground cumin to taste (optional)

Remove the papery husks from the tomatillos. Bring a quart of water to boil, add the tomatillos, onion, chilies, and garlic. Lower the heat and simmer just until the tomatillos change from bright to olive green. Don't boil or overcook, or the tomatillos may split.

Remove all the vegetables with a slotted spoon and transfer to a blender or food processor. Add the cilantro and process until you have a smooth sauce. If necessary, add a small amount of the cooking liquid so the consistency isn't too thick. Season with cumin to taste, if desired.

THE VEGETABLES

1½ to 2 pounds red potatoes
1 green bell pepper, diced in small squares

2 scallions or chives, thinly sliced
Radishes, scrubbed and chopped or left whole, as preferred

Unless the skins look fresh and unblemished, peel the potatoes and slice them into ¼-inch rounds. Set them in a steamer, cover, and steam until tender, about 25 minutes.

Remove them to a platter and gently mix with the other vegetables, reserving some of the scallions and radishes for garnish. Ladle the sauce over the salad and garnish with the remaining vegetables. If possible, dress the salad just before serving.

Serving size = 1 cup
134 calories
0.4 grams total fat
trace saturated fat
0 milligrams cholesterol

POTATOES COOKED IN WINE WITH BASIL

YIELD: ABOUT 2½ CUPS (2 TO 3 SERVINGS)   BY DEBORAH MADISON

This dish can be thought of as a warm potato salad with its mildly acidic sauce of vinegar and wine. If possible, use new potatoes or one of the buttery yellow-fleshed varieties such as the Finnish potatoes. Try it with different herbs and herb-flavored vinegars, such as tarragon with tarragon vinegar or dill with dill vinegar. Even among basil plants there are many to choose from—cinnamon basil, lemon basil, opal basil. Potatoes take kindly to all herbs and mixtures of herbs.

1 pound new potatoes or Finnish
   potatoes
1 clove garlic, finely chopped
2 shallots or ½ bunch scallions,
   finely chopped
1 cup dry white wine
¼ cup white wine, champagne, or
   basil vinegar

½ teaspoon dried basil or 1
   tablespoon fresh
Freshly ground black pepper
1 teaspoon Dijon mustard
1 tablespoon freshly chopped
   parsley or basil leaves

If the potatoes are new and fresh, leave the skins on and simply wash them well. Otherwise, peel, then quarter them lengthwise. Place the potatoes in a pan with the garlic, shallots, wine, vinegar, basil, and pepper, bring to a boil, then lower the heat and cook slowly until the potatoes are tender. Once they are sufficiently cooked, remove them with a slotted spoon to a serving dish and cover to keep warm. Continue to cook the sauce until it has reduced and thickened. Stir in the mustard and parsley or basil, then remove from the heat and pour over the potatoes.

VARIATION: Once the sauce has reduced, stir in 2 tablespoons nonfat yogurt to make a creamier dressing.

Serving size = 1 cup
181 calories
0.3 grams total fat
trace saturated fat
0 milligrams cholesterol

ORANGE-JICAMA SALAD WITH PICKLED ONIONS

YIELD: 8 CUPS (8 SERVINGS)   BY DEBORAH MADISON

This is based on a Mexican recipe, one of the few I've ever seen that doesn't use oil. Jicama, a large, spherical root vegetable with a pale, brown papery skin, is a leguminous tuber. Its white flesh, which doesn't discolor, is delightfully crisp and juicy, like a water chestnut. It goes well with oranges but you could use it mixed with other citrus fruit as well, such as tangerines, grapefruit, or lime. For the juice, use a mixture of juices, such as grapefruit, lime and orange, or orange juice, tarted with a squeeze of lemon. If you don't have pickled onions on hand, omit them or simply add some finely diced or sliced raw red onion.

4 navel oranges plus 1 for juice or other citrus juice
1 pound (or more) jicama root
½ cup mixed citrus juice (see note above)
1 teaspoon citrus zest

1 pinch red hot chili flakes
Approximately 1 cup freshly chopped cilantro
1 cup Pickled Red Onions (page 401)

First grate some of the orange peel, if using, then cut off all the peels, slicing beneath the white pith of the orange. Slice the oranges into rounds or segments and set on a platter.

Peel the jicama and cut it into cubes or strips, and add to the platter with the oranges.

Make a mixture of citrus juices or use only orange juice with a squeeze of lemon juice to taste. The juice should be tart enough to be lively. Mix with the zest, chili flakes, and cilantro, then pour over the fruit and jicama. Scatter the pickled onions over all, toss lightly and carefully with your hands, and serve.

VARIATIONS: Include sliced radishes and add them just before serving. Use fresh green chilies, minced or sliced in rounds and scattered over the top. Grate some ginger and mix it with the citrus for an entirely different flavor. If you don't like cilantro, try using parsley or a mixture of parsley and dill. Pomegranate seeds scattered over the top would make a beautiful jewel-like garnish.

Serving size = 1 cup
30 calories
0.05 grams total fat
trace saturated fat
0 milligrams cholesterol

WATERCRESS, FENNEL, AND ORANGE SALAD

YIELD: 4 CUPS (4 SERVINGS)   BY MARK HALL

Remove the outer leaves of the fennel bulb for this salad. Save them for use in your homemade vegetable stocks.

4 cups sliced fennel (2 to 3 bulbs)	*4 teaspoons rice wine vinegar*
2 oranges, sectioned	*2 teaspoons freshly chopped*
¼ cup watercress leaves	* Italian parsley for garnish*
Juice of 1 orange	*Lettuce*

Slice the fennel bulbs. Toss the orange sections with the fennel and watercress. Then season with the orange juice and rice wine vinegar. Garnish with parsley and place on a bed of lettuce.

Serving size = 1 cup
55 calories
0.3 grams total fat
trace saturated fat
0 milligrams cholesterol

JICAMA-CUCUMBER SALAD WITH LIME AND CHILI

YIELD: APPROXIMATELY 4½ CUPS (4 TO 5 SERVINGS)   BY DEBORAH MADISON

In Mexico one can buy paper cones of refreshing fruit and vegetable salads. They always include salt, but even without it, these taste good. The contrasting cool and hot of the crisp, wet vegetables and lime with the chili is what makes this interesting. Serve as an appetizer with tiny forks or, as they do in Mexico, with toothpicks. If possible, use a pure, fresh chili powder. Old chili powder will taste musty and dull. The New Mexican powders are excellent.

If you can get them, try using different varieties of cucumbers for their different colors, textures, and tastes.

½ pound jicama root	*Chopped cilantro leaves plus*
¾ pound firm cucumbers	* leaves for garnish or the finely*
* (English, lemon, Armenian, or*	* chopped leaves of lemon*
* whatever is available)*	* verbena (optional)*
Grated zest and juice of 2 limes	*Pure red chili powder to taste*

Peel and cube the jicama. If the cucumber has been waxed, remove the skin completely. Otherwise, leave it on. For a more interesting-looking dish, score the skin with a fork, then quarter and cube the cucumber. If the cucumber is very seedy, scrape out the seeds and cut it into spears.

Toss the vegetables with the lime zest and juice and cilantro or lemon verbena, if using. Pile into a dish and sprinkle with chili powder to taste. This dish can be made ahead of time and chilled, but only add the chili right before serving. Garnish if you like with a spray of cilantro or lemon verbena leaves.

Serving size = 1 cup
23 calories
0.1 grams total fat
trace saturated fat
0 milligrams cholesterol

WALDORF SALAD

YIELD: 6 CUPS (6 SERVINGS)   BY MARY CARROLL

½ cup no-oil Italian dressing or
   vinaigrette
2 tablespoons apple juice
   concentrate
2 tablespoons nonfat yogurt
1 teaspoon curry powder
¼ teaspoon white pepper
¼ teaspoon ground cumin

4 cups chopped red Delicious
   apples, cored but not peeled
1 cup raisins
1 cup chopped celery
Salt to taste
Freshly ground black pepper
Leaf lettuce

Whisk together the Italian dressing, juice concentrate, yogurt, curry, white pepper, and cumin. Toss with the apples, raisins, and celery. Add salt and black pepper to taste and serve on a bed of lettuce.

Serving size = 1 cup
139 calories
0.7 grams total fat
0.1 grams saturated fat
trace cholesterol

QUINOA SALAD

YIELD: 2 CUPS (4 SERVINGS)   BY DEBORAH MADISON

Quinoa is called "the wonder grain" because of its unusually high protein content. It is light and delicate, but must be rinsed well to remove any traces of bitterness. This dish can be eaten warm or cold.

1 cup quinoa
2½ cups water
4 dried apricots, finely diced
3 tablespoons currants, softened
  in hot water and squeezed dry
3 small scallions, sliced in rounds
¼ cup very finely diced
  various-colored bell peppers
1 stalk of celery, finely diced

The Dressing:

3 tablespoons cooking water from
  the quinoa

Grated zest of 1 lemon or lime
2 tablespoons lime juice, or lemon
  juice, if preferred
1 teaspoon orange flower water
1 tablespoon finely chopped
  parsley or cilantro
½ teaspoon paprika
¼ teaspoon ground cumin
¼ teaspoon ground coriander
Pinch cinnamon
2 pinches cayenne

Rinse the quinoa in several changes of water, then pour into a fine-meshed strainer and rinse once more under tap water. Bring the 2½ cups water to a boil, then stir in the quinoa. Cover and cook over a low heat for 15 minutes. By then the quinoa should be done. Drain into a colander, but reserve the liquid. When the excess water has come off the grain, give the colander a shake and put the quinoa in a bowl.

Add the apricots, currants, scallions, peppers, and celery, and toss together.

To make the dressing, whisk all the ingredients together. Taste and adjust as necessary. Since the dressing is going over the grain, it can be a little sharper than usual. Pour over the still-warm quinoa and toss.

Serving size = ½ cup
90 calories
1.1 grams total fat
trace saturated fat
0 milligrams cholesterol

TABBOULEH

YIELD: 5 CUPS (5 SERVINGS)   BY MARK HALL

This is a traditional Middle Eastern salad minus the oil. It is served as a salad and may be served on a bed of lettuce. It also goes well with other Middle Eastern-inspired dishes such as hummus with pita bread.

2¾ cup water
1½ cups bulgur wheat
1 cup seeded, chopped, and diced
    fresh tomato
1 cup diced red onions
1 teaspoon freshly minced garlic

1 tablespoon freshly minced
    parsley
2 tablespoons freshly minced mint
1½ teaspoons lemon juice
Salt
Freshly ground black pepper

Bring the water to a boil. Add the bulgur and stir. Cover with an airtight lid and let sit for at least 4 hours before opening again.

Drain the bulgur of any excess water or squeeze it out. Toss with the tomato, onions, garlic, parsley, and mint. Add the lemon juice and add salt and pepper to taste.

Serving size = 1 cup
102 calories
1.0 grams total fat
0.2 grams saturated fat
0 milligrams cholesterol

RICE SALAD WITH APRICOTS AND CURRANTS

YIELD: 3 CUPS (3 SERVINGS)   BY MARK HALL

This very colorful salad has a lot of texture and depth of flavor. You would expect it to be a little sweet because of the apricots and currants, but the savoriness is a surprise. It is actually a variation of the Quinoa Salad (page 418). Serve it at room temperature or slightly chilled.

¼ cup uncooked wild rice
½ cup uncooked basmati rice
2½ tablespoons minced dried
    apricots
⅓ cup dried currants
⅓ cup finely diced red onions
⅓ cup sliced scallions

½ tablespoon orange juice
½ teaspoon rice wine vinegar
Small pinch freshly ground black
    pepper
1 teaspoon orange zest
Salt
Freshly ground black pepper

Cook the wild rice and basmati rice separately. The free-boiling time is 40 minutes and 30 minutes, respectively. Alternatively, you can follow the package instructions, being sure not to add any salt or butter.

When they are done, toss with the apricots, currants, onions and scallions. Combine the orange juice, rice wine vinegar, black pepper and orange zest separately. Add the rice mixture, salt and more pepper to taste.

Serving size = 1 cup
218 calories
0.2 grams total fat
trace saturated fat
0 milligrams cholesterol

FRUITED GRAIN SALAD

YIELD: 10 CUPS (10 SERVINGS)   BY MOLLIE KATZEN

This is a simple, yet unusual-tasting salad. Each grain—barley, whole wheat berries, brown rice—has its own distinct personality, especially if you take the slight trouble to cook each of them correctly. The addition of golden raisins, chives, mint, and plums (and/or apples) makes it taste both exotic and yet homey and familiar. Do try to find fresh mint for this salad. It's an important component, and dried mint is not quite the same thing.

The grains need to cook separately. You can cook them in advance and store them in tightly covered containers until you are ready to make the salad. You can also prepare the salad a night or two before you plan to serve it. (Add everything except the fresh fruit, which should go in shortly before serving.) It takes very little work. Most of the preparation time is for cooking the grains, so you can easily make it during an evening when you are home doing other things.

This salad keeps very well and is great to have on hand for lunches and snacks.

1 cup uncooked wheat berries
1 cup uncooked pearl barley
1 cup uncooked short-grain brown rice
3 tablespoons cider vinegar
1 tablespoon lemon juice
1/2 teaspoon salt
1 1/2 cups packed golden raisins

3/4 cup packed freshly minced chives or finely minced scallions
6 to 7 large freshly minced mint leaves, or 1 to 2 teaspoons dried mint
4 or 5 ripe firm small red plums, sliced

1 or 2 tart green apples, sliced
(optional use in addition to, or
instead of, the plums)

Soak the wheat berries for about 30 minutes. Meanwhile, rinse the barley several times in cold water, until the water in which it is rinsed looks clear. Put the barley and 2½ cups water in a saucepan. Bring to a boil, partially cover, and simmer until tender, about 30 minutes.

Place the rice and 1¾ cups water in a small saucepan. Bring to a boil, partially cover, and simmer about 35 minutes, or until tender.

Drain the wheat berries and place in a saucepan with 2½ cups water. Bring to a boil, cover, and simmer until tender, about 1 to 1¼ hours. Check the water level and add just a little extra if it seems dry.

When all the grains are cooked, combine them in a large bowl. Stir to let excess steam escape. Add the remaining ingredients except the plums and/or apples. Cover and chill well before serving. This will keep up to 3 days. Add the plum and/or apple slices, and mix them in gently just before serving.

Serving size = 1 cup
260 calories
1.2 grams total fat
0.1 gram saturated fat
0 milligrams cholesterol

PASTA PRIMAVERA WITH DIJON VINAIGRETTE

YIELD: 8¼ CUPS (6 TO 8 SERVINGS)   BY JUDY TALBOTT

This very colorful salad tastes better warm or hot. The piquant flavor of the dressing works well with just a plate of steamed vegetables and is balanced here by the macaroni's bland taste. This recipe is also successful when cut in half to yield approximately four cups of salad.

1 pound macaroni, cooked
¾ cup finely diced carrots
2 cups chopped green onions
½ cup chopped celery
2 large tomatoes, seeded and
* diced*

4–5 tablespoons Dijon Vinaigrette
* (see below)*
1 cup Italian Dressing (page
* 397)*
2 tablespoons chopped fresh basil
Balsamic vinegar

Salt
Freshly ground black pepper

Dijon Vinaigrette:
YIELD: 3/4 CUP
4 tablespoons oil-free Dijon
   mustard
3 tablespoons red wine vinegar
1 tablespoon white wine vinegar

1/4–1/2 teaspoon salt
2 cloves freshly minced garlic
1/2 teaspoon dried basil
1/8 teaspoon freshly ground black
   pepper
2 drops of hot red pepper sauce
1 tablespoon grated onion
3 tablespoons soft tofu

To prepare the Dijon Vinaigrette, simply combine all ingredients and blend. Keep this in your refrigerator for several days. The ingredients may separate out.

Steam the carrots for 1 to 2 minutes. Toss the macaroni, carrots, green onions, celery and diced tomatoes with the Dijon Vinaigrette. Add the Italian Dressing and the fresh basil. Add the balsamic vinegar, salt and freshly ground black pepper to taste.

Pasta Primavera with Dijon Vinaigrette
Serving size = 1 cup
245 calories
0.6 grams total fat
trace saturated fat
0 milligrams cholesterol

Dijon Vinaigrette
Serving size = 2 tablespoons
16 calories
0.8 grams total fat
trace saturated fat
0 milligrams cholesterol

WHITE BEAN SALAD

YIELD: 4 CUPS (8 SERVINGS)   BY MARK HALL

The combination of these aromatic herbs and spices makes this especially delightful.

1 cup dry white beans
8 1/4 cups water

5 bay leaves
1 tablespoon dried sage

¼ cup finely diced carrots
¼ cup finely diced celery
⅓ cup seeded and diced tomato
1 cup freshly chopped Italian
   parsley
⅛ teaspoon freshly ground black
   pepper
⅛ teaspoon salt
Chopped Italian parsley (optional)
Lettuce

Dressing:
1 tablespoon Dijon mustard
1½ teaspoons freshly minced
   garlic
2½ tablespoons lemon juice
½ teaspoon salt
½ teaspoon freshly ground black
   pepper

Sort and rinse the beans, then soak overnight in water. Drain the beans and put 8¼ cups water in another pot with the beans, bay leaves, and sage. Cook the beans for about 40 minutes, until tender.

While the beans are cooking, combine the ingredients for the dressing. When the beans are cooked, remove the bay leaves and drain the water. Toss the diced raw vegetables and dressing with the beans. Garnish with some extra chopped parsley, if desired, and serve on a bed of varied lettuces.

Serving size = ½ cup
89 calories
0.5 grams total fat
0.1 grams saturated fat
0 milligrams cholesterol

FRENCH LENTIL SALAD

YIELD: 5 CUPS (5 SERVINGS)   BY MARK HALL

The very tiny lentils have a delicate appearance. They give a lot of flavor to this pretty salad. Serve at room temperature or slightly chilled.

1½ cups dry French lentils or 3
   cups cooked
6 cups water
3 bay leaves
½ cup finely diced carrots
½ cup finely diced celery
½ cup seeded and finely diced
   tomatoes
½ cup finely diced onions

2 tablespoons minced Italian
   parsley or fresh thyme, sage, or
   marjoram
⅛ cup sherry wine vinegar
1 teaspoon freshly minced garlic
Salt
¼ teaspoon freshly ground black
   pepper or to taste

If using dry, rinse and sort the lentils, then cook for 15 to 20 minutes in 6 cups of water with the bay leaves until done. Do not overcook, or the lentils may fall apart. When the lentils are done, drain and toss them with the vegetables, parsley, or other fresh herbs. Season with the sherry vinegar and garlic. Add salt and pepper to taste.

Serving size = 1 cup
204 calories
0.7 grams total fat
0.1 grams saturated fat
0 milligrams cholesterol

BABY LIMA BEAN SALAD

YIELD: 3 CUPS (3 SERVINGS)   BY MARK HALL

Lima beans make this an unusual salad. Serve this on a bed of lettuce with a light soup.

1 cup dry baby lima beans
4 cups water
4 bay leaves
1 teaspoon dried thyme
1 teaspoon dried sage
1/2 cup finely diced fresh tomatoes
1/2 cup finely diced celery

1 teaspoon freshly chopped
    parsley
1 tablespoon red wine vinegar
1/2 teaspoon freshly minced garlic
1/2 teaspoon salt
1/4 teaspoon freshly ground black
    pepper or to taste

Sort the lima beans, rinse, and then soak overnight in water. Cook the beans for 30 to 40 minutes in the water with the bay leaves, thyme, and sage. Cook until the lima beans are tender but are not falling apart. Remove the bay leaves and drain.

Toss the beans with the tomatoes, celery, parsley, vinegar, and garlic. Add salt and pepper to taste. Serve on a bed of tossed greens.

Serving size = 1 cup
232 calories
1.0 grams total fat
0.2 grams saturated fat
0 milligrams cholesterol

BLACK BEAN SALAD

YIELD: 4 CUPS (4 SERVINGS)   BY MARK HALL

The red hues of the peppers and onions are a nice contrast to the color of the black beans, and the taste of this vibrant salad retains the Latin flair that is associated with black beans.

1 cup dry black beans
5 cups water
3 bay leaves
1 cup finely diced red onion
1 cup finely diced red bell pepper
2 tablespoons freshly chopped
   cilantro
1/2 teaspoon ground cumin

1 to 2 tablespoons rice wine
   vinegar
1/2 teaspoon cayenne, or to taste
1 teaspoon freshly minced garlic
Salt
1/4 teaspoon freshly ground black
   pepper or to taste

Sort and rinse the beans, then soak overnight in water. Strain and rinse again just before cooking. Boil the 5 cups water with the black beans and bay leaves. Reduce the heat and cook until tender. This should take from 30 to 45 minutes. They should not be allowed to lose their shape. Drain the beans and remove the bay leaves.

Toss the vegetables with the black beans and season with the cilantro, cumin, vinegar, cayenne, and garlic. Toss again and add salt and pepper to taste.

Serving size = 1 cup
139 calories
0.8 grams total fat
0.1 grams saturated fat
0 milligrams cholesterol

SUNOMONO (JAPANESE NOODLE AND CUCUMBER SALAD)

YIELD: 4 CUPS (4 SERVINGS)   BY MOLLIE KATZEN

This salad is subtle and very refreshing. There is a variety of textures—chewy cold noodles, crunchy sesame seeds, and smooth cucumber slices. Sweet, salt, and vinegar combine harmoniously, each understated but very much present.

Everything except the cucumbers and toppings can be combined several days ahead of time. The cucumbers can be prepared ahead also and kept separate until serving.

5 to 6 ounces dry vermicelli or
bean thread noodles
6 tablespoons rice wine vinegar
4 teaspoons sugar
2 teaspoons soy sauce
1 teaspoon salt

1 medium-sized cucumber
1 tablespoon thinly sliced scallions
greens (optional)
1½ teaspoons sesame seeds for
garnish (optional)

Cook the noodles in boiling water until just tender. Drain and rinse in cold water. Drain thoroughly and transfer to a medium-sized bowl.

Add vinegar, sugar, soy sauce, and salt. Mix well. Cover and chill until cold.

Peel and seed the cucumber. Cut into quarters lengthwise, then into thin pieces. If not serving right away, wrap the cucumber pieces in a plastic bag or plastic wrap and refrigerate.

To serve, divide noodles among 4 serving bowls. Top with a small handful of cucumber slices, and, if desired, a few very thin slices of scallion greens and some sesame seeds. Serve cold.

Serving size = 1 cup
201 calories
1.9 grams total fat
0.3 grams saturated fat
0 milligrams cholesterol

SALSA PICANTE

YIELD: 1½ CUPS (6 SERVINGS)   BY MARY CARROLL

This spicy salsa has more of the consistency of a sauce and is wonderful with many Mexican dishes.

1½ tablespoons minced onion
3 cloves garlic, minced
2½ tablespoons dry red wine
(such as Cabernet)
½ teaspoon ground fresh
rosemary leaves
5 small Roma tomatoes, cored
and thickly pureed or 3 cups
chopped tomatoes
2½ tablespoons minced green
bell pepper
1 tablespoon freshly minced
cilantro

1 tablespoon freshly minced
Italian parsley
¼ teaspoon ground coriander
¼ teaspoon chili powder
¼ teaspoon ground cumin
⅛ teaspoon cayenne
Pinch ground cinnamon
2 tablespoons fresh lemon juice
Freshly ground black pepper
Salt

Heat the onion, garlic, and wine in a small saucepan on high heat for 5 minutes. Add the remaining ingredients. You may want to use only half as much cayenne at first to see if this is too "hot" for you. Refrigerate overnight before using for the best flavor. Serve at room temperature.

Serving size = ¼ cup or 4 tablespoons
26 calories
0.3 grams total fat
trace saturated fat
0 milligrams cholesterol

APPLE CHUTNEY

YIELD: 2 CUPS (16 SERVINGS)   BY MARY CARROLL

This cooked chutney is a delicious accompaniment to curries. The sweet and sour taste of this and the other chutneys make a nice contrast to other savory dishes as well.

4 tart apples, unpeeled, cored, and chopped
2 ripe pears, unpeeled, cored, and chopped
2 cloves garlic, minced
4 teaspoons freshly grated gingerroot
½ cup freshly squeezed orange juice
1 teaspoon each ground cloves, cinnamon, and cardamom
⅔ cup cider vinegar
1 cup apple juice concentrate
⅛ teaspoon cayenne

Combine everything in a saucepan and simmer over medium heat, covered, for 20 minutes. Remove from heat and let cool overnight to thicken.

Serving size = 2 tablespoons
65 calories
0.3 grams total fat
trace saturated fat
0 milligrams cholesterol

VEGETABLE SIDE DISHES

These vegetable dishes are simpler and lighter than the hearty ones on pages 490–504. They're meant to be eaten as side dishes along with grains, beans, or tofu, or for a light lunch or supper. That said, you could make a very simple meal of vegetable dishes alone—Mushrooms Braised with Herbs (page 430) served with Roasted Potatoes (page 442), for instance; or Yams with Ginger and Dried Apricots (page 429), served with Broccoli with Lemon Sauce (page 433). The colors of the vegetable dishes are beautiful on the plate, and you will love the combinations of flavors and textures.

In addition to the vegetable dishes here, don't forget about unadorned steamed vegetables. Nothing can beat a serving of bright green steamed broccoli, spinach, or green beans. In fact, most vegetables, when they're in season, are so inherently delicious that they require no other seasoning than perhaps a little lemon juice or pepper.

ONION CONFIT WITH CROUTONS

YIELD: 3 CUPS (16 SERVINGS)   BY MARK HALL

You can use any combination of red wine vinegars in equal amounts. The balsamic vinegar is a milder, sweeter variety that has less of an acid taste.

1 French sourdough baguette,
  egg- and oil-free
6 cups thinly sliced red onions
2 teaspoons freshly minced garlic
1 teaspoon dried thyme

1 teaspoon dried marjoram
½ cup medium dry red wine
¼ cup balsamic vinegar
½ teaspoon salt

Preheat the oven to 350°F. To prepare the croutons, thinly slice the baguette into rounds of a uniform thickness (¼- to ⅓-inch thick). Lay them on a baking sheet and bake for 10 minutes until they are completely dried.

Toss the onions, garlic, and herbs with the wine and vinegar. Cook over low heat for an hour. Stir frequently and allow the liquid to evaporate.

Place about 1½ tablespoons of confit on each crouton and serve.

Serving size = 2 croutons
56 calories
0.5 grams total fat
0.1 grams saturated fat
0 milligrams cholesterol

YAMS WITH GINGER AND DRIED APRICOTS

YIELD: 3 CUPS (3 SERVINGS)   BY DEBORAH MADISON

Apricots are quite delicious with yams. Leave the ginger in big pieces and pull it out later, or finely chop it and leave it with the yams, as you wish.

1 large yam (12 to 16 ounces)	1 ½ cups water
6 dried apricots, cut in quarters	
½-inch piece fresh ginger, left in large pieces or finely diced	

If the skin on the yam looks firm and smooth, scrub the yam. Otherwise, peel it.

Cut the yam into rounds slightly less than ½-inch thick, and cut each round into quarters, or sixths if it is very large. Combine all the ingredients in a small saucepan, cover with 1 ½ cups water, bring to a boil, then simmer, covered, for ½ hour. Check the pan and add more water, in small increments if necessary, until the yams are completely cooked, another 20 minutes or so. Allow whatever liquid is left to boil down until a small amount of sauce is left. Pile into a bowl and serve.

VARIATION: Whip the yam-apricot mixture briefly in a food processor to make a puree.

Serving size = 1 cup
173 calories
0.3 grams total fat
0.1 gram saturated fat
0 milligrams cholesterol

MUSHROOMS BRAISED WITH HERBS

YIELD: 2 CUPS (4 SERVINGS)   BY MARK HALL

Stir this into your favorite tomato sauce to serve over pasta.

1 pound domestic or other
  mushrooms, sliced
1/4 cup red wine
1 teaspoon minced garlic
1/2 teaspoon dried thyme

1 teaspoon dried marjoram
1/8 teaspoon freshly ground black
  pepper
Salt

Braise the mushrooms in the red wine with the garlic, thyme, and marjoram. Cover the pan until for about 5 minutes, until the mushroom juices have been released, then remove the lid. Cook further until the liquid is completely reduced. Add the pepper and salt to taste.

Serving size = 1/2 cup
42 calories
0.3 grams total fat
trace saturated fat
0 milligrams cholesterol

MUSHROOM GRAVY

YIELD: 2 CUPS (8 SERVINGS)   BY CAROL CONNELL

Because of the earthy, full flavor of the shiitake mushrooms, this pureed and strained brown sauce has the flavor and look of a rendered gravy. The seitan, a wheat product, gives it added texture.

1/2 cup hot water
1/2 cup dried shiitake mushrooms
1/4 cup sherry or dry white wine
1/4 cup apple juice
1/4 teaspoon dried thyme
1/8 teaspoon freshly ground black
  pepper

1/8 teaspoon dried sage
1/8 teaspoon dried oregano
1 cup thinly sliced seitan
Salt

Bring 1/2 cup water to a boil, add the dried mushrooms, and simmer for 30 minutes. Add more water as needed to keep the sauce from boiling dry. Strain the mushrooms out of the cooking liquid. Reserve the liquid. Cut off the woody stems and discard. Place the mushrooms, reserved stock, and other ingredients (except for the seitan) into a blender. Puree and strain through a fine mesh strainer. Pour into a saucepan and add the sliced seitan. Simmer for 15 minutes, or until the alcohol odor has evaporated. Add salt to taste, and then serve warm over rice, potatoes, or other vegetables.

Serving size = ¼ cup
119 calories
0.4 grams total fat
trace saturated fat
0 milligrams cholesterol

RATATOUILLE

YIELD: 8 CUPS (8 SERVINGS)   BY MARK HALL

This is a classic French vegetarian stew with all of the major elements except the olive oil.

1½ cups diced onion
1 tablespoon freshly minced garlic
1 tablespoon dried basil
1 tablespoon dried oregano
½ cup dry red wine
5½ cups tomato puree
2 cups sliced mushrooms
6 cups cubed eggplant

1 cup large-diced green bell
  pepper
1 cup large-diced red bell pepper
1¼ cups ¼-inch rounds zucchini
⅛ teaspoon cayenne
⅛ teaspoon salt
Freshly ground black pepper

Braise the onions, garlic, and dried herbs in the red wine. The herbs will rehydrate and release their flavor. When the onions are soft and start to turn translucent, add the tomato puree and the sliced mushrooms. Then stew together for about 10 minutes. Add the eggplant and the red and green peppers. When these are almost cooked, add the zucchini. Don't cook the squash too long or it will become mushy and lose its bright color.

When all the vegetables are cooked to the desired doneness, add the cayenne pepper. Then add salt and pepper to taste.

Serving size = 1 cup
125 calories
0.1 grams total fat
trace saturated fat
0 milligrams cholesterol

SCALLOPED POTATOES

YIELD: 5 CUPS (5 SERVINGS)   BY CAROL CONNELL

The creamy texture of this dish makes it hard to believe that it does not contain any dairy products. It owes this to the amasake, a nonalcoholic fermented rice drink whose texture is that of heavy cream. In the fermentation process, the rice becomes sweet. More rice, liquids, and flavorings are frequently added to the amasake.

4 large russet potatoes, unpeeled
2 large onions, peeled and thinly
* sliced*
1 tablespoon freshly minced
* rosemary*
1 tablespoon freshly minced
* thyme*

⅛ teaspoon salt
Freshly ground black pepper
3 cups plain amasake
Paprika

Preheat the oven to 350°F. If you do not have a nonstick pan, spray the baking dish with a vegetable oil spray. Slice the potatoes into ¼-inch rounds. Layer the onions and potatoes in the pan. Sprinkle with the chopped herbs, salt, and black pepper. Pour the amasake over it. Cover with a very light dusting of paprika, then cover with foil and bake for 45 minutes. Uncover and continue baking for 20 minutes, or until browned and crisp.

Serving size = 1 cup
255 calories
1.0 grams total fat
0.1 grams saturated fat
0 milligrams cholesterol

YAMS WITH LEMON

YIELD: 3 CUPS (3 SERVINGS)   BY MARK HALL

People frequently confuse yams with sweet potatoes. They are actually different root vegetables. In this country the word yam *is used to refer to the sweet potato, and not to any of the distinctively sharp-tasting root vegetables that people from the Caribbean or Africa know. This recipe calls for sweet potatoes.*

3 cups peeled and cubed yams
1 tablespoon fresh lemon juice
1 tablespoon freshly chopped
* Italian parsley*

Salt
Freshly ground black pepper

Preheat the oven to 375°F. Place the yams in a covered baking dish with just enough water to coat the bottom of the pan. After they've baked for 45 to 50 minutes, until tender, add the lemon juice and parsley. Add salt and pepper to taste, then serve.

Serving size = 1 cup
178 calories
0.3 grams total fat
0.1 grams saturated fat
0 milligrams cholesterol

BROCCOLI WITH HONEY AND MUSTARD SAUCE

YIELD: 2 CUPS (4 SERVINGS)   BY MARK HALL

For a variation, toss the sauce with other steamed vegetables, such as cauliflower, squash, zucchini or spinach.

2 cups broccoli florets
7 tablespoons water
1/4 cup Dijon mustard

7 tablespoons honey
1/4 teaspoon freshly ground black
   pepper

Blanch or steam the broccoli florets. To make the sauce, mix the water with the mustard, honey, and pepper. Toss 1/2 cup of sauce with the broccoli and serve.

Serving size = 1/2 cup broccoli + 2 tablespoons sauce
112 calories
0.7 grams total fat
0.1 grams saturated fat
0 milligrams cholesterol

Sauce only:
Serving size = 2 tablespoons
89 calories
0.5 grams total fat
trace saturated fat
0 milligrams cholesterol

KALE AND LEMON

YIELD: 2⅔ CUPS (2 TO 3 SERVINGS)   BY MARK HALL

This recipe is delicious with other green leafy vegetables such as spinach, mustard, and beet greens.

4 cups chopped fresh kale   *¼ teaspoon fresh lemon juice*
*   (approximately 10 ounces)*   *Salt*
½ teaspoon fresh minced garlic   *Freshly ground black pepper*

Steam the kale, then toss with the garlic. Add the lemon juice. Add salt and pepper to taste and serve.

Serving size = 1 cup
58 calories
0.8 grams total fat
0.2 grams saturated fat
0 milligrams cholesterol

BROCCOLI WITH LEMON SAUCE

YIELD: 2 CUPS (2 SERVINGS)   BY MARK HALL

This lemon sauce also works nicely with cauliflower, squash, or zucchini.

1 tablespoon cornstarch   *2 tablespoons fresh lemon juice*
2 tablespoons cold water   *2 tablespoons Dijon mustard*
½ cup water   *4 cups broccoli florets*

Dissolve the cornstarch in 2 tablespoons cold water. In a saucepan, whisk together the ½ cup water, lemon juice, and the Dijon mustard. Heat and add the cornstarch mixture. Continue heating and stirring until the sauce thickens. Add more lemon juice if desired.

Blanch the broccoli in boiling water or steam until done, then toss with the lemon sauce.

Serving size = 1 cup
71 calories
0.8 grams total fat
trace saturated fat
0 milligrams cholesterol

BRUSSELS SPROUTS WITH MAPLE SYRUP

YIELD: 3 CUPS (3 SERVINGS)   BY MARK HALL

The sweetness of the maple syrup makes this an unusually elegant dish.

3 cups Brussels sprouts   *Salt*
¼ cup maple syrup   *Freshly ground black pepper*

If they need to be trimmed, remove the outer leaves from the sprouts. Cut
the ends off, then slice them into halves and cook for about 15 to 20 minutes
in boiling water until tender. Drain and toss with the maple syrup. Add salt
and pepper to taste.

Serving size = 1 cup
128 calories
0.8 grams total fat
0.2 grams saturated fat
0 milligrams cholesterol

BUTTERNUT SQUASH WITH BROWN SUGAR

YIELD: 5 CUPS (5 SERVINGS)   BY MARK HALL

The brown sugar creates a gentle glaze for the squash.

2¾-pound butternut squash
½ cup brown sugar
Water

Peel the squash and remove the seeds, then cut it into chunks or cubes.
There should be 5 cups of squash chunks. Bake in a covered casserole dish
with a small amount of water and 3 tablespoons of brown sugar for 30 to
40 minutes at 375°F. Then sprinkle the top with the remaining brown sugar
and serve.

Serving size = 1 cup
123 calories
0.2 grams total fat
trace saturated fat
0 milligrams cholesterol

RED CABBAGE WITH APPLES

YIELD: 3 CUPS (6 SERVINGS)   BY MARK HALL

This tastes better if it sits for several hours to allow the flavors to develop.

2½ cups shredded red cabbage
1 large apple
3 tablespoons dry red wine
1 tablespoon balsamic vinegar

1 tablespoon red wine vinegar
1 bay leaf
¼ teaspoon salt

Using a large pot, combine the shredded cabbage with the apples, red wine, vinegars, and the bay leaf. Stir well, cover, and cook on low heat for 20 to 30 minutes, until the cabbage is wilted. When the cabbage has finished cooking, remove the bay leaf and add salt to taste.

VARIATION: Add ½ cup sliced onions and increase the balsamic vinegar to 2 tablespoons.

Serving size = ½ cup
33 calories
0.1 grams total fat
trace saturated fat
0 milligrams cholesterol

ZUCCHINI AND MUSHROOMS WITH ANCHO CHILI SAUCE

YIELD: 2½ CUPS (2 TO 3 SERVINGS)   BY MARK HALL

The chilies are sometimes not at all hot but you may want to add the pureed chilies gradually to be certain that this isn't too fiery.

2 cups sliced mushrooms
1 teaspoon freshly minced garlic
¼ teaspoon black pepper
2 teaspoons dried oregano

¼ cup dry white wine
2½ cups round-sliced zucchini
2 teaspoons Ancho Chili Puree
  (page 465)

Braise the mushrooms, garlic, black pepper, and oregano in the white wine. When the mushrooms release their own juices and are cooked through, add the thinly sliced zucchini. Just before the three vegetables are completely done add the Ancho Chili Puree. Even though the chilies do not actually need to cook, let this simmer for 5 to 10 minutes to combine the flavors.

Serving size = 1 cup
56 calories
0.5 grams total fat
trace saturated fat
0 milligrams cholesterol

ZUCCHINI PANCAKES

YIELD: 15 4-INCH PANCAKES (5 SERVINGS)   BY NORMA LEONARDOS

Serve these pancakes hot with your favorite tomato sauce and basil, or with salsa and a cilantro garnish. They can also be eaten cold and make a good sandwich filler.

3 cups shredded zucchini
1 cup all-purpose white flour
6 ounces Egg Beaters
3 tablespoons dried onions
¾ tablespoon Mrs. Dash extra spicy powder, or 1 teaspoon dried dill or tarragon

2 cups water
Salt to taste

Combine all ingredients. If the batter is too thick, gradually add more water. Use a nonstick frying pan and/or a little vegetable oil spray on the surface of a regular pan. Heat the frying pan, then ladle several tablespoons per pancake onto the pan. When the edges of the pancakes have browned, flip and cook for another minute or so. Serve.

Serving size = 3 4-inch pancakes
120 calories
0.4 grams total fat
trace saturated fat
0 milligrams cholesterol

PLANTAIN PANCAKES WITH RED PEPPER–JALAPEÑO SAUCE

YIELD: 15 5-INCH PANCAKES (5 SERVINGS)   BY SHIRLEY BROWN

These pancakes can also be eaten without the sauce for breakfast with fruit and yogurt. For later in the day, serve with a crisp legume-based salad or soup.

PANCAKE

3 medium-sized ripe plantains
3/4 cup whole wheat pastry flour
3/4 cup unbleached all-purpose
   flour
2 teaspoons baking powder
1 teaspoon baking soda
1/2 teaspoon salt

1 1/2 cups nonfat milk
1 tablespoon apple juice
   concentrate
2 egg whites
Fresh cilantro, Italian parsley, or
   minced scallions for garnish

Peel 3 medium plantains, slice into thirds and steam for 30 minutes, or cook in a pressure cooker for 8 minutes, then mash them. There should be 1 1/4 cups.

Sift together the whole wheat and white flours with the baking powder, baking soda, and salt. In a separate bowl, combine the nonfat milk, apple juice, and the egg whites. Stir the mashed plantain into the liquids. Then stir the dry ingredients into the plantain-milk mixture until just combined.

Pour 1/4 cup of pancake batter onto the nonstick pan and agitate the pan to spread the batter over the skillet. It will need to be at least 5 inches in diameter to cook thoroughly. Cook over very low heat. About 2 minutes after the surface has stopped bubbling, flip the pancake and cook for several minutes more.

RED PEPPER SAUCE

6 shallots, minced
1 teaspoon dried thyme or 1 sprig
   of thyme
1/4 cup dry white wine
3/4 large red bell pepper, chopped
2 tablespoons tomato puree
1/2 cup vegetable broth

1 teaspoon minced jalapeño
   pepper
2 tablespoons nonfat milk
1 teaspoon Butter Buds
Salt
Freshly ground black pepper

Braise the shallots and thyme in the white wine. When the garlic looks cooked, add the red pepper, tomato sauce, and the broth. Cover and simmer until the red pepper is a little softened.

When the pepper is done, transfer the stock with the vegetables to a food processor or blender. Remove the sprig of thyme, if used, and add the jalapeño pepper. Puree until very smooth. Pour through a strainer into a saucepan and add the milk. Simmer for 3 to 5 minutes. Whisk in the Butter Buds and add salt and pepper to taste. There should be 1 cup sauce.

Top the pancakes with the red pepper sauce and and garnish with fresh cilantro, Italian parsley, or scallions.

Serving size = 3 pancakes
222 calories
0.9 grams total fat
0.2 grams saturated fat
1 milligram cholesterol
213 milligrams sodium

Serving size = 2 tablespoons sauce
17 calories
trace total fat
trace saturated fat
trace cholesterol

BROCCOLI WITH TERIYAKI SAUCE

YIELD: 5 CUPS (5 SERVINGS)   BY MARK HALL

Because of the soy sauce, the sodium content of the teriyaki sauce is very high (1031 milligrams per ⅓ cup) and may be unsuitable for those persons with a history of congestive heart failure and/or hypertension. One cup of broccoli with the sauce contains 222 milligrams of sodium.

5 cups broccoli florets

Teriyaki Sauce:

2 teaspoons arrowroot
½ cup water

2 tablespoons soy sauce
½ teaspoon freshly minced garlic
1 tablespoon freshly minced
    ginger
2 tablespoons honey
Pinch freshly ground black pepper

Blanch the broccoli and plunge into ice cold water to stop the cooking. Drain and set aside.

To prepare the teriyaki sauce, dilute the arrowroot in 2 tablespoons of cold water. Heat the remaining water, soy sauce, garlic, and ginger. Add the honey and stir to dissolve. Add the arrowroot mixture and the pepper. Continue stirring to thicken. There should be about ⅔ cup sauce.

Toss the broccoli with ⅓ cup of sauce and serve.

Refrigerate the remaining sauce and use with other steamed or stir-"fried" vegetables.

Serving size = 1 cup broccoli
64 calories
0.4 grams total fat
trace saturated fat
0 milligrams cholesterol

Sauce only:
⅓ cup = 91 calories
0.1 grams total fat
trace saturated fat
0 milligrams cholesterol

POTATO PANCAKES

YIELD: 2⅔ CUPS (4 SERVINGS)   BY PHYLLIS GINSBERG

The Butter Buds add just a slight taste of butter for those who like it. It has negligible amounts of fat, doesn't "fry," and doesn't prevent the pancake from sticking to some pans. It does have some fat and cholesterol. For a serving of 2 pancakes it adds 1 milligram of cholesterol and 17 calories. The saturated fat and total fat are not increased.

2 egg whites
1½ cups finely minced onions
2 tablespoons unbleached
   all-purpose white flour
1 teaspoon salt
½ teaspoon freshly ground black
   pepper

About 1¼ pounds peeled potatoes
2 tablespoons Butter Buds
   (optional)
Applesauce

Preheat the oven to 450°F. and have a nonstick or vegetable oil-sprayed baking sheet ready.

Measure out all the ingredients besides the potatoes. (If using, combine the Butter Buds with the flour.) Then grate the potatoes; there should be 3 cups. Squeeze out all of the excess moisture and combine with the other ingredients. (It's important to have all the other ingredients ready because the potatoes will quickly turn gray upon exposure to the air.)

Using ⅓ cup of the mixture, form into thin flat cakes on the baking sheet. Bake for 14 minutes, then turn the pancakes over and bake an additional 2 minutes until golden brown. Serve with applesauce.

Serving size = 2 pancakes
150 calories
0.3 grams total fat
trace saturated fat
0 milligrams cholesterol

BEETS WITH ORANGE AND DILL

YIELD: 1½ CUPS (3 SERVINGS)   BY MARK HALL

The orange and dill make this a refreshing dish.

*5 medium beets (about 1½
    pounds)
¼ cup orange juice*

*½ teaspoon orange zest.
1 teaspoon freshly chopped dill*

Put the beets with enough water to cover the bottom of the dish to a depth of ½ inch, in a covered casserole. Bake at 375°F. 1 hour. Slip the skins off easily, then slice or dice the beets. Toss with orange juice, orange zest, and dill. Cool and serve.

Serving size = ½ cup
104 calories
trace total fat
trace saturated fat
0 milligrams cholesterol

ROASTED POTATOES

YIELD: 3 CUPS (3 SERVINGS)   BY MARK HALL

These potatoes should be crispy when done.

*1 ½ pounds unpeeled new
    potatoes
½ head garlic, whole cloves*

*¼ cup chopped fresh rosemary
Salt
Pepper*

Preheat the oven to 375°F.

Cut the potatoes in halves or quarters and place them in a baking pan with the whole cloves of garlic and a small amount of water. Toss with the rosemary. Cover pan and bake for for 20 minutes, then remove the cover and roast for another 10 to 15 minutes. Add salt and pepper to taste.

Serving size = 1 cup
224 calories
0.5 grams total fat
trace saturated fat
0 milligrams cholesterol

GRAINS AND LEGUMES

Most of the delicious grains and bean dishes here make hearty main courses. Some will be adaptations of familiar dishes, like the Red Bean Chili (page 445), the Black Bean Chili (page 447), and the Black Bean Burritos (below). Lovers of Italian food will find Risotto (page 451) and a number of polenta dishes.

There are also a number of side dishes. Some of the grain and bean dishes go well together and provide complete protein when they're served in combination. They also make filling meals.

When cooking grains and beans, think about menus for the whole week. You might want to double the amount and use the extra for salads or stir-fry. Cooked beans and grains also freeze well.

BLACK BEAN BURRITOS

YIELD: 3 CUPS (6 SERVINGS)   BY MARK HALL

If you have the black beans already made, this is a very quick meal to pull together. The "guacamole" is a surprise for those who have given up avocados because of their fat content. Serve this crowd pleaser with a tossed green salad and a bowl of chopped jalapeños on the side.

1 ½ cups dry black beans
6 cups water
4 bay leaves
1 cup chopped onions
½ cup dry white wine
2 teaspoons freshly minced garlic
2 teaspoons ground cumin
¼ teaspoon freshly ground black
  pepper
1 teaspoon Ancho Chili Puree
  (page 465) (optional)

¼ cup orange juice
⅛ teaspoon cayenne pepper
Salt
Green Pea "Guacamole" for
  garnish
Salsa Cruda for garnish
Chopped lettuce, scallions, or
  tomatoes for garnish (optional)
6 oil-free flour tortillas

For the *filling,* sort and rinse the beans, then soak overnight in plenty of water. Drain and rinse. Cook the beans in a separate pot with the 6 cups of water and bay leaves for about 1 hour. In another pot, braise the onions in ½ cup white wine with the garlic, cumin, and black pepper. When the black beans are cooked, remove the bay leaves and drain, leaving about ¾ cup of liquid in the beans. Add the beans to the onions and stir. (If desired, add the Ancho Chili Puree at this stage and let stew for 5 to 10 minutes to let the flavors mesh.) Add the orange juice and cayenne to the beans. Then add the salt to taste.

GREEN PEA "GUACAMOLE"

3 cups green peas, fresh or frozen	¼ teaspoon freshly ground black
2 tablespoons lemon juice	pepper
1 cup red onions	⅛ teaspoon cayenne
2 teaspoons freshly minced garlic	Salt
1 teaspoon ground cumin	

Steam the peas if fresh. Do not overcook. They should still have their bright green color. If using frozen peas, just defrost them.

Puree the peas in a blender or food processor with the lemon juice, onions, garlic, cumin, and black pepper. Add cayenne and salt to taste.

SALSA CRUDA

2 cups seeded and diced tomatoes	1 teaspoon rice wine vinegar
½ cup peeled and diced cucumbers	2 tablespoons freshly chopped cilantro
½ cup diced onions	1 teaspoon fresh lime juice
½ cup diced green bell peppers	⅛ teaspoon cayenne
1 teaspoon freshly minced garlic	Salt

Mix the tomatoes with the cucumber, onions, green peppers, and garlic. Season with vinegar, cilantro, lime juice, and cayenne. Salt to taste and serve. There should be about 4 cups salsa. (By diluting this, you can also make a soup.)

To *assemble the burrito,* place about ½ cup of the black beans, an equal volume of "guacamole," and ¼ cup of the salsa in the center of the tortillas. Fold the opposite ends of the tortilla inward and roll. You can also add some chopped lettuce, onions, tomatoes, or cilantro before rolling the tortilla.

Ladle some salsa over the tortilla, garnish with whole cilantro sprigs or chopped leaves, and serve.

Serving size = 1 burrito
303 calories
4.0 grams total fat
0.6 grams saturated fat
0 milligrams cholesterol

Beans only:
Serving size = 1 cup
299 calories
1.8 grams total fat
0.1 grams saturated fat
0 milligrams cholesterol

Serving size = ¼ cup "guacamole"
41 calories
0.3 grams total fat
0.1 grams saturated fat
0 milligrams cholesterol

Serving size = ¼ cup salsa cruda
8 calories
0.1 grams total fat
trace saturated fat
0 milligrams cholesterol

RED BEAN CHILI

YIELD: 8 CUPS (8 SERVINGS)   BY DEBORAH MADISON

Use your favorite red beans with this chili recipe—pinto, pinquito, or kidney beans. You might like to experiment with other varieties as well, such as anasazi or black beans. All are good and have their own special qualities. The canned chipotle chilies, which can frequently be found in the Mexican part of your supermarket or in Mexican groceries, give a rich, smoky flavor to this dish. They are hot, though. The best way to use them is to puree them first, then add the puree gradually, tasting as you go.

This will keep well in the refrigerator for several days. In fact, the flavors will keep improving. Check the seasoning when you reheat it and add an extra splash of vinegar, if desired.

This chili can be used in various ways. Thin it out and serve it as a soup. If cooked thick, or left to thicken, the spicy beans can be used in enchiladas.

Fortunately, beans can be frozen, so you might want to double the amount and freeze portions in freezer bags.

2 cups beans
1 teaspoon cumin seeds
1 teaspoon dried oregano,
   preferably Greek or Mexican
1 to 2 tablespoons mild chili
   powder
2 bay leaves
1 onion, finely diced
2 cloves garlic, minced
2 cups chopped tomatoes
3 tablespoons freshly chopped
   cilantro

About 1 teaspoon pureed chipotle
   chilies
1 green bell pepper, diced in
   small squares
Vinegar to taste
Freshly chopped cilantro for
   garnish
Roasted green chilies (such as
   Ortega), cut in strips or diced
Nonfat yogurt

Sort and rinse the beans, then soak overnight in water. Pour off the soaking water from the beans and cover them generously with fresh water in a large pot to at least a few inches above the beans. Bring to a boil and boil vigorously for about 5 minutes. Usually a lot of scum will rise to the surface. Skim off what you can, then lower the heat.

Toast the cumin seeds and the oregano very briefly in a dry pan, then grind them in a mortar to break up the seeds or briefly in an electric spice mill. Add them to the beans along with the chili powder, bay leaves, onion, and garlic. Cook over a medium heat until the onions are soft, about 15 minutes, then add the chopped tomatoes with their juice and the cilantro. Stir in about a teaspoon of chipotle chili, let it cook for a minute or so, then taste and add more if you wish. (You can continue to taste and add while the beans cook, since the balance of flavors will keep altering.) Add the diced pepper, then lower the heat and allow the beans to simmer gently until they are well cooked, about an hour, or longer, if necessary.

Once the beans have cooked, the flavor of the chili will continue to soften and develop. Just before you serve it, stir in some vinegar to sharpen the taste. Garnish with cilantro and green chilies. Or stir the cilantro and chilies into ½ cup nonfat yogurt and serve the chili with a spoonful on top.

Serving size = 1 cup (without yogurt)
161 calories
1.0 grams total fat
0.2 grams saturated fat
0 milligrams cholesterol

BLACK BEAN CHILI

YIELD: 6 CUPS CHILI (6 SERVINGS)   BY MARK HALL

Instructions are given for preparing it on the stove as well as using a pressure cooker. The pressure cooker will reduce the preparation time and the sauce will have a smoother consistency.

2 cups dry black beans
8 cups water
4 bay leaves
½ teaspoon ground cumin
1 tablespoon rice wine vinegar
1 teaspoon Ancho Chili Puree
  (page 465)
Salt
2 tablespoons freshly chopped
  cilantro
½ teaspoon cayenne
Chopped chilies or cilantro for
  garnish

Chili-Tomato Sauce Base:

1 28-ounce can chopped tomatoes,
  drained
1⅔ cups chopped onions
1 teaspoon freshly minced garlic
5 tablespoons water
1½ teaspoons ground cumin
2 teaspoons dried oregano
2 teaspoons paprika

Sort and rinse, then soak the beans overnight in water. Bring a pot of water containing the beans and the bay leaves to a boil and then simmer for 1 to 1½ hours.

For the chili-tomato sauce, reserve the liquid from the can of tomatoes if you plan to use the pressure cooking method. Braise the onions and garlic in the water with the 1½ teaspoons cumin, oregano, and paprika. Add the tomatoes and stew for about 30 minutes, until the sauce is thickened. There should be approximately six cups.

When the beans have cooked, drain any excess liquid and set aside the bean stock. Add the beans and 1 cup of the reserved bean stock to the chili-tomato sauce. Cook for about 30 minutes, until the sauce is thickened. If it is too thick, gradually add more bean stock until the right consistency is achieved. Add the ½ teaspoon cumin, vinegar, and 1 teaspoon Ancho Chili Puree. Add salt to taste, and add the cilantro. If more "fire" is desired, add some cayenne. Garnish with fresh chopped chilies or more cilantro.

VARIATION: Prepare the beans in a pressure cooker.

PRESSURE COOKING METHOD

2 cups black beans, sorted and rinsed

8 cups water (including the juice from a 28-ounce can of tomatoes)

6 cups Chili-Tomato Sauce (see above)

Put the beans and liquid in a pressure cooker and cook for 40 minutes. Meanwhile, prepare the Chili-Tomato Sauce as described. Drain the stock from the beans and reserve. Mix the sauce and the beans. Add stock to achieve a desired consistency. Add 1 teaspoon Ancho Chili Puree, 1 teaspoon ground cumin, 1 tablespoon rice wine vinegar, ½ teaspoon cayenne, and 2 tablespoons chopped cilantro. Add salt and pepper to taste. Garnish with fresh chopped chilies or more cilantro.

Serving size = 1 cup
205 calories
1.5 grams total fat
0.2 grams saturated fat
0 milligrams cholesterol

TAMALE PIE

YIELD: 7½ × 12-INCH LASAGNA PAN (6 SERVINGS)   BY CAROL CONNELL

This makes a very hearty meal. Serve with a light citrus-based salad to cleanse the palate.

Crust:

½ cup cornmeal
½ cup unbleached all-purpose flour
1½ teaspoons baking powder
¼ teaspoon salt
½ cup nonfat yogurt
¼ cup water
1 teaspoon sugar
½ teaspoon cayenne
¼ cup cooked corn kernels

Filling:

1 cup chopped onions
6 cloves garlic, minced
1 tablespoon ground cumin
½ tablespoon chili powder
¼ teaspoon coriander powder
¼ cup apple juice concentrate
¼ cup tomato paste
1 cup chopped tomato
3 tablespoons diced jalapeño peppers

2 cups cooked kidney beans
1/4 cup fresh green peas
1/4 cup corn kernels
1/2 cup finely chopped carrots
1/2 cup chopped red bell pepper
3 tablespoons freshly chopped
    parsley

Vegetable stock
4 tablespoons freshly chopped
    cilantro
1/8 teaspoon salt

For the crust, mix together the cornmeal, flour, baking powder, and salt. Gradually add the yogurt and water, then mix until smooth. Stir the sugar, cayenne, and corn kernels into the batter. Set aside under a damp cloth.

Preheat the oven to 350°F. For the filling braise the onions, garlic, cumin, chili powder, and coriander in the apple juice concentrate in a large skillet or a heavy pot. Add the tomato paste, chopped tomato, and diced jalapeño peppers. Then add the beans, peas, corn, carrots, bell pepper, and parsley. Braise for about 10 minutes, adding vegetable stock as needed to keep the vegetables from sticking. Add the cilantro and salt. Pour into a 7½ × 12-inch lasagna pan that is nonstick or coated with vegetable oil spray.

To assemble, spread the batter over the vegetables as evenly as possible. Bake for about 30 minutes, until the top is bubbling and the crust is just beginning to brown at the edges.

Serving size = 1 cup
233 calories
1.7 grams total fat
trace saturated fat
trace cholesterol

CHICK-PEA AND VEGETABLE STEW WITH COUSCOUS

YIELD: 8 CUPS (4 SERVINGS)   BY DEBORAH MADISON

The basis of this stew is the chick-pea and its cooking broth. You can vary the vegetables according to the season, using winter squash in the winter and zucchini in the summer, for example. You can also increase or lessen the amount of vegetables, according to your own taste. The cooking liquid is important for it lends a certain viscosity that is reminiscent of oil but which is absent in water. It gives the stew more body and a richer texture.

This is easy to multiply.

1 cup dry chick-peas (about 2½ cups cooked), plus the cooking broth
1 large onion, diced in ¼-inch squares
2 cloves garlic, minced
1½ teaspoons paprika
¼ teaspoon ground cinnamon
¼ teaspoon cayenne
½ teaspoon ground cumin
½ teaspoon freshly ground black pepper
½ teaspoon ground ginger
1 green bell pepper, diced slightly larger than the onions
1 cup cubed zucchini or other summer squash
1 can (about 2 cups) canned tomatoes, chopped, and their juices
2 tablespoons golden or black raisins
1 teaspoon safflower stamens (these are available in the Mexican part of your grocery) or 2 pinches saffron (optional)
2 tablespoons freshly chopped parsley
2 tablespoons freshly chopped cilantro
1 cup fresh or frozen peas
8 ounces couscous
Fresh cilantro branches or freshly minced parsley or cilantro for garnish

Sort and rinse the chick-peas, then soak overnight in water. Drain and cook in 5 cups water until tender, about 2 to 3 hours. Drain, reserving the broth, and set aside.

Warm a cup of the chick-pea broth in a skillet or soup pot and add the onion, garlic, and the dried spices. Simmer gently until the onions have begun to soften, about 7 minutes. Don't let the pan dry out or the spices will burn. Add more liquid as needed instead.

Once the onions are soft, add the chick-peas, pepper, squash, the juice from the tomatoes and the chopped tomatoes, the raisins, safflower or saffron, if using, the parsley, and cilantro. Add enough chick-pea broth or water to cover, bring to a boil, then simmer until the vegetables are done and the liquid has reduced, making a nice sauce. Add the green peas during the last 5 minutes.

Make the couscous and serve with the vegetables and their sauce. Garnish with cilantro or parsley.

COUSCOUS

If using packaged couscous, follow the directions on the box. Otherwise bring 1½ cups of water to a boil, pour in the precooked couscous and turn off the heat. Cover and let stand until the couscous has absorbed the moisture, about 5 minutes.

Serving size = 2 cups stew
272 calories
3.6 grams total fat
0.5 grams saturated fat
0 milligrams cholesterol

Serving size = 1 cup stew + 1 cup couscous
244 calories
2.8 grams total fat
0.5 grams saturated fat
0 milligrams cholesterol

RISOTTO

YIELD: 2½ CUPS (5 SERVINGS)   BY DONNA NICOLETTI

You will not miss the chicken stock in this risotto. Stir to keep the grains separate and to distribute the stock well. You do not need to stir continuously.

1 teaspoon freshly minced garlic   *2 tablespoons chopped scallions*
2 cups vegetable stock   *1 teaspoon dried oregano*
1 cup Arborio rice   *1 teaspoon saffron threads*
1 cup tomato juice

In a sauté pan, braise the garlic with ⅓ cup vegetable stock. When softened, add the rice and another cup of the stock and let cook on a low flame, uncovered, for 10 minutes, stirring occasionally. Add the rest of the stock. Continue to cook.

When most of the liquid has evaporated, add the tomato juice, scallions, oregano, and saffron. Cook for another 10 minutes, stirring occasionally as before until the rice is slightly firm to the bite. You can let the cooking liquid completely evaporate or let the rice stay a little wet. The total cooking time is about 30 minutes.

Serving size = ½ cup
158 calories
0.2 grams total fat
trace saturated fat
0 milligrams cholesterol

SPANISH BULGUR

YIELD: 6 CUPS (6 SERVINGS)   BY CAROL CONNELL

Since the bulgur and the sauce are essentially cooked separately and then mixed together, this recipe can be prepared with whatever grain you prefer.

4½ cups water
3 cups bulgur
1 cup finely diced scallions
1 cup chopped green bell pepper
1½ teaspoons paprika

2 cups tomato sauce
1 cup salsa
Salt
Minced fresh cilantro

Bring the water to a boil. Pour the bulgur into the water, stirring as you do so. Turn down the heat to very low, then let simmer 20 minutes. Combine the remaining ingredients in a separate pot and let simmer for 10 minutes, then stir into the cooked bulgur, mixing thoroughly. Add salt to taste. Garnish with a small amount of cilantro and serve.

Serving size = 1 cup
177 calories
0.8 grams total fat
0.3 grams saturated fat
0 milligrams cholesterol

STUFFED RED PEPPER WITH SPANISH RICE AND TOMATILLO SAUCE

YIELD: 4 STUFFED PEPPERS (4 SERVINGS)   BY MARK HALL

This very pretty dish, made special by the tomatillo sauce and the roasted red pepper, is well worth the effort to prepare.

4 red peppers, roasted
½ cup uncooked brown rice
5 cups water
2 bay leaves
1 cup chopped onions
½ teaspoon freshly minced garlic
1½ teaspoons dried oregano
½ cup dry red wine
1⅓ cups finely diced green bell peppers

1 cup canned tomato puree
½ teaspoon ground cumin
Salt
Freshly ground black pepper
Cayenne
Cilantro or Italian parsley sprigs (optional)
1½ cups Tomatillo Sauce (page 413)

To prepare the peppers for stuffing, start by roasting them in the oven on flat pans until the skins have blackened. Rotate the peppers frequently. They can be moved from the top shelf to bottom depending on how quickly each side is charring.

Alternatively, you can broil the peppers on top of the stove right over an open flame or in a wood-burning fireplace. They will need to be cooked until the skins have completely blackened.

Put the peppers into a bowl, cover with a plate, and let them steam for at least 15 minutes to soften the flesh and make the peels easier to remove. Slit the side of each pepper open and take the seeds out, being careful that the peppers don't fall apart. Leave the stem on and set aside. The peppers are now ready for stuffing.

Soak the rice in 3 cups of water for 30 minutes, then drain. Bring 5 cups of water to a boil. Add the rice and 2 bay leaves to the water, stir, cover, and cook at a slow boil for 25 to 30 minutes, until tender. Strain and remove the bay leaves. This makes 1½ cups.

Braise the onion, garlic, and oregano in the red wine. When the onions have softened a bit, add the green pepper. When the pepper is almost completely cooked, add the tomato puree. Let stew for 15 to 20 minutes, until the vegetables are tender. Add the cumin and rice when the vegetables are cooked. Add salt and pepper to taste. If you want it spicier, add some cayenne pepper.

To assemble, use approximately ¾ cup filling per pepper. Make a bed of tomatillo sauce and put the peppers on top. Bake at 350°F. for 20 to 30 minutes or microwave the filled peppers until they're hot. Garnish with the fresh sprigs of cilantro or Italian parsley.

Serving size = 1 pepper + ¾ cup filling + ½ cup sauce
217 calories
1.7 grams total fat
0.3 grams saturated fat
0 milligrams cholesterol

WILD AND ARBORIO RICE

YIELD: 3 CUPS (3 SERVINGS)   BY MARK HALL

The two grains are cooked separately and tossed together when done. There are no added seasonings except for salt and pepper, if desired.

Each rice will be prepared in a manner different from the way we usually resort to when cooking rice. The Arborio rice and the wild rice are both "free-boiled." This means cooking so that the water isn't completely absorbed or evaporated. The pot will need to be well covered and more water to be added if it begins to evaporate. The goal is to keep each grain freely moving and separate within the boiling water. This method will give you well-cooked, completely separate grains to be used in salads or pilafs when the grains to be mixed have much different cooking times.

4 cups water	*¹/₃ cup wild rice*
³/₄ cups uncooked Arborio rice	*Salt*
1¹/₂ cups water	*Freshly ground black pepper*

Bring 4 cups of water to a boil and add the Arborio rice. Cover the pot and continue boiling for about 30 minutes, until the rice is tender. Occasionally check the pot and add more water if it is evaporating.

To prepare the wild rice, bring 1½ cups of water to a boil, then add the wild rice. Keep this at a rolling boil for about 30 to 40 minutes, until the grains crack. Add more water if needed.

When the Arborio rice and wild rice are tender, drain them and toss together with the salt and pepper to taste.

Serving size = 1 cup
249 calories
0.4 grams total fat
0.2 grams saturated fat
0 milligrams cholesterol

GOLDEN RICE PILAF

YIELD: 6 CUPS (6 SERVINGS)   BY CAROL CONNELL

The water chestnuts, carrots and celery add more crunch to this already highly textured dish.

3¹/₂ cups water or vegetable stock	*1¹/₂ teaspoons curry*
1¹/₂ cups long-grain uncooked	*¹/₄ teaspoon freshly grated ginger*
* brown rice*	*1 tablespoon Butter Buds*
¹/₄ cup minced carrots	*¹/₈ teaspoon salt*
¹/₄ cup minced celery	*¹/₄ cup chopped scallions for*
¹/₂ cup sliced water chestnuts	* garnish*
1 teaspoon saffron threads	

Bring the water or vegetable stock to a rolling boil. Add the rice and cook on high heat until the water begins to boil again. Reduce the heat, cover, and let the rice simmer for 1 hour. Sauté the minced carrots in a small amount of water or vegetable stock for about 5 minutes before adding the other vegetables and spices except for the Butter Buds and salt. Continue braising the vegetables for about 10 minutes, adding more water or stock as needed to prevent burning or browning. Add the Butter Buds to the rice and toss this with the vegetables. Add salt to taste and garnish with the scallions.

Serving size = 1 cup
195 calories
1.1 grams total fat
0.2 grams saturated fat
trace cholesterol

POLENTA WITH TOMATO SAUCE

YIELD: 2½ CUPS (4 SERVINGS)   BY MARK HALL

Polenta is very coarse cornmeal that is slowly cooked and then served as a soft "mush" or allowed to solidify so that it can be cut into various shapes and served as is, broiled, or even fried. Frequent stirring is necessary as it cooks. If it is being served with a savory topping or sauce, the polenta can be served simply with a little salt. Alternatively, you can cook the polenta with fresh or dried herbs, or with onions and garlic.

1 cup polenta
4 cups water or vegetable stock

Tomato Sauce:

2 cups chopped canned tomatoes
1 cup chopped onions
½ cup red wine
2 tablespoons freshly minced garlic
2 tablespoons freshly chopped basil

2 tablespoons dried oregano
Salt
Freshly ground black pepper
Chopped fresh basil or Italian parsley for garnish

Gradually add the polenta to the 4 cups of water or stock, stirring as it is added to prevent lumps from forming. Cook over low heat, stirring frequently, about every 5 minutes for about 30 to 40 minutes. The polenta burns easily. It has finished cooking when the mixture is hard to stir and the stirring spoon is able to stand within the polenta. Before it becomes too thick, you may want to add salt to taste. Add small amounts of liquid if the cornmeal is not cooked and too much liquid has evaporated. Once cooked, transfer the polenta to a baking dish or cookie sheet and smooth out until it is a uniform height. Allow to cool somewhat. While this is cooling prepare the tomato sauce.

To start the sauce, puree the tomatoes with their canned liquid. Set aside. Braise the onions in red wine with the garlic, basil, and oregano. When the wine has been reduced and the onions are tender, add the pureed tomatoes. Cook for approximately an hour, stirring frequently, until the sauce is thick and with little visible liquid. Season with salt and pepper to taste. There should be about 1½ cups sauce.

Serve the polenta with tomato sauce ladled over the top. Garnish with basil or Italian parsley.

Serving size = 1 cup polenta with sauce combined
195 calories
0.8 grams total fat
0.2 grams saturated fat
0 milligrams cholesterol

POLENTA WITH TOMATO SAUCE AND ZUCCHINI

SERVES 4   BY MARK HALL

1 cup polenta
Tomato Sauce (page 464)
¾ cup thinly sliced zucchini
1 tablespoon freshly minced garlic
1½ teaspoons freshly chopped
    basil

½ tablespoon chopped dried
    oregano
Salt
Freshly ground black pepper

Preheat the oven to 375°F. Prepare 1 cup of polenta and the tomato sauce as per the instructions for Polenta with Tomato Sauce. Set the polenta out in a pan. Toss the sliced zucchini with the garlic, basil, oregano, and salt and pepper to taste, place on a nonstick baking sheet and bake for about 15 minutes. After the polenta has been assembled, ladle the tomato sauce evenly over the polenta and arrange the zucchini over the sauce. Bake for 15 minutes more.

Serving size = approximately 1⅛ cup
207 calories
0.8 grams total fat
0.2 grams saturated fat
0 milligrams cholesterol

QUINOA MEXICAN STYLE

YIELD: 6 CUPS (6 SERVINGS)   BY PHYLLIS GINSBERG

Washing the quinoa well is absolutely necessary. Otherwise this dish will be spoiled by the harsh and disagreeable taste of its natural coating.

½ pound onions, chopped
1 teaspoon freshly minced garlic
1 cup vegetable stock
1 cup quinoa, well rinsed
1 cup canned Italian plum tomatoes, drained

1 cup tomato juice from canned tomatoes
½ to 1 whole jalapeño or serrano pepper, seeded and chopped
2 tablespoons freshly chopped cilantro for garnish

Braise the onions and garlic in about ¼ cup vegetable stock. When the onions are soft, add the quinoa, remaining vegetable stock, the plum tomatoes, tomato juice, and chili. Bring to a boil. Then reduce the heat, cover, and cook for about 20 minutes, until the quinoa is tender. Sprinkle the cilantro over the quinoa and serve.

Serving size = 1 cup
167 calories
2.2 grams total fat
trace saturated fat
0 milligrams cholesterol

REFRIED BEANS

YIELD: 3 CUPS (6 SERVINGS)   BY MARK HALL

This dish also goes well with rice or any of the Latin-inspired dishes. Serve with corn tortillas that have been cut into wedges, steamed to cook, and then baked for crispness.

1 cup dry pinto peans, or 2 cups cooked
4 cups water
3 bay leaves
2½ cups tomato puree
1 cup chopped red onion
1 teaspoon freshly minced garlic
½ cup finely diced cucumber
½ cup finely diced red bell pepper

½ cup finely diced green bell pepper
2 teaspoons rice wine vinegar
½ teaspoon lemon juice
¼ teaspoon cayenne
¼ teaspoon freshly ground black pepper
2 tablespoons freshly minced cilantro
Salt

If using dried beans, sort and rinse them, then soak them overnight in 4 cups of water. Drain and bring 4 cups of water to a boil. Add the beans and the bay leaves. Simmer for 2 to 2½ hours, until tender. Drain and reserve ½ cup of the cooking liquid. Remove the bay leaves. Puree 1 cup of the beans with the tomato puree and set aside.

Braise the onions and garlic in ½ cup of the reserved bean stock. When the onions have softened, add the cucumber and red and green pepper. Continue cooking until the peppers have softened. Add the whole and pureed beans with the remaining ingredients. Stir and add salt to taste. Garnish with chopped cilantro and serve.

Serving size = ½ cup
103 calories
0.5 grams total fat
trace saturated fat
0 milligrams cholesterol

KAPPA MAKI

YIELD: 2 ROLLS 8 INCHES EACH   BY MARK HALL
(4 SERVINGS OF 4 1-INCH SLICES)

This is best made with Japanese white rice, which is more glutinous and sticky and helps to keep the roll together. Kappa Maki is traditionally served with a soy-based sauce. Take into account that there is some salt already in the roll. It can be served with the Chinese Dressing (p. 398), a hot Japanese mustard, or wasabi (horseradish).

1 cup uncooked rice or 2 cups
   cooked
2 cups water
2 tablespoons rice wine vinegar
2 tablespoons mirin
1/2 teaspoon freshly minced garlic

2 teaspoons freshly shredded
   ginger
1 teaspoon salt
1/3 English cucumber
2 8 × 10-inch sheets toasted Nori
   seaweed

Cook the rice, covered, in 2 cups water for about 30 minutes, or until tender and the liquid is absorbed. After the rice is done, season with the vinegar, mirin, garlic, ginger, and salt. You can add more vinegar to taste.

Peel and seed the cucumber, then slice into long thin strips. Set aside.

The assembly can be done without a Japanese bamboo rolling mat. Lay out a sheet of the toasted seaweed and cover with a thin layer of rice about 1/4-inch thick. Wet your hands to prevent the rice from sticking to them. Pack down the rice evenly on the seaweed, leaving a 1-inch border around the seaweed that is free of the rice. In the center of the rice bed lay strips of cucumber so that they line the entire length of the roll. Beginning with the side of the seaweed parallel to the cucumber strips, make a compact roll. If the roll falls apart and the seaweed isn't sticking, moisten the end of the roll with your fingers and then press the seaweed onto the roll. With a sharp knife, cut the roll into uniform 1-inch lengths.

VARIATIONS: You can make this roll with any other vegetables, such as carrots or scallions.

Serving size = 4 1-inch rolls
180 calories
0.3 grams total fat
0.1 grams saturated fat
0 milligrams cholesterol

RICE PILAF WITH SAFFRON PEPPERS

YIELD: 4–6 CUPS (3 TO 6 SERVINGS)   BY DEBORAH MADISON

Use the Roasted Peppers with Saffron to give this pilaf a special flavor and rich color. If you have peppers on hand, this won't take long to prepare. For a fuller dish, you could combine this with already cooked chick-peas or large white beans, using some of the bean broth for the liquid.

1 cup long-grain rice
1 recipe for Roasted Peppers with
    Saffron (p. 407)
1 large ripe tomato
1 small onion, finely diced
1 clove garlic, sliced
1 bay leaf
1 tablespoon chopped parsley

1 tablespoon chopped fresh basil,
    or 1 teaspoon dried basil
2 teaspoons chopped marjoram
    leaves, or ½ teaspoon dried
    marjoram
2½ cups water, vegetable stock,
    or bean broth
Chopped herbs for garnish

Cover the rice with hot tap water and set it aside while you assemble the rest of the ingredients. Prepare the peppers, if you haven't any on hand. Peel, seed, and finely dice the tomato, reserving the juice.

Drain the rice and put it in a pot with a tight-fitting lid with the onion, garlic, bay leaf, and herbs. Turn on the heat and stir the rice until the moisture has evaporated, then add the tomato, juice, and peppers. Add the water, vegetable stock, or bean broth, bring to a boil and cook over a medium-high heat for five minutes. Lower the heat, cover, and cook until all the liquid has been absorbed, another ten minutes or so. (The time will depend on the type of rice used. If it is not done after all the water has been absorbed, add more water successively in small amounts, a few tablespoons at a time, until it is done.) Once the liquid has been absorbed, lay a clean cloth napkin or towel over the rice, return the lid to the pot and allow it to sit undisturbed for a half-hour.

To serve, gently loosen the rice with a fork and put it in a serving dish. Garnish with fresh herbs and serve.

Serving size = 1 cup
220 calories
0.6 grams total fat
0.1 grams saturated fat
0 milligrams cholesterol

PASTA

You will see from the recipes that follow that meatballs and Alfredo sauce are not the only things with which to toss pasta. Restaurants specializing in pasta have flourished in America over the past decade. Bookstores stock pasta cookbooks by the dozen. Most of the restaurant fare and traditional recipes contain more oil than our guidelines allow. But all that oil isn't really necessary. The combinations on these pages prove the point. The most important thing about a pasta sauce is that it coats the noodles and adds flavor to the dish. You don't need oil for that; tomatoes alone would do the trick, and they really come alive when they're mixed with the ingredients you'll find in these recipes—fresh basil, garlic, and balsamic vinegar, to name just a few. Cooked tomato sauces can be simmered with no addition of oil, and none of the flavors will be sacrificed.

Some of the dishes here are piquant with hot pepper flakes or cayenne. Roasted red peppers come up often, because they are so good tossed with pasta. One of the most intriguing and satisfying sauces here is a Red Pepper and Lentil Sauce (page 467), which is also high in protein. Beans and pasta, in fact, are a traditional combination in Italy. These dishes are quite lovely to look at, with their bright combinations of lively colored vegetables and herbs contrasted with the neutral shades of the pasta.

Dry packaged pasta (as opposed to fresh pasta containing eggs) is a perfect food for this diet. Made from either semolina flour or whole wheat flour and water, it is a healthful, high-carbohydrate food. Many no-oil products are widely available. It's no wonder that Italians have a low incidence of heart disease.

PASTA WITH ASPARAGUS AND ASPARAGUS CREAM

YIELD: 6 CUPS SAUCE (6 SERVINGS)   BY DEBORAH MADISON

Pureed asparagus and other spring vegetables make the sauce for this pasta, while more asparagus is cooked separately, then mixed in with the pasta for texture. Serve with either whole wheat or spinach pasta.

1½ pounds asparagus
1 bunch scallions, rinsed and
*   chopped including the firm*
*   parts of the stems*

1 bay leaf
½ teaspoon dried marjoram or
*   basil or 1 tablespoon fresh*
3 parsley branches

1 cup frozen peas
Grated zest of 1 lemon plus juice
  to taste
½ jalapeño pepper, seeds and
  veins removed, minced
  (optional)

2½ ounces spaghetti or fettuccine
  per person
A mixture of finely chopped
  parsley or chervil, chives, basil,
  marjoram, or lemon thyme for
  garnish

Snap off the toughest ends of the asparagus and discard them. Take half the asparagus and chop into small pieces. Bring 8 cups of water to a boil, add the chopped asparagus, scallions, bay leaf, marjoram, parsley, and peas. Simmer until the asparagus is tender, then remove the bay leaf. Drain, reserving the cooking liquid. Put the cooked vegetables in a food processor and process until smooth, gradually adding 1½ cups of the cooking water to make the sauce whatever consistency you like. To make the sauce extra fine, pass it through a sieve or a food mill. Stir in the lemon zest and add the jalapeño, if using. Set aside.

Slice the rest of the asparagus either into rounds or into long, thin diagonals. If the heads are thick, slice them in half lengthwise. Bring 3 quarts of water to a boil, add the asparagus, and cook until tender. Remove from the water and set aside. Add the pasta and cook according to package directions without using salt until al dente—tender but firm to the bite. Drain.

Just before the pasta is finished, heat the vegetable puree gently and season with the lemon juice to taste. (Just warm it, don't let it boil.) Have a warm serving bowl ready. Pour in the sauce, then the hot pasta. Garnish with the cooked asparagus and a handful of fresh herbs. Toss right away and serve.

VARIATION: If your diet allows, warm ½ cup nonfat yogurt with the vegetable sauce, then proceed as above.

Serving size = 1 cup sauce + 1 cup pasta
461 calories
0.5 grams total fat
trace saturated fat
0 milligrams cholesterol

Variation with yogurt sauce:
serving = 1 cup sauce + 1 cup pasta
471 calories
0.5 grams saturated fat
trace saturated fat
trace cholesterol

LINGUINI WITH ROASTED RED PEPPER AND HERBED TOMATO SAUCE

YIELD: 3 CUPS SAUCE (3 SERVINGS)   BY PAMELA MORGAN

This is a very simple, fresh tomato sauce, but the addition of the peppers and balsamic vinegar adds a unique flavor.

2 red bell peppers
10 ripe plum tomatoes, peeled,
    seeded, and chopped
6 cloves garlic
1/2 cup chopped yellow onion
1 tablespoon balsamic vinegar
1 teaspoon salt
Freshly ground black pepper to
    taste
1 teaspoon sugar

1/2 teaspoon red hot chili flakes
1 tablespoon freshly chopped basil
1 tablespoon freshly chopped
    parsley
Fresh basil leaves and freshly
    cracked black pepper for
    garnish
2 1/2 ounces dry linguini or other
    pasta per person

Roast the peppers under the broiler, turning frequently until the skins are charred and blackened. Place in a plastic bag and close tightly for 10 to 15 minutes. When the peppers are cool, remove from the bag and peel. The skin will come off easily. Make a slit in the pepper. Cut out the stem and remove the seeds. Place the peppers in a food processor with 1 cup of the tomatoes.

Roast the garlic cloves in the oven at 350°F. for 15 to 20 minutes. Remove the skins and place the garlic in a food processor with the onions, balsamic vinegar, salt, and pepper. Process for 20 seconds.

Transfer the mixture to a medium-sized saucepan. Add the rest of the tomatoes, the sugar, and red chili flakes, and simmer for 5 minutes. Add the fresh basil leaves and parsley, then remove from the heat immediately.

Cook the pasta in a large pot of boiling water, according to package directions, without using salt, al dente—tender but firm to the bite. Drain and toss, while still warm, with the sauce. Garnish with basil leaves and pepper.

Serving size = 1 cup sauce + 1 cup pasta
313 calories
1.3 grams total fat
0.3 grams saturated fat
0 milligrams cholesterol

EGGPLANT LASAGNA

YIELD: ONE 8 × 6½-INCH PAN (4 SERVINGS)   BY MARK HALL

A few strips of grilled eggplant placed over the last layer of pasta before baking makes this dish a visual treat.

Tomato Sauce:

1 28-ounce can whole tomatoes, undrained
1⅔ cups chopped onion
4 tablespoons red wine
2 cloves garlic, minced
1 teaspoon dried marjoram
2 teaspoons dried oregano
1 to 2 bay leaves

2 medium Japanese eggplants (approximately ½ pound total)
1 teaspoon freshly chopped Italian parsley
5 ounces egg-free, oil-free spinach lasagna sheets, cooked
Freshly chopped basil for garnish

To start the sauce, puree the tomatoes and set aside. Braise the onions in red wine with the garlic, marjoram, oregano, and bay leaves. When the wine has been reduced and the onions are tender, add the pureed tomatoes. Cook for approximately 1 hour, stirring frequently. The sauce should become thick and there should be little visible liquid. There should be 3 cups of sauce.

Cut the eggplant into ½-inch slices. Lay these out on a nonstick baking sheet with a small amount of water. Sprinkle with parsley, cover, and bake at 350°F. for about 12 to 15 minutes, until the eggplant is soft throughout.

Preheat the oven to 350°F. Ladle ½ cup sauce on the bottom of an 8 × 6½ inch pan. Top with a layer of noodles, more sauce, and a layer of the eggplant. Repeat the layer of lasagna sheets, sauce, and eggplant. Add another layer of pasta and sauce. Garnish with fresh basil. Cover the pan and bake for 20 to 30 minutes until the sauce is bubbling.

Serving size = ¼ pan
261 calories
0.7 grams total fat
0.1 grams saturated fat
0 milligrams cholesterol

PASTA WITH CREOLE SAUCE

YIELD: 3¼ CUPS SAUCE (3 TO 4 SERVINGS)   BY MARK HALL

This tomato-based sauce is very spicy. The cayenne pepper is not meant to give it heat, but to contribute to the overall balance of flavors. This sauce is also delicious served over rice.

½ cup dry kidney beans or 1⅓ cups cooked
5 cups water
6 bay leaves
1½ cups chopped onion
⅓ cup dry red wine
½ cups thinly sliced green bell peppers
2 cups canned tomatoes, pureed

1 teaspoon freshly minced garlic
1 tablespoon dried oregano
½ teaspoon dried thyme
⅛ teaspoon cayenne
1 teaspoon rice wine vinegar
Salt
¼ teaspoon freshly ground black pepper or to taste
2½ ounces dry pasta per person

If you are using cooked beans omit this step. Sort and rinse the beans, then soak overnight in water. Drain and cook the kidney beans in a separate pot with 5 cups of water and 4 bay leaves. Cook for 1½ hours until tender. When the kidney beans are done, remove the bay leaves, drain, and set aside.

In another pot braise the onions in the red wine. When the onions are soft, add the green pepper. Before the peppers are completely softened, add the tomatoes, garlic, oregano, thyme, and 2 bay leaves. Stew all of this together for 20 to 25 minutes. Add the kidney beans, cayenne, and rice wine vinegar. Stir, then add salt and pepper to taste.

Cook the pasta in a large pot of boiling water, according to package directions without using salt, until al dente—tender but firm to the bite. Drain. Top with creole sauce.

VARIATION: Add 1 teaspoon Ancho Chili Puree with the tomatoes.
NOTE: To make *Ancho Chili Puree,* remove the seeds and soak 1 dried ancho chili in water for about 1 hour until it is soft and plump. Use enough water to cover the chili. Drain it and reserve the liquid. Place the chili in a food processor or blender and puree. Add whatever reserved liquid is necessary to give the puree a smooth consistency and to yield 1 tablespoon of puree. It should not require more than a little water.

Serving size = 1 cup sauce + 1 cup pasta
375 calories
1.0 grams total fat
0.2 grams saturated fat
0 milligrams cholesterol

PASTA WITH EGGPLANT–RED PEPPER SAUCE

YIELD: 2 CUPS SAUCE (2 TO 4 SERVINGS)   BY MARK HALL

While eggplant is thought of as an alternate filling for lasagna, it does not usually come to mind when one thinks of pasta "sauces," so this dish is particularly special.

1 large red bell pepper	¾ cup chopped onions
3½ cups cubed Globe eggplant (about ½ pound)	½ teaspoon freshly minced garlic
	1 cup vegetable stock
½ cup dry red wine	5 or 6 basil leaves
⅛ teaspoon freshly ground black pepper	Salt
	2½ ounces pasta per serving

Roast the peppers in the oven on a flat pan until the outer skin is blackened and charred. Rotate frequently. Remove and set in a bowl and cover with a plate. Let them steam for 15 minutes to soften the flesh and make the peels easier to remove. Seed the peppers and then slice into matchsticks or julienne. You will need ½ cup of thinly julienned strips. Set aside.

Puree the eggplant. Put the puree into a pot with ¼ cup of the wine and the black pepper. Cook for 30 minutes, until the puree is completely soft and mushy. Set aside.

Cook the onion and garlic in the remaining red wine. When the onion has softened, add the pureed eggplant, sliced red peppers and vegetable stock. Simmer for about 15 minutes. To chiffonade the basil, roll the leaves tightly and slice the basil into thin ribbons. You will need 1 tablespoon. Add this to the sauce. Add salt and more pepper, if desired, to taste.

Cook the pasta in a large pot of boiling water, according to package directions without using salt, until al dente—tender but firm to the bite. Drain and ladle the sauce over it.

Serving size = ½ cup sauce + 1 cup pasta
273 calories
0.4 grams total fat
trace saturated fat
0 milligrams cholesterol

PASTA WITH RED PEPPER AND LENTIL SAUCE

YIELD: 2 CUPS SAUCE (4 SERVINGS)   BY MARK HALL

Any variety of pasta shapes can be used for this. The sauce is a combination of lentils and pureed red peppers and onions. Most of the texture in this red-pepper-based sauce comes from the lentils. The two make a very unexpected combination.

½ cup dried lentils
4 cups water
2 bay leaves
1½ cups diced onions
2 cloves garlic, minced
1 tablespoon dried basil
¼ cup plus 2 tablespoons
  burgundy or other red wine
2 cups chopped sweet red bell
  peppers

1 teaspoon balsamic vinegar
Salt to taste
Freshly ground black pepper
2½ ounces uncooked pasta per
  person
¼ cup freshly chopped basil for
  garnish

Rinse and sort the lentils. Boil the 4 cups water. Add the lentils and bay leaves and simmer until the lentils are tender but have not lost their shape. Strain and remove the bay leaves.

Combine the onions, garlic, and dried basil, and braise them in the red wine. Seed, core, and chop the red peppers and add them to the onions. Let them stew with the onions until they are soft, about 25 to 30 minutes. Then transfer these vegetables to a blender or food processor and puree until smooth. Stir the lentils into the sauce. (Do not puree the lentils.) Add the vinegar. Add salt and pepper to taste.

Cook the pasta in a large pot of boiling water, according to package directions without using salt, until al dente—tender but firm to the bite. Drain and ladle the sauce over it. Garnish with fresh chopped basil.

Serving size = ½ cup sauce + 1 cup pasta
345 calories
0.9 grams total fat
0.1 grams saturated fat
0 milligrams cholesterol

JAPANESE BUCKWHEAT NOODLES WITH VEGETABLES

YIELD: 6 CUPS SAUCE AND 6 CUPS NOODLES (6 SERVINGS)   BY MARK HALL

This is an Asian dish in which the vegetables are "sautéed," then mixed with some aduki beans and served over the noodles in a gingered sauce. One serving contains 190 milligrams sodium.

½ cup dry aduki beans
3½ cups water
1 cup diced onions
1 teaspoon freshly minced garlic
1 tablespoon freshly minced ginger
1 cup diced carrots
1½ cups thinly sliced purple or Napa cabbage

2 cups sliced-on-the-diagonal bok choy
2 teaspoons arrowroot
1 tablespoon soy sauce
5½ ounces Japanese buckwheat noodles, cooked

Sort and rinse the aduki beans, then soak overnight in water. Drain and cook in 2 cups of water for 45 to 60, minutes until tender. Drain and set aside.

Braise the onions, garlic, and ginger in ½ cup water until the onions are soft. Add the carrots. Continue braising, and after a few minutes, when the carrots are nearly cooked, add the cabbage. When the cabbage begins to soften, add the bok choy. The vegetables should remain a bit crisp. All of the liquid should not be allowed to evaporate as it will form the stock for the sauce. Mix the arrowroot into the soy sauce and add this to the vegetables with 1 cup of water. Stir until the sauce thickens.

Toss the vegetables with the beans and ladle over the noodles.

Serving size = 1 cup sauce and vegetables + 1 cup pasta
296 calories
0.4 grams total fat
trace saturated fat
0 milligrams cholesterol

PASTA WITH TOMATO-LENTIL SAUCE

YIELD: 2¾ CUPS SAUCE (3 TO 5 SERVINGS)   BY MARK HALL

This very hearty sauce works with lasagna as well.

1 cup diced onion
1½ teaspoons freshly minced
  garlic
1½ teaspoons dried basil
1½ teaspoons dried oregano
¼ cup dry red wine
½ cup dry lentils or 1 cup
  cooked

4 bay leaves
1½ cups water
1½ cups tomato puree
Salt
Freshly ground black pepper
2½ ounces dried pasta per
  serving

Braise the onions, garlic, basil, and oregano in red wine. (If you are using cooked lentils, ignore the information regarding lentil preparation and omit the bay leaves.) While the onions are cooking, put the lentils and bay leaves into a separate pot with 1½ cups water and cook for 30 minutes, until done. Do not overcook the lentils because they will need to retain their shape.

After the onions have softened, add the tomato puree. Let cook for approximately 20 minutes, until some of the liquid is reduced and the sauce has thickened.

When the lentils have finished cooking, remove the bay leaves. Drain the lentils and add them to the sauce. Add salt and pepper to taste.

Cook the pasta in a large pot of boiling water, according to package directions without using salt, until al dente—tender but firm to the bite. Drain. Serve the sauce over the pasta.

Serving size = 1 cup pasta + 1 cup sauce
422 calories
0.9 grams total fat
0.1 grams saturated fat
0 milligrams cholesterol

SOUPS

Some of the soups here are hearty meals in themselves, such as the Minestrone Soup (page 483), the Spanish Chick-Pea and Garlic Soup (page 485), and the Lentil-Hominy Soup with Lime and Chili (page 487). Others, such as the Gazpacho (pages 477), make lighter meals or first courses. Accompany them with whole-grain bread and a salad, and you will be very satisfied indeed. Soups are filling, and as you will see here, they need not be thickened with cream or fattened up with cheese or meat stocks. The pureed vegetable soups in this section are sometimes thickened with potato, and the bean soups are partially or thoroughly pureed in a blender to make rich, creamy, elegant potages, full of surprising flavors and textures.

Many of these soups, especially the bean soups, freeze well. You may wish to double quantities for the freezer.

SOUP STOCKS

A good soup stock serves to deepen flavors and provide an aromatic background for a few predominant vegetables. For stocks to work well, they need to be made of enough different ingredients to provide a clear, complex flavor that is greater than any of its parts. No one vegetable or herb should predominate. This kind of stock is very useful to make when you want a soup that is otherwise fairly simple and delicate, such as a soup of leeks and rice, or when you want to have a flavorful base for a sauce or gravy.

Here are two recipes for soup stocks, one based on summer flavors and the other on stronger, heartier winter tastes. These are suggestions. If you don't have an ingredient on hand or one isn't easily available to you, such as leeks or celery root, then omit it and substitute something else, such as an extra onion or some celery seeds. On the other hand, if you have some other aromatic elements, such as the cooking broth from beans or trimmings of other vegetables you're using that you think would be good, include them.

There are a few things to keep in mind when making stocks of any kind. The first is that the stock won't be any better than what goes into it. The ingredients should be as nice as those you would plan to cook in another dish. A stock is not for leftover, tired vegetables, but for fresh, firm produce.

Everything should be well washed and cut in small pieces to help the flavors to come out more quickly and thoroughly. Don't overcook a vegetable stock. Unlike meat stocks, the flavors will have been drawn out of the vegetables after only forty minutes or so. It's best to strain the stock then, and if you want a more concentrated taste, reduce it further by simmering. It's important to strain the stock soon after it has cooked as certain herbs and vegetables will impart a bitter taste if allowed to sit for long periods of time.

Avoid using brassica, or members of the cabbage family such as cabbage, cauliflower, Brussels sprouts, broccoli, turnips, or rutabagas. These vegetables tend to take on a dominating and rank taste if they cook for very long and can spoil a stock.

Get to know your ingredients—herbs, vegetables, legumes, dried mushrooms—and find out how they work. There are many unexpected sources of flavor in the foods we cook with, and by paying attention and experimenting, you can quickly become adept at building a wide range of flavors to work with.

MAKING SOUPS WITHOUT A SEPARATE STOCK

While soup stocks are a great aid in the kitchen for deepening flavors, they require some special thought and a little planning since they rely on a variety of ingredients to make them strong and complex. However, there is another way to look at soup making and stocks which is much more simple, and that is to make a stock, as you're making a soup, that parallels the soup by including the trimmings of the very vegetables in the recipe.

For example, if you are making a leek, potato, and mushroom soup, take the roots and greens of the leeks, the potato peelings and maybe even an extra potato, and the mushroom ends. Cover them with 5 or 6 cups cold water, add a bay leaf, some parsley branches, and a pinch of thyme, bring to a boil, then simmer for 20 minutes or longer, if you have the time. Or with an asparagus-pea soup, use the ends of the asparagus, the pea pods, some parsley, bay leaves, and maybe a few onion slices, and make a quick stock.

You might not want to take the full 30 or 40 minutes to cook the trimmings, but even 15 minutes on the stove, using just 5 or 6 cups of water instead of the 8 or 9 suggested in the soup stock recipes, will draw out some extra flavor. Usually this simple stock can be cooking while the rest of the vegetables are being prepared for the soup, adding virtually nothing to the time you are spending in the kitchen.

When making this kind of simple stock, there are many possibilities for ingredients that might be overlooked since they are somewhat unusual. For example, the seeds and stringy material that gets scraped out of a winter squash as well as the hard skins have plenty of flavor. So do corn cobs, when the corn has been scraped off. Also try pea pods, the gnarled skins of celery roots, the scarred outer leaves of fennel bulbs as well as the stalks, the roots of leeks, the hard ends of asparagus stalks, the leafless stems of plucked parsley branches, the stems of chard and spinach, and so forth. The outer leaves of lettuce which you might not want to include in a salad also have a surprising amount of taste, as do the leaves and stems of many herbs. Try everything. If you're not sure about how something will work, try cooking it alone and see what kind of a flavor it produces. You will find there are numerous resources for flavor that you may not have imagined!

SUMMER VEGETABLE SOUP STOCK

YIELD: 6 CUPS   BY DEBORAH MADISON

This stock is made with summer vegetables and is intended to have the light flavors most appropriate for the soups one makes from late spring into early autumn. Be sure to include trimmings of any other vegetables and herbs you are using at the time, unless they are strongly flavored members of the cabbage family, like broccoli, cauliflower, or Brussels sprouts.

1 medium-sized potato
2 medium-sized carrots
1 cup chopped leek trimmings, the roots and the firm, inner green leaves
1 onion
2 celery stalks plus a handful of celery leaves
3 ripe tomatoes
3 medium-sized summer squash (zucchini or yellow squash)
3 ounces green beans
Approximately 1 cup diced eggplant

6 leaves of chard or spinach
8 whole stalks of parsley
1 teaspoon dried basil or several large fresh basil leaves
1 teaspoon dried marjoram or several branches fresh marjoram
2 bay leaves
Pinch thyme
1 teaspoon nutritional yeast
9 cups water

Wash all the ingredients well. Peel the potato and the carrots if the skin doesn't look fresh. Chop everything in pieces about ½-inch square and put them in a pot with 9 cups cold water. Bring to a boil, then lower the heat and simmer for 30 minutes. Strain and reserve the liquid.

1 cup = 23 calories
0.2 grams total fat
trace saturated fat
0 milligrams cholesterol

WINTER VEGETABLE STOCK

YIELD: 6 CUPS   BY DEBORAH MADISON

This stock has stronger, deeper flavors that go better with hearty cold-weather soups. As with the Summer Vegetable Soup Stock (page 472), be sure to include the trimmings of other vegetables you may be using at the time, such as parsnips or fennel, perhaps substituting them for some of the hard-to-find ingredients, like celery root. This stock can also be reduced and used as the liquid base for gravies in vegetable stews.

1 cup chopped leek trimmings, the roots and the firm, inner green leaves	*¹/₄ cup lentils*
	Several chard stems
	Several chard leaves (or lettuce)
1 onion	*10 whole stalks parsley*
2 medium carrots	*5 cloves garlic*
3 celery stalks plus a handful of celery leaves	*¹/₂ teaspoon dried thyme*
1 cup cubed winter squash, or the squash seeds and skins	*¹/₂ teaspoon dried sage, or 4 to 5 sage leaves*
2 medium-sized potatoes	*2 bay leaves*
¹/₂ small celery root or the parings of 1 whole root	*1 to 2 teaspoons nutritional yeast*

Wash all the ingredients and peel the carrots and the potato, unless the skin looks fairly fresh and is without blemishes. Chop everything into pieces no larger than ½-inch square. Put them in a pot with 9 cups cold water, bring gradually to a boil, then simmer for 40 minutes and strain, reserving the liquid.

If you wish to intensify the flavor of the stock, continue to simmer after it has been strained until it has reduced as much as you want.

---

1 cup = 30 calories
0.2 grams total fat
trace saturated fat
0 milligrams cholesterol

NOTES ON DRIED MUSHROOMS FOR SOUPS

Cepes or porcini (species *Boletus eduli*) are extremely flavorful and not particularly difficult to find. Their presence, in a broth or stock, can lend considerable depth and character to a soup, a stew, or a sauce, so it is worth the effort to find them. Check in Italian markets, big delicatessens, specialty foodshops and some supermarkets.

There are generally two grades you can buy. The finest grade, which is naturally the most expensive, consists of mushrooms imported from Italy or France. Not only can these mushrooms be used in stocks, but once soaked, they can be cooked and eaten as well, and should be! The other grade consists of mushrooms from South America. They are also very flavorful, but they have been treated in such a way that their texture is not particularly pleasant to eat. Accordingly, they are much less expensive. They contribute so much to the flavor of broths and stocks, the fact that they have to be discarded after cooking is not that important. But be sure you know what you're getting. If the mushrooms are sold in bulk, ask where they are from and if they can be eaten or only boiled. Usually, the more expensive French and Italian mushrooms will be in small glass jars, behind the counter, not out in huge boxes where you can go through them.

Other dried mushrooms that have good flavor are shiitake, easy to find in the Oriental sections of supermarkets or in any Japanese or Chinese market. As with cepes, there are different grades. In Chinese stores those referred to as "fragrant mushrooms" have caps that are thin, flat, and smooth. They are used for their flavor and fragrance and are less expensive than the varieties with thick, succulent caps, which beg to be eaten. This more expensive variety is referred to as "flower mushrooms."

Morels, imported from France, are perhaps the best mushrooms, but very, very expensive. They should be used with special consideration.

All in all, it is the cepes imported from South America that are the most useful and economical for everyday use.

MUSHROOM BROTH

YIELD: 6 CUPS (6 SERVINGS)   BY DEBORAH MADISON

Dried, wild mushrooms, such as morels or cepes, make this thin broth very flavorful. If you have fresh wild mushrooms, use them to whatever degree you can afford, as well. This consomme would make a good opening to a meal of many courses. It can also be used as a stock for cooking rice, barley, and other grains. Serve it clear and unadorned, or garnish with cooked rice, pasta shapes, fresh herbs, or thinly sliced mushrooms.

1 ounce dried mushrooms, such as morels or cepes	*1 yellow onion, cut in ¼-inch dice*
2 small bay leaves	*1 large leek, white part and roots, washed and sliced*
Pinch thyme	
5 full branches parsley	*6 cloves garlic, roughly chopped*

2 pounds fresh mushrooms, finely
    chopped by hand or in a food
    processor
2 quarts water

Lemon juice, to taste
¼ cup Madeira, or to taste
Freshly ground black pepper

Combine all the ingredients except the lemon juice and Madeira in a large saucepan and cover with 2 quarts cold water. Gradually bring to a boil, then lower the heat, cover the pan, and simmer slowly for 1½ hours. Strain the broth, pressing all the vegetables to extract as much liquid as possible, then to clarify it, pour it carefully through a large coffee filter or a double layer of cheesecloth. Store in the refrigerator until ready to use.

To serve, slowly reheat the soup without bringing it to a full boil. Stir in the lemon juice, to taste, and the Madeira. Serve plain, in heated bowls, or with any of the garnishes plus a grating of pepper.

Serving size = 1 cup
20 calories
0.1 grams total fat
trace saturated fat
0 milligrams cholesterol

VEGETABLE STOCK

YIELD: 2½ QUARTS   BY WOLFGANG PUCK

This savory stock comes alive with the flavor of garlic and ginger.

1 pound (1 large) onion, cut into
    large chunks
¾ pound (2 large) carrots, cut
    into chunks
½ pound (3 or 4) celery stalks,
    cut into chunks
2 ounces (about 1 whole head)
    garlic, separated into cloves

1 ounce fresh ginger, sliced
1 tablespoon chopped fresh thyme
1½ teaspoons peppercorns
1 bay leaf
3 quarts cold water

In a large saucepan, combine all the ingredients and bring to a boil. Lower heat and simmer for about 3 hours. Strain into a clean bowl and use as needed.

1 cup = 22 calories
0.1 grams total fat
trace saturated fat
0 milligrams cholesterol

LIGHT TOMATO SOUP

YIELD: 3 CUPS (3 SERVINGS)   BY MOLLIE KATZEN

This tomato soup is mostly tomatoes. It also features several of the tomato's best friends and closest associates: garlic, basil, parsley, and dill. A touch of sugar cuts the acidity, so there is no need for any oil or dairy products. This soup can be made several days in advance and reheats nicely.

3 pounds fresh and perfectly ripe tomatoes, cut into chunks
4 cloves garlic, chopped
6 to 8 fresh basil leaves or 2 teaspoons dry

2 tablespoons brown sugar
1 teaspoon salt
Freshly ground black pepper
Freshly minced parsley and/or dill for garnish (optional)

Place tomatoes, garlic, and basil in a kettle, large saucepan, or Dutch oven. Cover and cook over medium heat for 10 to 15 minutes, or until tomatoes are quite liquefied.

Remove from heat, and cool to the point at which you feel confident about pureeing it. (Dodging hot splatters is not a lot of fun.) Fish out the basil, and puree the tomatoes and garlic in a food processor or blender until quite smooth.

Strain through a medium-fine strainer back into the kettle, and season with brown sugar, salt, and freshly ground black pepper to taste.

Heat just before serving. If desired, sprinkle each bowlful with a light touch of parsley and/or dill.

Serving size = 1 cup
131 calories
1.0 grams total fat
0.3 grams saturated fat
0 milligrams cholesterol
756 milligrams sodium

GAZPACHO

YIELD: 6 CUPS (6 SERVINGS)   BY MARK HALL

There is no cooking involved and this soup can be served chilled or at room temperature.

1 cup finely diced red onion
1 1/2 cups seeded and finely diced
   cucumber
3/4 cup seeded and finely diced
   red bell pepper
1/2 cup seeded and finely diced
   green bell pepper
1 28-ounce can tomato puree
1 teaspoon freshly minced garlic

1/4 cup rice wine vinegar
1/8 teaspoon cayenne
1/2 teaspoon freshly ground black
   pepper
1/4 cup dry red wine
2 teaspoons fresh lime juice
1/4 cup water
1/4 cup freshly chopped cilantro
Salt

Add the diced vegetables to the tomato puree. Stir in the garlic, rice wine vinegar, cayenne, black pepper, red wine, lime juice, water, and cilantro. Add salt to taste, then serve.

Serving size = 1 cup
82 calories
0.5 grams total fat
trace saturated fat
0 milligrams cholesterol

CARROT SOUP WITH GINGER, ORANGE, AND CILANTRO

YIELD: 4 CUPS (4 SERVINGS)   BY MARK HALL

Even though the soup can be served warm or hot, the ginger gives this a very cooling effect.

1 1/2 cups roughly chopped onion
1/4 cup water
3 cups peeled and diced carrots
1 tablespoon freshly minced
   ginger

1 1/2 cups vegetable stock or water
1/2 cup orange juice
Chopped cilantro for garnish
Salt
Freshly ground black pepper

Cook the onions in 1/4 cup of water, adding the carrots when the onions are translucent. Add the ginger and stock or water (just enough to cover the carrots), and cook until tender. When the carrots are done, puree the entire mixture and add the orange juice. Add more stock or water until you achieve a desired consistency. Garnish with cilantro and add salt and pepper to taste.

Serving size = 1 cup
81 calories
0.4 grams total fat
trace saturated fat
0 milligrams cholesterol

SPICY CARROT AND TOMATO SOUP

YIELD: 8 CUPS (8 SERVINGS)   BY JUDY TALBOTT

The savory flavor of this very pretty soup actually improves with age.

1 large onion, chopped
2 cups water
5 cups carrot rounds, ¼-inch thick, about 2 pounds
6 cups peeled and chopped ripe tomatoes
¼ teaspoon Tabasco sauce or to taste

¼ cup freshly chopped dill or 2 teaspoons dried
2 teaspoons dried tarragon
Salt
Freshly ground black pepper
1 cup nonfat yogurt for garnish

Braise the onions in a large soup pot with ¼ to ½ cup of water. When the onions become translucent, add the carrots and remaining water. Simmer for 30 minutes. Add the tomatoes and continue cooking for another 30 to 45 minutes, until the tomatoes have broken down completely and you are satisfied with the taste and texture. Remove from the heat and puree in food processor or blender. Return the soup to the pot and add the Tabasco sauce, dill, and tarragon. Add the salt and pepper to taste, with more Tabasco, if desired. Serve hot or cold with a large dollop of yogurt.

Serving size = 1 cup
82 calories
0.6 grams total fat
0.1 grams saturated fat
trace cholesterol

TOMATILLO SOUP WITH CORN AND CILANTRO

YIELD: 4 CUPS (4 SERVINGS)   BY MARK HALL

Both salsa verde and enchiladas suizas in your local Mexican restaurants rely heavily on the tomatillo for their distinctive color and taste. If you have had either of these, then this soup should rekindle fond memories of mariachis and sombreros.

1 1/4 pounds whole tomatillos (approx. 1 cup puree)
2 large ears fresh corn
1 1/2 cups chopped red onions
1/4 cup + 2 teaspoons dry white wine
1 1/2 teaspoons freshly minced garlic
1 cup finely diced red bell pepper

1 cup vegetable stock
1/8 teaspoon cayenne pepper
1/2 teaspoon freshly ground black pepper
2 tablespoons chopped cilantro
Salt
Cilantro, green onions, and tortilla chips for garnish

Husk and then rinse the tomatillos. Blanch them in boiling water until the color changes to olive green. Drain, then puree in a blender or food processor. Set aside.

Shave the kernels off the ears. Take the back of the knife and rub it against the ear to remove any of the leftover corn and juice. There should be 2 cups.

Braise the onions in the white wine with the minced garlic. When the onions are translucent, add the corn and red pepper and cook until tender. Add the vegetable stock, pureed tomatillos, cayenne, and black pepper. Simmer for about 15 minutes to allow the flavors to blend. Add the cilantro, salt to taste, garnish, and serve.

Serving size = 1 cup
145 calories
1.5 grams total fat
0.2 grams saturated fat
0 milligrams cholesterol

HOT CABBAGE BORSCHT

YIELD: 4 CUPS (4 TO 5 SERVINGS)   BY MARY CARROLL

This soup will always be thought of as classically Russian. There are many variations on this theme, and also part of this soup's wide tradition is to throw in some cooked white kidney beans.

2 tablespoons sherry
2½ cups vegetable stock
1 cup diced onions
½ cup peeled and finely diced beets
½ cup finely diced carrots
1½ cups thinly sliced purple cabbage
½ cup cubed potatoes
¼ cup diced celery
½ teaspoon crushed caraway seed
¼ teaspoon freshly ground black pepper
⅛ teaspoon dill weed
2 tablespoons apple cider vinegar
2 tablespoons apple juice concentrate
1½ teaspoons minced raisins
½ cup tomato puree
Salt
Nonfat yogurt for garnish

Place the sherry and ¼ cup vegetable stock in a soup pot with the onions and simmer for 10 minutes. Add the beets, carrots, cabbage, potatoes, celery and 1 cup vegetable stock and then cook for 10 minutes over medium heat. Stir frequently. Add the remaining stock, the spices, vinegar, juice concentrate, raisins, and tomato puree. Bring this to a boil, then lower the heat and simmer for 40 minutes. Serve warm with yogurt as a garnish.

Serving size (without the yogurt) = 1 cup
102 calories
0.3 grams total fat
trace saturated fat
0 milligrams cholesterol

POTATO SOUP

YIELD: 5 CUPS (5 TO 6 SERVINGS)   BY MARK HALL

This is a very tasty and attractive soup. The diced vegetables actually look like confetti sprinkled onto the soup.

1¼ pounds potatoes, peeled and quartered
1½ cups diced onions
1 tablespoon freshly minced garlic

1 tablespoon freshly minced basil
1/2 cup dry white wine
1/2 cup finely diced carrot
1/2 cup finely diced red pepper
1/2 cup finely diced zucchini

3 1/2 cups vegetable stock
1/8 teaspoon salt
1/8 teaspoon freshly ground black
   pepper

In a large pot, boil the potatoes. In another pot, braise the onions, garlic, and basil in the white wine. Add the carrots. When they are partially cooked, add the red pepper. Add the zucchini when the peppers have softened.

Drain the potatoes and reserve the liquid to add to the soup later if necessary. Puree the potatoes with a food mill, processor, or blender and add to the other vegetables. Stir. Add all of the vegetable stock to thin the soup. If it is still too thick, gradually add some of the potato liquid to a desired consistency. Do not let the soup become too thin or it will lose most of its flavor. Add salt and pepper.

Serving size = 1 cup
160 calories
0.4 grams total fat
trace saturated fat
0 milligrams cholesterol

GARLIC-HERB SOUP

YIELD: 6 CUPS (6 SERVINGS)   BY DEBORAH MADISON

This soup is easy to make, requiring only that you simmer in water plenty of garlic with herbs—namely, sage and parsley. The flavor of the garlic softens considerably as it cooks. As we are not including the traditional salt and olive oil, it is important that you use good quality herbs, preferably fresh ones. This broth can be drunk by itself as a pick-me-up or used as a thin soup garnished with large or small pasta shapes, diced potatoes, cooked chick-peas or white beans, rounds of scallions or leeks, and so forth. It also makes an excellent soup stock or cooking liquid for the same kinds of ingredients, imparting its flavors to the otherwise bland starches.

If you are planning to add the same items to the broth, however, be sure to cook them separately so that they don't absorb all the liquid.

1 large or 2 small heads of garlic,
   broken apart and peeled

10 full branches of parsley
2 bay leaves

12 large, fresh sage leaves or 1
    teaspoon dried
5 cloves
4 thyme branches or a generous
    pinch of dried

8 cups water
A generous pinch saffron threads
Freshly ground black pepper
Finely chopped parsley or chervil
    for garnish

When peeling the garlic, look to see that the cloves are fresh, firm and ivory colored. When garlic is discolored with brown spots, it does not taste good. (It's best to discard any garlic heads that are partially spoiled, as the spoiled flavor of one clove generally permeates the entire head.)

Put the first six ingredients into a pot with the water, bring gradually to a boil, then simmer 30 minutes. Strain well and return the broth to the pot. Add the saffron threads and let them sit in the hot broth for at least 5 minutes before serving. Serve with pepper and parsley or chervil sprinkled on top.

VARIATIONS: If using pastina (tiny pasta shaped like stars or *o*'s) cook ¼ to ½ cup directly in the saffron-flavored broth until they are done, a few minutes at most. If using rounds of leeks, simmer them directly in the broth when you add the saffron. Scallions, thinly sliced, can be added uncooked. Rice, potatoes, large pasta shapes, and beans, as mentioned, should be cooked before being warmed in the broth.

Serving size = 1 cup
19 calories
0.1 grams total fat
trace saturated fat
0 milligrams cholesterol

BLACK BEAN SOUP

YIELD: 3 CUPS (3 SERVINGS)   BY MARY CARROLL

Although this isn't a traditional black bean soup for Brazilian feijoadas, you couldn't tell by the rich flavor of this soup. Starting out with cooked black beans make this a surprisingly easy and fast soup to make.

¾ cup chopped onion
3½ cups vegetable stock
3 cloves freshly minced garlic
1 large carrot, chopped
1 stalk celery, chopped
1 teaspoon ground coriander
1 teaspoon ground cumin

2 cups cooked black beans
½ cup freshly squeezed orange
    juice
¼ cup dry sherry
¼ teaspoon freshly ground black
    pepper
¼ teaspoon cayenne

½ teaspoon lemon juice
½ cup apple juice

*Freshly chopped cilantro for
garnish*

Place the onion and ½ cup of vegetable stock in a heavy soup pot and bring to a boil. Lower the heat and simmer, stirring, until the onion becomes soft and transparent. Then stir in garlic, carrot, and celery. Cook 5 minutes over medium heat, stirring occasionally. Add coriander and cumin and cook an additional 5 minutes. If the mixture dries out, add more vegetable stock as needed. Add the black beans, remaining stock, orange juice, and sherry and let cook 20 minutes over medium heat, covered, stirring occasionally. Add the peppers, lemon juice, and apple juice before serving. Taste and adjust seasonings. Put a half of the soup in a blender to make a thick puree. Add back to soup. Garnish with cilantro.

Serving size = 1 cup
312 calories
1.3 grams total fat
0.1 grams saturated fat
0 milligrams cholesterol

MINESTRONE SOUP

YIELD: 6 CUPS (6 SERVINGS)   BY RIYA RYAN

Use any variety or combination of beans that you want for this soup. You could also substitute some corn, rice or another grain for the macaroni.

1 cup chopped onions
3 tablespoons freshly minced
  garlic
1 cup minced carrots
¼ cup freshly minced parsley
1 teaspoon dried oregano
1 teaspoon dried basil
½ teaspoon dried thyme
¼ cup dry red wine
½ cup chopped celery
1 cup sliced cabbage
¼ cup chopped green bell pepper
1–2 cups vegetable stock or water

1 cup cooked Great Northern
  beans
1½ cups chopped tomatoes
¼ teaspoon ground cloves
¼ cup salt-free tomato paste
1 cup apple juice
2 cups unsalted vegetable juice
  cocktail
1 cup sliced zucchini
¼ cup egg-free, oil-free macaroni
Salt
Freshly ground black pepper

Braise the onions, garlic, carrots, and herbs in the wine until the onions are soft. Add the celery, cabbage, bell pepper, and 1 cup of the stock or water and simmer for 5 minutes, stirring occasionally. Add the beans, tomatoes, cloves, tomato paste, apple juice, and vegetable juice and bring to a boil. Lower the heat and simmer for 15 minutes, then add the zucchini and simmer for another 2 minutes. Add the macaroni and cook 8 minutes more. Add salt and pepper to taste.

Serving size = 1 cup
154 calories
0.6 grams total fat
0.1 grams saturated fat
0 milligrams cholesterol

TOMATO AND LENTIL SOUP

YIELD: 4 CUPS (4 SERVINGS)   BY MARK HALL

All that is needed to turn this richly satisfying soup into a meal is some french bread and a salad.

½ cup dried lentils	*1 cup diced carrots*
1 bay leaf	*1 cup diced red bell peppers*
5 cups water	*1 tablespoon dried basil*
1⅔ cups diced onions	*1 tablespoon dried oregano*
1½ teaspoons freshly minced garlic	*1½ cups tomato puree*
	2 cups vegetable stock
¼ cup dry red wine	*Salt*
1 cup diced celery	*Freshly ground black pepper*

In a separate pot, cook the lentils for about 35 to 45 minutes with the bay leaf in the water until the lentils are tender. Remove the bay leaf from the lentils, drain the liquid, and reserve at least ¾ cup of the cooking liquid for the soup.

Braise the onions and garlic in the red wine. Add the celery, carrots, bell peppers, basil, and oregano, being careful to cook only until the carrots are tender. Add the lentils and tomato puree to the vegetable mixture, and gradually increase the volume with ¾ cup of the reserved cooking liquid and 2 cups of vegetable stock until the soup reaches the desired consistency. Let the soup simmer for 15 minutes. Add salt and pepper to taste.

Serving size = 1 cup
198 calories
1.1 grams total fat
trace saturated fat
0 milligrams cholesterol

SPANISH CHICK-PEA AND GARLIC SOUP

YIELD: 6 CUPS (6 SERVINGS)   BY MARK HALL

This heavenly soup is a garlic lover's delight.

1 ½ cups dry chick-peas
  (garbanzos)
6 cups water
6 bay leaves
1 cup chopped onions
1 cup finely diced celery
½ cup dry white wine
⅛ teaspoon crushed saffron
  (about 10 threads)

1 cup tomato puree
4 heads garlic
1 cup vegetable stock
Salt
Freshly ground black pepper
2 tablespoons freshly chopped
  basil

Sort and rinse the chick-peas, then soak overnight in water. Cook them in 6 cups of water in a separate pot with the bay leaves for 1 ½ hours, or until soft.

While the chick-peas are cooking, braise the onions and celery in wine until the onion is softened. Mix the saffron into the onion and celery. Add the tomato puree and let simmer for about 30 minutes.

Prepare each head of garlic by cutting the root end off. Place the flat end of each head in a baking pan with the vegetable stock. Cover the pan with foil and bake at 375°F. for about 40 minutes, until the garlic is soft and can easily be removed from its skins. Some cloves will be mushy but most will still be intact. There should be about 1 cup. Mash the cloves that haven't fallen apart.

When the chick-peas are done, drain them and reserve the bean stock. Add the chick-peas to the onion, celery, saffron, and tomato mixture. Then add the garlic and any residual vegetable stock from its baking pan. Simmer this mixture for about 15 to 20 minutes. If a thinner consistency is desired, add some of the reserved bean stock. Add salt and pepper to taste. Garnish with basil.

Serving size = 1 cup
255 calories
2.9 grams total fat
0.3 grams saturated fat
0 milligrams cholesterol

WHITE BEAN AND TOMATO SOUP WITH FRESH HERBS

YIELD: 9 CUPS (9 SERVINGS)   BY DEBORAH MADISON

*This bean soup is appropriate for warmer weather as it's made with fresh
tomatoes and herbs. Since beans yield a flavorful broth on their own, you can
make this without a stock, but for a soup with more depth, use the Summer
Vegetable Stock (page 472). Although the freshness of the tomato and herbs
is part of the charm of this soup, it also tastes good when leftover and reheated
the next day. The flavors will be less sparkly but more blended. If you find
you have more soup than you want, strain it, puree the beans, and reseason
with fresh garlic and lemon to make a spread for bread or crackers.*

The Stock:
Use the broth from the beans alone or in combination with the Summer
Vegetable Stock.

The Soup:

*1 cup dry white beans, such as
   baby limas or navy beans*
*11 cups water or a mixture of
   water and Summer Vegetable
   Stock*
1 large onion, finely diced
2 carrots, finely diced
10 sage leaves
3 bay leaves
5 parsley branches, chopped
*4 cloves garlic, thinly sliced or
   minced*
*2 pinches dried thyme, or several
   thyme branches*

*3 or 4 medium-sized ripe
   tomatoes*

The Garnish:

1/2 cup packed parsley leaves
*1/2 cup mixed fresh herbs,
   marjoram, thyme, lovage, basil,
   and/or chives*
2 cloves garlic
*Peel of 1 lemon, plus juice to
   taste*
Freshly ground black pepper

Sort and rinse the beans, then soak for 6 hours or overnight in water.

The next day, pour off the soaking water and cover the beans with 11 cups
fresh water or stock. Bring to a boil and skim off the foam that rises to the
surface, then lower the heat to a simmer. Add the onion, carrots, sage, bay
leaves, parsley, garlic, and thyme. Simmer until the beans are tender, an
hour or longer depending on the type of bean. The beans can be cooked a
day or two in advance of serving, if desired.

Just before serving, prepare the tomatoes and the garnish. Bring a small pot
of water to a boil and drop in each of the tomatoes for 20 seconds or so,
to loosen the skins. Remove the skins, halve the tomatoes crosswise and

gently squeeze out the juice and the seeds. Strain the juice and return it to the soup. Dice the tomatoes and stir them into the soup.

To make the garnish, strip all the leaves from the stems of the herbs. If you only have parsley, then use a cup rather than ½ cup. Finely chop the herbs along with the garlic and the lemon peel or chop everything separately, then pound together in a mortar with enough lemon juice to make a paste. Either way, stir the mixture into the soup as you serve it. Season to taste with lemon juice and plenty of pepper.

Serving size = 1 cup
101 calories
0.4 grams total fat
0.1 grams saturated fat
0 milligrams cholesterol

LENTIL-HOMINY SOUP WITH LIME AND CHILI

YIELD: 9 CUPS (9 SERVINGS)   BY DEBORAH MADISON

Hominy is unusual and delicious in this soup. If you live in a part of the country where it's possible to buy fresh, chopped cactus (nopales), use it in place of the green peppers. Cook the diced cactus in water until barely tender, then drain and add it to the soup toward the end.

1 cup lentils
6 cups water
2 bay leaves
2 large cloves garlic, peeled
1 tablespoon freshly chopped
  cilantro
1 teaspoon cumin seeds
1 teaspoon dried Mexican or
  Greek oregano
1 teaspoon New Mexico chili
  powder or paprika
1 yellow onion, finely chopped
1 medium carrot, finely diced

1 celery stalk, finely diced
1 large green bell pepper, or ¼
  pound fresh nopales, diced in
  ¼-inch squares
2 tomatoes, peeled and chopped
1 clove garlic, minced
1 15-ounce can hominy, drained
Pureed chipotle chilies, to taste
  (approximately 1 teaspoon) or 2
  jalapeño chilies, seeds and veins
  removed, chilies minced
Juice of 1 or 2 limes
Fresh cilantro for garnish

Rinse the lentils and put them in a pot with 6 cups water, the bay leaves, whole garlic cloves, and cilantro. Bring to a boil, then lower the heat and simmer 15 minutes, or until the lentils are just barely cooked. Set aside, but don't drain.

In a small skillet, roast the cumin seeds over medium heat, constantly shaking the pan back and forth. After a minute, add the oregano. Remove the pan from the heat but continue shaking. As soon as you can smell the oregano, add the paprika. Shake the pan another few seconds, then turn the spices out onto a plate. Grind in a mortar or electric spice mill and set aside.

Sauté the onion in water, starting with ¼ cup and adding more as needed to keep it from sticking to the pan. Once the onion starts to color some, add the garlic, carrot, celery, green pepper, tomatoes, and the toasted, ground spices. Stir to combine and simmer for 5 minutes. Add the cooked lentils, minced garlic, and hominy. Add the chipotle chilies or jalapeños. Additional water may be needed to bring the soup to a desired consistency. Cover and cook slowly until the lentils are completely done, another 20 minutes or so. If you are using the nopales, add them during the last 5 minutes of cooking.

Season the finished soup with lime juice and serve garnished with cilantro leaves.

Serving size = 1 cup
121 calories
0.3 grams total fat
trace saturated fat
0 milligrams cholesterol

GREEN SPLIT PEA SOUP WITH CARROTS AND CELERY

YIELD: 4½ CUPS (4 TO 5 SERVINGS)   BY MARK HALL

1 cup dry green split peas
5 cups water
4 bay leaves
1 cup diced onions
½ cup white wine
2 teaspoons freshly minced garlic
1 tablespoon dried thyme
½ teaspoon dried rosemary, slightly crushed
¼ teaspoon freshly ground black pepper

1 cup diced carrots
1 cup diced celery
1 cup diced red bell peppers
½ cup vegetable stock
1 tablespoon freshly chopped basil
1 tablespoon freshly chopped Italian parsley
Salt

Cook the split peas in the of water with the bay leaves until most of the water has been absorbed. This will take about 45 minutes.

While the split peas are cooking, braise the onions in a separate pot in the white wine. Add the garlic, thyme, rosemary and black pepper to the pot with the onions. When the onions become translucent, add the carrots and celery. Continue to cook until the vegetables are done but retain some firmness. Add the red pepper and cook for 2 to 3 minutes. Turn off the heat and set the pot aside until the peas are cooked.

When the peas are done, remove the bay leaves and run the peas through a blender or food processor. Combine this with the vegetables and stir. Gradually add the vegetable stock until you are satisfied with the texture. Add the fresh basil and parsley. Salt to taste.

Serving size = 1 cup
213 calories
0.9 grams total fat
0.2 grams saturated fat
0 milligrams cholesterol

HEARTY VEGETABLE DISHES

Most of these dishes are combinations of vegetables that are slowly cooked, either in the oven or on top of the stove, into savory, comforting stews. They can be served over grains or in wide soup bowls by themselves, in their own fragrant juices. Root vegetables—potatoes, turnips, rutabagas, carrots, parsnips—lend themselves well to this kind of dish, and you will find some delicious winter vegetable stews here. Mushrooms, both fresh and dried, often provide the base for sauces. The Red Pepper Coulis as a sauce for the Vegetable Cakes (below) will prove a delightful surprise. Serve these as an appetizer or in larger portions as an entree.

You will also find lots of southwestern flavors here, in the pungent Southwestern Vegetable Stew (page 500), the Tomato and Okra Stew (page 497) and the Enchiladas with Tomatillo Sauce (page 498). The spicy flavors of India are in the Indian Vegetable Stew (page 495), which you may accompany with a chutney on page 490, for a perfect combination of sweet and pungent tastes.

For lighter, more summery meals, try the Mushroom and Artichoke Frittata (page 502) or the Zucchini "Pasta" with Yogurt Sauce (page 504). If you haven't been convinced yet, these recipes should prove once and for all what a satisfying basis for a meal vegetables can be, and what beautiful dishes they make.

VEGETABLE CAKES WITH RED PEPPER COULIS

YIELD: 12 CAKES (6 SERVINGS)   BY WOLFGANG PUCK

*1 pound (2 medium) baking
   potatoes
1 cup diced celery
1 cup diced carrots
1 cup diced onion
1 medium peeled, seeded and
   diced tomato
Vegetable stock, if necessary
   (page 475)*

*1 cup fresh peas
3 tablespoons chopped fresh basil
1 teaspoon ground cumin
1/2 teaspoon turmeric
Pinch of red pepper flakes
3 large egg whites
3 tablespoons nonfat milk
About 1 cup dried bread crumbs
Red Pepper Coulis (page 400)*

Bake the potatoes until tender.

In a large nonstick skillet, slowly sauté the celery, carrots, onion and tomato until the vegetables are tender, 10 to 15 minutes. If the tomatoes are not juicy, add a little vegetable stock. Transfer to a large mixing bowl and add the peas, basil, cumin, turmeric and red pepper flakes. Set aside to cool.

Scrape the potato from the shell into a mixing bowl and mash.

In a small bowl whisk together the egg whites and the milk. Stir into the mashed potatoes until smooth. Add to the vegetables and combine thoroughly. Form into 12 patties, about 2 ounces each.

Pour the dried bread crumbs onto a large plate and lightly coat both sides of each patty. For firmer patties stir the crumbs into the potato-milk mix until distributed evenly.

Spray 1 or 2 large skillets with a vegetable oil spray and sauté the patties until browned, about 5 minutes per side.

Presentation: Nap each of 6 plates with the red pepper coulis and set 2 vegetable cakes on the sauce. Serve immediately.

Serving size = 2 vegetable cakes with ¼ cup Red Pepper Coulis
145 calories
1.3 grams total fat
0.1 gram saturated fat
0 milligrams cholesterol

WINTER VEGETABLE STEW

YIELD: 8 CUPS (8 SERVINGS)   BY DEBORAH MADISON

In this recipe you begin by making a flavorful stock from dried wild mushrooms. Or use the Mushroom Broth (page 474), with or without the Madeira. Cook this in a clay pot or a Crockpot. (If using a clay pot, soak both halves in cold water for at least 15 minutes before using.) Both will leave you free for at least a couple of hours while dinner cooks.

The vegetables listed are merely suggestions. You may want to include celery root, onions, fresh mushrooms, Brussels sprouts, etc., which will cook in roughly the same amount of time. If you add fresh mushrooms, broccoli or cauliflower, do so during the last 40 minutes. You may find the cooking times vary from the directions, but that is to be expected: different sizes, tough, or tender produce will make a difference. It's up to you, the cook, to check now and then and see how things are going, then adjust accordingly.

The sauce will be flavorful but thin. However, it can be thickened just before serving, if you wish. Instructions for thickening and flavoring are included.

THE MUSHROOM STOCK

1 yellow onion, roughly diced
6 juniper berries
4 fresh sage leaves or 1/2 teaspoon
    dried
2 bay leaves
2 pinches dried thyme
4 branches parsley
2-inch piece fresh rosemary, or 1/2
    teaspoon dried

1/2 cup dry red wine
1/2 to 1 ounce dried cepes
    (porcini)
1 cup finely chopped fresh
    mushrooms
3 cups water
Juice from tomatoes (from the
    vegetables)

Heat a few spoonfuls of water in a wide saucepan, add the onion, and cook over medium-high heat, stirring continually for about 7 minutes and adding more water as needed, until the onions are browned. They can get as dark as you have time for (and without their burning) as this caramelizing helps enrich the flavor.

When done, add the herbs and the wine, bring the mixture to a boil, and let it reduce for several minutes.

Rinse the dried mushrooms briefly in cold water to get rid of any sand, then add them to the pot along with the fresh mushrooms, water, and juice from the tomatoes. Cook at a slow boil while you are preparing the vegetables or until the liquid has reduced to about 2 to 2 1/2 cups. Strain the stock and set aside. Reserve the mushrooms if they are of good quality to use in this dish.

THE VEGETABLES

4 parsnips (8 ounces), cut in
    2-inch lengths
5 carrots (14 ounces), cut in
    2-inch lengths
8 ounces small white potatoes,
    halved lengthwise
5 stalks celery (5 ounces), cut in
    2-inch lengths
2 or 3 leeks, white part only (5 to
    6 ounces), halved lengthwise
    and cut in 1-inch pieces
2 medium rutabagas (6 to 8

ounces), peeled and cut in
    1/2-inch wedges
1 medium turnip (3 to 4 ounces),
    peeled and cut in 1/2-inch
    wedges
4 cloves garlic, left whole and
    unpeeled
1 15-ounce can whole tomatoes,
    quartered, juice reserved for
    Mushroom Stock (see above)
2 pinches dried thyme
1/2 teaspoon dried sage leaves

2 small bay leaves
Dash of red wine or sherry
* vinegar to taste*

Dijon mustard to taste (optional)
Freshly chopped parsley
Freshly ground black pepper

Prepare all the vegetables as described. Peel the parsnips and the carrots, but leave the skins on the potatoes if they look clean and fresh. Cut the parsnips in half lengthwise and remove the woody cores. Halve or quarter the thicker pieces of carrot so that they are roughly the same size as the thin ends.

Put all the vegetables into a Crockpot or bottom half of a clay pot along with the herbs, and add the Mushroom Stock. If you have used French or Italian mushrooms for the stock, add them as well. If using a Crockpot, cover and cook on low for about 3 hours. If using a clay pot, cover, put into a 350°F. oven, and cook for about an hour, check, and continue cooking, if necessary.

When the vegetables are cooked, thicken the sauce, as described below, if you want more of a gravy. Otherwise, taste, add a dash of vinegar and mustard to sharpen the tastes, if necessary, and serve the vegetables in soup plates with the sauce. Garnish with some parsley and plenty of pepper.

VARIATION: To thicken the sauce, pour off the sauce into a measuring cup and note how much there is. For every cup, measure 2 teaspoons arrowroot. Dissolve the arrowroot in some of the broth in a small bowl, then add it to the whole amount. Heat over a medium-high flame until the sauce has thickened. Taste and season with vinegar to brighten the flavors, and add plenty of pepper. You could also stir in a couple of teaspoons of mustard. Cook at least 5 minutes, stirring constantly, then return to the vegetables and serve.

Serving size = 1 cup
117 calories
0.6 grams total fat
trace saturated fat
0 milligrams cholesterol

MUSHROOM AND LEEK CRÊPES

YIELD: 14 CRÊPES (7 SERVINGS)   BY MARK HALL

If you like your crêpes to have a lot of sauce within the crêpe itself, then double the recipe and ladle several tablespoons of sauce over the filling before folding the crêpe and baking.

Filling:

3 cups sliced leeks
½ cup dry white wine
2½ cups thinly sliced or
  small-diced domestic
  mushrooms
2¼ ounces fresh shiitake
  mushrooms
1 teaspoon balsamic vinegar
Salt
Freshly ground black pepper
1 tablespoon Italian parsley or
  mixed herbs

Crêpe Batter:

½ cup unbleached all-purpose
  flour

½ cup whole wheat pastry flour
⅓ cup masa harina
2 cups water

Sauce:

5 ounces dried shiitake
  mushrooms
4 large onions, rough chopped
4 cups domestic mushrooms
6 cups water
2 cups dry red wine
6 tablespoons semolina flour
Freshly chopped parsley or other
  herb for garnish

For the filling, braise the leeks in the white wine for 20 minutes. Add the domestic and fresh shiitake mushrooms. Add the balsamic vinegar to the mushrooms and cook until all of the liquid has been released and is mostly reduced. Add salt and pepper to taste before the mushrooms are completely cooked. Toss with the parsley or mixed herbs. There should be 5 cups filling.

For the crêpe batter, sift the flours and masa harina together. Mix in the water until the batter forms a light cream that can coat a wooden spoon. If the batter is lumpy, you can blend it in a blender. Make a test crêpe. Ladle about 3 ounces of batter onto a nonstick skillet. Cook until golden on both sides. The crêpe should be wafer-thin and malleable; if not, add more water and mix again. There should be about 3 cups batter, enough for 14 crêpes.

For the sauce, add the shiitake mushrooms, onions, and domestic mushrooms to the water. Cook for 30 to 45 minutes, until the onions become soft and some of the liquid is reduced. Use a slotted spoon to remove the onions and mushrooms, reserving the liquid. There should be about 1½ cups remaining. Add 2 cups of red wine to the stock and cook for a few minutes on a very high flame to reduce the alcohol. Gradually whisk the semolina flour into the simmering hot stock until thickened but still pourable. There should be about 2⅔ cups sauce.

Preheat the oven to 375°F. For each crêpe, fill with one-third cup filling and top with 1½ tablespoons sauce. Roll and place in a baking pan. Repeat until you've made all 14 crêpes. Ladle more sauce over the crêpes in a baking dish and bake for 10 minutes, or just until hot. Use chopped parsley or chopped fresh herbs as a garnish.

Serving size = 2 crêpes
325 calories
1.3 grams total fat
0.1 grams saturated fat
0 milligrams cholesterol

INDIAN VEGETABLE STEW

YIELD: 4½ CUPS (4 TO 5 SERVINGS)   BY MARK HALL

This is a curry-flavored stew of coarsely chopped vegetables with a thick gravy made from yellow split peas.

½ cup dry yellow split peas
3 cups water
1 cup large broccoli florets
1 cup chopped onions
1 cup vegetable stock
2 cloves garlic, minced
¼ teaspoon turmeric
1½ tablespoons freshly minced
   ginger
1 teaspoon whole black mustard
   seeds
1 cup canned tomatoes, chopped

1 cup large cauliflower florets
1 cup chopped carrots
1 cup chopped red bell pepper
2 teaspoons ground cumin
2 teaspoons ground coriander
½ teaspoon freshly ground black
   pepper
Pinch cayenne pepper
1¼ cups vegetable stock
Salt
2 tablespoons freshly chopped
   cilantro for garnish (optional)

Put the yellow split peas into a large pot and cover with 3 cups water. Cook for about 40 minutes, until the peas are tender. When they are done, puree them in a food processor and set aside.

Blanch the broccoli separately and then plunge into ice cold water to stop the cooking and retain its color. Set aside.

While the peas are cooking, braise the onions in the vegetable stock with the garlic, turmeric, ginger, and black mustard seeds. When the onions have softened, add the tomatoes, cauliflower, and carrots. When the carrots are partially cooked, add the red pepper, cumin, coriander, black pepper, and cayenne, then continue simmering until the vegetables are cooked.

When the stew is ready, pour the processed peas into the onion-tomato mixture. Gradually add the vegetable stock until you reach a desired consistency. Add the broccoli. Salt to taste and garnish with cilantro.

Serving size = 1 cup
153 calories
1.7 grams total fat
0.2 grams saturated fat
0 milligrams cholesterol

HEARTY BEAN AND VEGETABLE STEW (OR SOUP)

YIELD: 12 CUPS (12 SERVINGS)   BY LENORE LEFER

This stew/soup is very versatile and can use any fresh or leftover ingredients. It consists of three or four kinds of beans such as black, red kidney, pinto, baby lima, lentils, and green and/or yellow split peas. Cooked pasta and rice are added to the cooking liquid, which contains the diced vegetables and seasonings, after the beans are cooked. It freezes well.

Lenore prefers this dish as a stew served in the center of a bowl and rimmed with rice. As a soup, serve it with a hearty bread and salad for a winter's lunch or dinner.

1 pound assorted dry beans	*1 onion, diced*
2 cups vegetable juice	*1 teaspoon dried basil*
½ cup dry white wine	*1 teaspoon dried parsley*
⅓ cup soy sauce	*1 teaspoon garlic powder or 3*
⅓ cup apple or pineapple juice	*cloves fresh garlic*
Vegetable stock or water	*1 bay leaf*
½ cup diced celery	*1 teaspoon freshly ground black*
½ cup diced carrots	*pepper*
½ cup diced parsnips	*1 cup cooked rice or pasta*
½ cup diced mushrooms	

Sort and rinse the beans, then soak overnight in water. Drain and place in a Crockpot. Add the vegetable juice, wine, soy sauce, and apple or pineapple juice. Cover with vegetable stock or water; the amount added depends on whether you prefer a soup (more liquid) or a stew (less). The juice adds just a tad of sweetness and the soy sauce adds depth and the tang of salt.

Cook for several hours on high. (You can also cook it on "low" overnight and finish it in the morning. The soup benefits from slower cooking.)

Add the vegetables herbs, and spices and cook for several more hours until the carrots and parsnips are tender. (In a slow Crockpot this could take almost half a day and is good for people who go off to work or want to take a long hike.) When tender, but not overcooked, add the rice or pasta and heat for 1 hour more.

Serving size = 1 cup
170 calories
0.3 grams total fat
trace saturated fat
0 milligrams cholesterol

TOMATO AND OKRA STEW

YIELD: 4 CUPS (4 SERVINGS)   BY MARK HALL

Serve this stew over Wild and Arborio Rice (page 453) or another grain dish.

⅔ cup chopped onions
2 tablespoons freshly minced garlic
2 tablespoons dried oregano
1 cup water
1½ cups fresh corn kernels (2 to 3 large ears)
¼ cup dry red wine
¼ teaspoon ground cumin

1½ cups diced green bell pepper
1½ cups thinly sliced okra
3 cups chopped tomatoes
¼ teaspoon plus 1 pinch cayenne pepper
Salt
⅛ teaspoon freshly ground black pepper or to taste

Braise the onions, garlic, and oregano in the 1 cup water. When the onions begin to soften, add the corn kernels and red wine. Continue braising for 10 minutes after adding the corn.

Add the cumin, green pepper, okra, and tomatoes. Cover and stew for 45 to 60 minutes, until the vegetables are soft. Stir in the cayenne and add salt and pepper to taste.

Serving size = 1 cup
139 calories
1.6 grams total fat
0.3 grams saturated fat
0 milligrams cholesterol

ENCHILADAS WITH TOMATILLO SAUCE

YIELD: 10 ENCHILADAS (5 SERVINGS)   BY MARK HALL

*The vegetable filling bursts with the robust flavors of the cumin and chili.
Serve with the Orange-Jicama Salad with Pickled Onions (page 415) and the
Refried Beans (page 458).*

Tomatillo Sauce:

1 ¼ pounds tomatillos (to make 1
    cup tomatillo puree)
½ cup diced onions
1 teaspoon freshly minced garlic
¼ cup vegetable stock
¼ teaspoon rice wine vinegar
½ cup fresh tomatoes, seeded
    and diced
1 tablespoon freshly chopped
    cilantro
Salt
Freshly ground black pepper to
    taste, or pinch of cayenne

Filling:

2 cups chopped onions
2 tablespoons freshly minced
    garlic

2 teaspoons dried oregano
2 teaspoons ground cumin
⅔ cup dry red wine
5 cups sliced mushrooms
2½ cups chopped red bell pepper
2½ cups chopped zucchini
1 cup cooked black beans
    (optional)
Salt
Approximately 1 teaspoon Ancho
    Chili Puree (page 465)
1 cup tomato sauce
10 6-inch oil-free corn tortillas,
    steamed
Cilantro sprigs for garnish

For the tomatillo sauce, remove the papery husk from the tomatillos and
rinse. Cook them in boiling water for 5 minutes until their color is drab
olive. Remove from the cooking water, place in a food processor or blender,
and puree. Set aside.

Braise the onion and garlic in vegetable stock until the onions have softened.
Add the pureed tomatillos and cook for another 20 minutes. Add the rice
vinegar, tomatoes, cilantro, and salt and pepper to taste. Set aside. There
should be 1½ cups sauce.

For the filling, braise the onions, garlic, oregano, and cumin in the red wine
until the onions have softened. Add the mushrooms and red peppers and
continue cooking. When these are almost done, add the zucchini. (Add the
beans also if you are using them.) Cook for a few minutes longer.

When the vegetables are tender, add salt to taste and 1 teaspoon Ancho Chili Puree. Since these chilies tend to vary in heat, taste and add more in small increments if necessary. There should be 5 cups of filling (6, if using the beans).

To assemble, preheat the oven to 350°F. Pour the tomato sauce into a baking dish or pan. If using more than one pan divide the sauce equally for each pan. Put ½ cup vegetable-chili filling onto each tortilla. Roll up and place in the baking pan with the seam side downward. Cover the enchiladas with aluminum foil and bake for 15 minutes, or until hot. For each serving, ladle ¼ cup tomatillo sauce over two enchiladas and garnish with sprigs of cilantro.

VARIATION: Bean Enchiladas with Tomatillo Sauce. Use the bean filling for the Black Bean Burritos (page 443) to substitute for the vegetable filling.

Serving size = 2 vegetable enchiladas
279 calories
3.7 grams total fat
0.3 grams saturated fat
0 milligrams cholesterol

Serving size = 2 vegetable enchiladas with beans
324 calories
3.9 grams total fat
0.3 grams saturated fat
0 milligrams cholesterol

Serving size = 2 bean enchiladas
472 calories
4.2 grams total fat
0.4 grams saturated fat
0 milligrams cholesterol

SOUTHWESTERN VEGETABLE STEW

YIELD: 3 CUPS (3 SERVINGS)   BY MARK HALL

Before reheating, add just a little vegetable broth to the leftovers (if there are any) to turn this into a hearty soup. Serve the stew or the soup with crisp corn tortillas crumbled on top.

1 ½ cups chopped red onions
½ cup water
2 teaspoons freshly minced garlic
2 teaspoons dried oregano
2 teaspoons ground cumin
2 cups thick-sliced mushrooms
½ cup diced carrots
1 cup chopped red peppers
1 ½ cups canned tomatoes, or 2
   cups fresh, chopped

2 cups canned tomato, puree
1 cup ½-inch sliced zucchini
1 teaspoon Ancho Chili Puree
   (page 465)
¼ teaspoon cayenne pepper
1 tablespoon freshly chopped
   cilantro
1 tablespoon freshly chopped mint
Salt

Braise the onions in ½ cup water with the garlic, oregano, and cumin. When the onions have softened, add the mushrooms and carrots. When the mushrooms have softened and the liquid is somewhat reduced, add the red peppers and tomatoes. Stew for about 10 minutes, then add the zucchini. Cook for 5 minutes (be careful not to overcook or the squash will lose its color).

When the vegetables are done, add the Ancho Chili Puree and the cayenne. Stir and add the cilantro and mint. Add salt to taste. If you want to make the dish hotter, add more cayenne.

Serving size = 1 cup
105 calories
1.7 grams total fat
0.2 grams saturated fat
0 milligrams cholesterol

WILD MUSHROOM FLAN

YIELD: 2½ CUPS (6 SERVINGS)   BY WOLFGANG PUCK

This elegant dish is perfect for your next dinner party.

1 pound button mushrooms,
  rinsed quickly and dried
  thoroughly
3 ounces shallots
4 garlic cloves
Juice of ½ lemon
2 ounces black trumpet
  mushrooms, coarsely chopped

4 large egg whites
½ cup nonfat milk
Freshly ground white pepper to
  taste
3 cups assorted greens of your
  choice (arugula, limestone,
  endive, etc.)
3 tablespoons balsamic vinegar

Preheat oven to 450°F.

Grind together the button mushrooms, shallots and garlic. Place in a heavy saucepan with the lemon juice and cook over medium heat until all the liquid has evaporated, 6 to 8 minutes. Transfer to a bowl and cool.

Sauté the trumpet mushrooms in a nonstick pan for 3 to 4 minutes. Stir into the ground mixture.

In a small bowl, whisk together the egg whites and milk. Pour into the mushroom mixture and combine thoroughly. Season with white pepper to taste.

Spray six ¾-cup soufflé dishes with vegetable oil spray. Cut rounds of parchment paper to fit the bottom of the dishes and place inside the cups. Divide the mushroom mixture evenly and spoon into the cups. Arrange in a shallow baking pan and pour boiling water into the pan halfway up the sides of the cups. Bake 20 minutes. Remove from the oven and let sit in the water bath while preparing the salad.

Toss the salad greens with the vinegar and arrange on 6 plates. Loosen each flan by running a sharp knife around the sides of the cup and unmold in the center of the greens. Remove the paper on top and serve immediately.

Serving size = 1 soufflé cup
61 calories
0.3 grams total fat
0.1 grams saturated fat
1.0 milligram cholesterol

MUSHROOM AND ARTICHOKE FRITTATA

YIELD: 4 CUPS (5 TO 6 SERVINGS)   BY MYRNA MELLING

There are several egg substitutes available in the market and just because the label says "egg substitute" does not mean that the product is going to promote good health. While the major constituents of such substitutes are egg whites, there are differences in cholesterol and salt content, as well as in taste. Some also contain hydrogenated oils. Read all labels to be sure the product doesn't contain ingredients you want to avoid.

2 cups sliced mushrooms
1 cup drained and chopped
   artichoke hearts packed in
   water
1/2 teaspoon dried tarragon
1 teaspoon dried basil
1 teaspoon dried marjoram
1 teaspoon dried thyme

1 teaspoon fresh chives
1/2 teaspoon ground sage
2 teaspoons Butter Buds
1/2 cup dry vermouth
1 4-ounce carton Egg Beaters
4 egg whites
Paprika

Preheat the oven to 375°F. Braise the mushrooms, artichokes, tarragon, basil, marjoram, thyme, chives, sage, and Butter Buds in the vermouth until the liquid is reduced by one half, approximately 5 to 10 minutes. Cool and drain, reserving the liquid. Combine the Egg Beaters and the egg whites in a separate bowl. Add the drained wine sauce to the egg mixture. Divide the mushrooms and artichokes evenly among five 1-cup custard dishes or ramekins. Pour the egg mixture over the vegetables. Lightly dust the tops with paprika.

Bake 30 to 35 minutes until the tops of the frittatas are browned.

VARIATIONS: Any combination of an equal volume of vegetables can be substituted for the artichokes and mushrooms.

Serving size = 3/4 cup
66 calories
0.1 milligrams total fat
trace saturated fat
trace cholesterol

STUFFED ZUCCHINI WITH TOMATO SAUCE AND FENNEL SEEDS

YIELD: SERVES 4 AT ½ PER PERSON TO 8   BY MARK HALL
AT ¼ PER PERSON

Serve this as an appetizer or in larger portions as an entrée. It is particularly nice with polenta, a salad, and a bean-based soup.

Tomato Sauce with Fennel Seeds:

½ cup diced onions
½ teaspoon minced garlic
2 teaspoons dried oregano
½ teaspoon fennel seeds
½ cup dry red wine
1 12-ounce can chopped tomatoes,
   drained, or 1 ¾ cups chopped
   tomatoes
½ teaspoon freshly ground black
   pepper
Salt
Fresh minced Italian parsley for
   garnish

2 9-ounce zucchinis
¼ cup dry red wine
1½ cups minced mushrooms
½ cup minced onions
½ teaspoon minced garlic
1 tablespoon dried basil or 1
   tablespoon minced fresh basil
1 tablespoon dried oregano
3 tablespoons minced tomatoes
3 tablespoons minced seedless
   raisins
Freshly ground black pepper
Salt

Preheat the oven to 350°F. To start the sauce, stew the onions, garlic, oregano and fennel in the red wine. Add the tomatoes when the onions have softened and cook for about 10 minutes, then puree in a food mill, processor, or blender.

Cut the zucchinis in half. Scoop out the insides with a spoon or melon baller. Reserve the insides of the zucchini for the filling. Place the zucchini shells on a baking sheet in a little water. Cover the zucchinis with foil and bake for 20 minutes at 350°F.

Braise the zucchini flesh in the red wine and puree when it is cooked. Return the zucchini to the pan and cook with the mushrooms, onion, garlic, and dried herbs over medium heat.

When the mushrooms are cooked add the minced tomatoes and raisins. If you are using fresh basil instead of dried, add it at this point. Add salt and pepper to taste.

Fill the zucchini halves and bake on a baking sheet at 375°F. until hot. Serve with about ¼ cup tomato sauce per person. The zucchini halves can be cut into quarters to serve as appetizers.

Serving size = ½ stuffed zucchini + ⅜ cup sauce
116 calories
1.0 grams total fat
0.1 grams saturated fat
0 milligrams cholesterol

ZUCCHINI "PASTA" WITH YOGURT SAUCE

YIELD: 3½ CUPS (2 TO 4 SERVINGS)   BY DEBORAH MADISON

This is good served hot or at room temperature as a salad. It is also delicious tucked inside whole wheat pita bread with a squeeze of lemon juice or served as a spread to eat with crackers or black bread.

1 firm zucchini, approximately 1
  pound
2 tablespoons water
½ cup nonfat yogurt
1 clove garlic, finely minced
2 teaspoons finely chopped fresh
  dill or mint leaves

1 teaspoon white wine vinegar, or
  more to taste
Freshly ground black pepper
Additional herbs for garnish

Cut the zucchini in half and grate it into coarse shreds either in a food processor or by hand, or cut the zucchini in diagonal slices, then into strips. Make sure the strips are not too fine or the dish will be mushy.

Warm a wide nonstick frying pan and add 2 tablespoons water and the zucchini. Cook gently over a medium flame, turning occasionally until the zucchini has cooked and the moisture has evaporated, about 7 to 10 minutes. If the zucchini threatens to stick, add small amounts of water as needed.

While the squash is cooking, mix the yogurt with the garlic, herbs, vinegar, and pepper. As soon as the zucchini is done, add the yogurt mixture and gently toss together over a medium flame until the yogurt is warm. Serve with a dusting of pepper and a garnish of fresh herbs.

Serving size = 1 cup
40 calories
0.3 grams total fat
0.1 grams saturated fat
1 milligram cholesterol

TOFU DISHES

Tofu is one of the most versatile of foods. It can be stir-fried, braised or mashed, blended and baked, broiled, steamed, or grilled. It absorbs the flavors of the foods with which it is cooked, blended, or mashed, transforming it from the somewhat bland food that it is in its original state into a truly fragrant and satisfying ingredient. Here you will find spicy Mexican dishes such as Lydia's Mexican Casserole (page 508), hearty and pungent stews, and vegetable/tofu mixtures such as Tofu Stew with Miso (page 509) and Chinese Eggplant and Tofu (page 511), and light, simple dishes such as Tofu Cheese with Fresh Herbs (below) and Marinated Tofu (page 507).

Tofu is very high in protein and the perfect substitute for cheese and eggs. Keep it on hand in your refrigerator for quick, nutritious meals. The dishes on these pages will help you develop a taste for this miracle food if you haven't discovered it already.

All of the recipes listed here contain more than 10 percent fat. As mentioned in the introduction to the recipes, tofu is relatively high in fat, as are all of the soybean products. However, the actual amount of total fat in tofu is low in comparison to other comparable sources of protein, and since that small amount of fat is mostly polyunsaturated, it is allowed in this diet.

We have recommended to our study participants that they limit their intake to ½ cup of tofu three times per week. At this level of intake, the total dietary fat over a several days should remain under 10 percent.

TOFU CHEESE WITH FRESH HERBS

YIELD: 1 CUP (4 SERVINGS)   BY DEBORAH MADISON

This is a very aromatic and pretty dish, flecked with green and garnished, if you desire, with herb blossoms. Serve with crackers on fresh, raw vegetables, or toss with hot noodles.

If you have the choice, use "silken" tofu, which has a very fine, smooth texture. If you can't find "silken" use firm tofu. Tofu is now available in sealed boxes which keep for a long time refrigerated. With this type of packaging, the tofu doesn't need to be packed in water, nor does it seem to spoil, and its texture is particularly creamy.

*8 ounces tofu, drained if
    previously kept in water
2 tablespoons white wine
1 shallot or 4 scallions, finely
    diced
1 large clove garlic, minced or
    pounded to a puree
2 tablespoons finely chopped fresh
    herbs, such as parsley,
    marjoram, dill, lemon thyme,
    lovage, tarragon, basil*

*Herb vinegar to taste
Freshly ground white pepper to
    taste
1/2 to 1 teaspoon mustard
Herb blossoms, nasturtium leaves,
    or watercress for garnish
    (optional)*

Process the tofu in a food processor with the wine until very smooth, 1 or 2 minutes. It may be necessary to stop the processor and scrape down the sides. If the tofu is very dry, add a little more wine to moisten it.

Transfer the tofu to a bowl and mix in the rest of the ingredients, except for the herb blossoms, if using. Taste and adjust the seasonings. Different herbs will contribute different strengths and qualities, which may affect the other seasonings you use. Don't forget, the garlic and onion flavors, as well as the herbal flavors, will get stronger as this sits.

Heap the tofu in a serving bowl, cover, and set aside, if possible, for several hours to allow the flavors to develop. Just before serving, garnish with more fresh herbs, chopped or whole, or with blossoms snipped with scissors or carefully cut, so as not to bruise them. Nasturtium and chive blossoms, or any other herb blossoms you might have, such as rosemary, sage, hyssop, or thyme will make attractive garnishes. Wreath, if desired, with nasturtium greens or watercress, both of which have strong peppery tastes.

NOTE: If for some reason your tofu cheese isn't firm enough (perhaps it didn't drain enough), you can correct this. Rinse out a piece of cheesecloth, line a strainer with it, double or triple thickness, put in the cheese and set over a bowl. After a few hours the excess liquid will have drained out. If left overnight, it should be firm enough to turn out onto a plate.

Serving size = 1/4 cup
51 calories
2.4 grams total fat
0.3 grams saturated fat
0 milligrams cholesterol

MARINATED TOFU

YIELD: 1 CUP (2 SERVINGS)   BY MARK HALL

Because of the soy sauce, the sodium content of this dish is a bit high (523 milligrams per 1/2 cup) and may be unsuitable for those persons with a history of congestive heart failure and/or hypertension.

Marinade:

2 tablespoons medium dry red
  wine (such as Burgundy)
1 tablespoon soy sauce
1 1/2 teaspoons water
1 teaspoon rice wine vinegar

1 teaspoon freshly grated ginger
1/2 teaspoon freshly minced garlic
1/8 teaspoon freshly ground black
  pepper

7 ounces firm tofu, cubed

Combine all of the marinade ingredients in a saucepan. Bring to a boil and pour over the tofu. Let this sit overnight. Alternatively, you can let the tofu and marinade simmer for 15 minutes, then drain and serve.

Serving size = 1/2 cup
96 calories
4.2 grams total fat
0.6 grams saturated fat
0 milligrams cholesterol

SCRAMBLED TOFU AND VEGETABLES

YIELD: 4 CUPS (4 SERVINGS)   BY MARY CARROLL

If you like tofu you may consider having this as a breakfast item with toast, with or without the vegetables.

1/2 cup minced carrots
1/3 cup sherry
1/2 cup diced onions
1/2 cup fresh, cooked corn kernels
1/2 cup minced red bell pepper
2 tablespoons diced jalapeño chili
1 cup fresh green peas
1/2 cup chopped celery
1 1/2 cups crumbled firm tofu (12
  ounces firm tofu)

1 tablespoon tumeric
1 teaspoon curry powder
1/4 teaspoon white pepper
1/2 teaspoon dried dill
1/2 teaspoon dried thyme
1 1/2 teaspoons fresh chives
Salt
Chopped scallions for garnish

Steam the carrots for 5 to 8 minutes until tender and set aside. Heat the sherry in a saucepan and cook the onions until soft, adding more sherry as necessary. Add the remaining vegetables, cover, and cook for about 5 to 10 minutes. Mix the tofu in a bowl with the spices, add it to the vegetables, and sauté until just heated through. Add salt to taste and garnish with chopped scallions. Serve with salsa, garlic toast, or fruit salad.

Serving size = 1 cup
155 calories
4.3 grams total fat
0.6 grams saturated fat
0 milligrams cholesterol

LYDIA'S MEXICAN CASSEROLE

YIELD: 8 CUPS (8 SERVINGS)   BY LYDIA KARPENKO

The green chilies are not necessarily very hot. If you like very hot food you may want to put in an extra red chili or add a pinch of cayenne pepper.

*1 dozen 6-inch corn tortillas,
   oil-free, uncooked
1 medium onion, chopped
2 cups diced tomatoes
2 cups tomato salsa
Ground cumin
1 red chili pepper or 1 jalapeño
   chili, chopped
3 cloves garlic, minced*

*1 27-ounce can whole green
   chilies
12 ounces firm tofu, mashed
32 ounces nonfat yogurt
1 tablespoon dry no-oil vinaigrette
   salad dressing mix.
Freshly chopped cilantro for
   garnish*

Preheat the oven to 350°F. Using a nonstick baking dish, line the casserole with six of the tortillas. Mix together the onion, tomatoes, salsa, 1 teaspoon cumin, chopped red chili pepper, and garlic. Pour about three-fourths of this mixture into the casserole. Lay the green chili peppers flat over this, then the mashed tofu. Cover with the remainder of the tortillas. Add the remaining chopped tomato and salsa mixture. Mix the yogurt with the dry salad dressing mix and pour over the chopped tomato and salsa. Sprinkle a little ground cumin over this and bake for about 35 to 45 minutes. Garnish with the cilantro.

VARIATION: Substitute some cooked beans for the tofu.

Serving size = 1 cup
269 calories
4.3 grams total fat
0.6 grams saturated fat
2 milligrams cholesterol

TOFU STEW WITH MISO

YIELD: 5½ CUPS (5 TO 6 SERVINGS)   BY MARK HALL

Miso is a soybean product to which a variety of grains have been added. It is salted and then fermented. Because of its soybean derivation, it also is high in protein and relatively high in polyunsaturated fat. There are many kinds of miso, and they vary in color, sweetness, savoriness, textures, aromas, and salt content. It can be very high in salt. The two misos here are combined to balance out the salt load. The sweet white shiro miso *has less salt than the darker* aka *variety. While it is not a problem here because very little is used in the total recipe, should there be a problem with hypertension or a history of congestive heart failure, then miso in general may not be suitable for liberal use. One serving of this stew provides 80 milligrams sodium.*

1 cup large-diced zucchini
½ cup mung bean sprouts
7 dried shiitake mushrooms
(approximately 1 ounce)
2½ cups water
1 cup diced onion
2 teaspoons freshly minced garlic
1 cup chopped carrot
1 teaspoon freshly minced ginger

1½ kabocha squash, cubed, or
any other winter variety, such
as butternut, acorn, or banana
1 cup diced red bell pepper
8 ounces cubed firm tofu
1 teaspoon sweet white shiro miso
1 teaspoon aka miso
Freshly ground black pepper

Blanch the zucchini (3 to 5 minutes) and sprouts (1 minute) separately. Plunge them into ice cold water to stop the cooking and put aside. Put the dried mushrooms in a bowl and cover with 2½ cups water. Put aside to soak for 1 hour. When finished soaking, remove the stems and mince or slice into ½-inch strips. Reserve the mushroom stock.

Braise the onions and garlic in ½ cup of the mushroom stock. When the onions begin to soften add the carrots, mushrooms, and ginger. Continue braising. When the carrots are partially cooked, add the cubed squash and the remaining mushroom stock. Add the red pepper when the squash is almost soft. After adding the pepper, stew for a total of about 25 minutes.

Add the zucchini and continue cooking for about 5 minutes longer. Toss in the tofu and then the sprouts. Stir in the miso. Add pepper to taste.

Serving size = 1 cup
107 calories
2.1 grams total fat
0.2 grams saturated fat
0 milligrams cholesterol

SWEET AND SOUR WOK-COOKED VEGETABLES WITH TOFU

YIELD: 4 CUPS VEGETABLES (4 SERVINGS)   BY CAROL CONNELL

Not all of the sweet and sour sauce will be used for this recipe. What isn't needed may be refrigerated for several days.

Sweet and Sour Sauce:

1 1/4 cups plain tomato sauce
2 teaspoons freshly minced garlic
1/2 teaspoon dried basil
1/2 teaspoon celery seed
4 teaspoons rice wine vinegar
1/4 cup apple juice concentrate
1/2 teaspoon tamari sauce
1/4 teaspoon ground cardamom
1/2 teaspoon coriander
1/3 cup water

1 ounce dried black mushrooms
1/4 cup dry sherry

1 cup thinly sliced onions
1/4 cup dry white wine
1/2 cup sliced chanterelles
1/4 cup julienned red bell peppers
1/4 cup julienned carrots
1/2 cup broccoli florets
1/2 cup whole snow peas, ends
  snapped off
1/4 cup shredded Napa cabbage
1/4 cup fresh pineapple chunks
1 cup firm tofu, cubed
1/4 cup mung bean sprouts
1 teaspoon whole sesame seeds
Salt
Cooked white or brown rice

First make the sauce, by combining all the sauce ingredients and simmering for 15 minutes. There should be 2 cups sauce.

Soak the mushrooms in the sherry for 10 minutes. Drain, remove the stems and thinly slice the mushrooms. Reserve the sherry to use if more liquid for braising is needed.

In a wok or large pan, braise the onions in the white wine for about 10 minutes until soft. Add the chanterelles and soaked black mushrooms and cook for 5 minutes at high heat, stirring frequently. Add the red pepper and carrots, cover, and steam for 5 minutes. Add the broccoli, snow peas, cabbage, pineapple, and tofu. Cover again and steam for 2 minutes more. Add the sprouts and cook for 1½ minutes.

Toss with one cup of the sweet and sour sauce and the sesame seeds. Add salt to taste, then serve over rice.

Serving size = 1 cup vegetable + sauce
169 calories
3.2 grams total fat
0.5 grams saturated fat
0 milligrams cholesterol

Serving size = 1 cup vegetable + sauce + ½ cup white rice
280 calories
3.3 grams total fat
0.6 grams saturated fat
0 milligrams cholesterol

Sweet and Sour Sauce
Serving size = ¼ cup
30 calories
0.2 grams total fat
0.03 grams saturated fat
0 milligrams cholesterol

CHINESE EGGPLANT AND TOFU

YIELD: 5 CUPS (5 SERVINGS)   BY MARK HALL

This can be served over pasta or rice. It contains more salt than usual and will not be appropriate for everyone. One serving contains 430 milligrams sodium.

2 cups chopped onion
1 cup medium dry red wine
7 cups diced eggplant
  (approximately 1 pound)
1½ cups water
2 teaspoons freshly minced garlic
¼ teaspoon red hot chili flakes

14 ounces firm tofu, diced or
  cubed
1 teaspoon arrowroot
2 tablespoons soy sauce
1 cup sliced scallions
2 teaspoons rice wine vinegar
Freshly chopped cilantro

Braise the onions in the red wine. When the onions are softened add the eggplant, ½ cup water, garlic, and chili flakes. Cover the pan and stew until the eggplant is completely cooked. Then add the tofu. Dilute the arrowroot in the soy sauce, then add to vegetable mixture with 1 cup of water. Stir until the sauce is thickened. Add the scallions and rice wine vinegar. Toss. Garnish with a little cilantro and serve.

Serving size = 1 cup
159 calories
3.7 grams total fat
0.6 grams saturated fat
0 milligrams cholesterol

STEAMED FRESH VEGETABLES AND TOFU WITH SOBA NOODLES

YIELD: 14 CUPS (14 SERVINGS)   BY MOLLIE KATZEN

This dish contains 171 milligrams sodium per serving.

1 large bunch broccoli
   (approximately 1½ pounds)
2 large carrots
1 medium-sized red or yellow
   onion
1 small head cauliflower

12 to 15 large mushrooms
About ¾ pound firm tofu
8 ounces uncooked soba noodles
1 cup Misoyaki Sauce (page 513)

Fill a medium-large saucepan with water and bring to a boil. Place a vegetable steamer over water in another saucepan and bring this to a boil also.

Cut off 3 inches from the base of the broccoli stalks and discard. Shave off the tough outer skin from the remainder of the stalks, and cut the broccoli into approximately 2-inch spears. Set aside.

Peel or scrub the carrots and cut into diagonal slices about ¼ inch thick. Set aside.

Cut the onion into 1-inch chunks, and break the cauliflower into 1-inch florets. Set aside in separate bowls.

Clean the mushrooms and trim off the bottoms of the stems. Quarter the mushrooms and set aside.

Cut the tofu into 1-inch cubes.

Arrange the vegetables in the steamer over the boiling water and cover. Cook over medium heat for 3 to 4 minutes. Then add the soba noodles to the boiling water in the other saucepan, partially cover, and turn heat to medium.

The vegetables and the soba noodles should be done at about the same time, in about 6 to 8 minutes. Drain the noodles in a colander over the sink, and transfer to a bowl. Add about ½ cup Misoyaki Sauce and mix well. Remove the vegetables from the steamer, either by lifting the entire basketful out from the saucepan or by picking the vegetables out with tongs.

Serve the vegetables on top of the lightly sauced noodles. Ladle additional sauce all over the vegetables.

Serving size = 1 cup
127 calories
1.6 grams total fat
0.2 grams saturated fat
0 milligrams cholesterol

MISOYAKI SAUCE

YIELD: 2 CUPS (16 SERVINGS)   BY MOLLIE KATZEN

Mixed together, miso and mirin create this delicious sauce used for broiled vegetables and tofu. It is so easy and satisfying, you will find yourself making it over and over again.

There are many varieties of miso that can be found at most Asian groceries and natural food stores. Mirin is also usually available at Asian grocery stores.

One 2-tablespoon serving of this sauce contains 249 milligrams sodium.

½ cup yellow, barley, or Hatcho   1 cup mirin
  miso   2 tablespoons cornstarch
1 cup water

Place miso in a medium-sized bowl. Heat ½ cup water, add to miso, and mash together with a spoon to make a uniform paste. Add ½ cup mirin to the paste and mix in thoroughly. Place cornstarch in a small saucepan. Whisk in remaining ½ cup water and ½ cup mirin until smooth. Heat cornstarch mixture over medium heat, whisking constantly. When hot, cook it, still whisking, until thickened, about 5 to 8 minutes. Remove from heat and stir into miso mixture. Mix thoroughly.

Serve at room temperature or warm (heat gently—without cooking!—in a microwave or on the stovetop) over hot broiled vegetables, tofu, and rice.

Serving size = 2 tablespoons
24 calories
0.4 grams total fat
0.1 grams saturated fat
0 milligrams cholesterol

STUFFED MANICOTTI

YIELD: 4 CUPS (8 STUFFED NOODLES)   BY JUDY TALBOTT
PLUS 3 CUPS SAUCE (4 SERVINGS)

This will keep well refrigerated or frozen until ready to use.

8 dry manicotti noodles
16 ounces soft tofu
1/2 teaspoon dried oregano
1/2 teaspoon dried thyme
1 teaspoon freshly minced basil
2 teaspoons freshly minced garlic
1/3 cup freshly minced Italian
    parsley

1/4 teaspoon white pepper
Salt
3 cups Marinara Sauce (page
    515)
Fresh Italian parsley or basil for
    garnish

Preheat the oven to 375°F. Cook the pasta for 5 minutes in boiling water, rinse in cold water, and set aside, making sure that the manicotti are not stacked or overlapping.

In a large bowl mix the tofu, oregano, thyme, basil, garlic, parsley, and white pepper. Add salt to taste. Stuff the manicotti noodles with the filling and place into a shallow 8 × 8-inch nonstick baking dish. Pour the Marinara Sauce over the manicotti and bake for 30 minutes, or until the sauce is bubbling. Garnish with the fresh herbs and serve.

Serving size = 2 manicotti (1 cup) + 3/4 cup sauce
367 calories
5.4 grams total fat
0.9 grams saturated fat
0 milligrams cholesterol

MARINARA SAUCE

YIELD: 4 CUPS (4 SERVINGS)   BY JUDY TALBOTT

The carrots lend a subtle sweetness to this very versatile sauce. It appears in the Stuffed Manicotti (p. 514) and the Wild Mushroom Pizza (p. 522). You can also pour it over pasta.

2 cups coarsely chopped onion
½ cup vegetable stock or water
2 cloves garlic, minced
1½ cups diced carrots
4 cups chopped tomatoes
1 teaspoon sugar

2 tablespoons freshly chopped basil
2 tablespoons freshly chopped Italian parsley
Salt
Freshly ground black pepper

Braise the onions in the vegetable stock until translucent. Add the garlic and cook further for about 1 minute. Add the carrots, continue cooking for about 5 minutes, and then add the tomatoes and the sugar. Cover and simmer over low to medium heat for 20 minutes, stirring occasionally. Add the basil and simmer, uncovered, for another 10 minutes. Transfer the sauce to a food processor, blender, or food mill and puree. If you prefer a chunkier sauce, puree only part of the sauce. Add the parsley and salt and pepper to taste. Serve.

VARIATION: Add your choice of fresh mushrooms when you add the tomatoes.

Serving size = 1 cup
94 calories
0.8 grams total fat
0.2 grams saturated fat
0 milligrams cholesterol

BREADS AND PIZZAS

Good bread is one of the most satisfying of foods, and there is plenty of room for it in this diet. Breads don't have to have added fat, and contain lots of energy-rich complex carbohydrates. Most of the breads here are whole-grain breads made with combinations of whole wheat and white, or whole wheat, white and rye flours. Their flavors are generous and hearty, and they have a moist, chewy crumb, even though they contain no additional oils.

If you don't have time to bake yeast breads, try the quick Corn Bread (page 518) or even speedier Garlic Bread. You can also find wholesome breads at natural food stores, bakeries, and supermarkets. But make sure you read labels, to check the fat content. Bread doesn't need fat, but bakers often add it anyway.

Bread also doesn't need to be spread with butter to taste good. In European restaurants butter usually isn't even put on the table. If you really want something on your bread, dip it into your salad dressing, soup, or the sauce of your main dish. Or top it with Hummus (page 410), Eggplant Puree (page 411), or Green Pea "Guacamole" (page 444). At breakfast, spread unsweetened jam or applesauce on toast.

CHEZ PANISSE BREAD

YIELD: 8 BAGUETTES (64 SERVINGS)   BY ALICE WATERS

3 1/4 pounds all-purpose flour (or
    bread flour with 12% to 13%
    gluten)

5 teaspoons salt
3 tablespoons dry yeast
4 cups water (70° to 80°F.)

Mix 3 1/4 pounds all-purpose flour with 5 teaspoons salt. In a large mixing bowl, dissolve 3 tablespoons dry yeast in 4 cups lukewarm water. Add the flour mixture, 2 cups at a time, whisking it smooth until it is thick enough to require mixing with a wooden spoon or paddle. The last cup or so of flour will have to be kneaded in. Turn the mass of dough, which will be shaggy, onto a floured surface and knead hard and rhythmically for 5 to 10 minutes, until the dough is smooth and elastic. Allow the dough to rise once in a large, covered bowl; punch down, and refrigerate, covered, overnight. The dough should be refrigerated in a container that allows for its triple expansion.

Let the dough stand at room temperature for 3 or 4 hours, until it is warm and rising. Punch down the dough and divide it into eight 10-ounce balls. Pound the air from the balls and roll them into baguette shape. This you should do in two stages. Press each ball into a roughly square, bubble-free sheet, and fold toward yourself, from the top, until you have a cylinder an inch or so in diameter and 6 to 8 inches long. Allow the dough to rest for 3 to 5 minutes. Then, placing your fingers (not your palms) on the dough, press moderately and roll back and forth, gradually moving your hands apart until the loaf you are shaping is 12 inches (or the width of your pan) long. Don't push too hard or stretch too fast or you'll tear the loaves.

Put the dough on baking sheets which have been lined with bakers' parchment and lightly floured. Cover the dough with light cloths and leave it in a warm place where there is no air movement for about 1½ hours, until the dough has doubled in size and a finger impression remains when the dough is poked lightly.

Slash the loaves or snip them into a wheat-stalk shape, and spray them thoroughly with a light mist of water. Put the loaves into a preheated 475°F. oven on the middle rack and immediately lower the heat to 425°F. once the loaves are baking. (Ideally, line the lower shelf with thick tiles and bake the loaves directly on them, using an oven temperature of 425°F. all the way through.) Spray very quickly after 2 minutes. Spray again quickly after 5 minutes, and again after another 5 minutes. After the final spraying the loaves should be glossy and beginning to brown. Turn the baking sheets around if necessary for even browning. The baguettes will be done in 15 to 20 minutes, when they are evenly brown and sound hollow when rapped.

Serving size = 1 ounce (⅛ baguette)
85 calories
0.2 grams total fat
trace saturated fat
0 milligrams cholesterol
169 milligrams sodium

BRIOCHE

YIELD: 1 LOAF (9″ × 5″) (10 SERVINGS)   BY CHRISTIAN JANSELME

This is an elegant bread, perfect for a special brunch.

1 package active dry yeast
½ teaspoon sugar
⅔ cup warm water
2⅔ cups all-purpose flour
½ tablespoon salt

1 tablespoon orange blossom
   water
3 egg whites
1 egg white for glaze

Dissolve the yeast and sugar in the water. Let it rest for 5 to 6 minutes until bubbles have formed on the top. Mix the flour and salt together and set aside. Whisk the orange blossom water into the 3 egg whites. With a mixer, add the egg white mixture to the yeast until incorporated. Slowly add the flour-salt mixture. If you have a dough hook for your mixer, put it on and knead the dough for 10 minutes on medium speed. Otherwise, knead by hand for approximately 20 minutes. If the dough seems sticky, add a little more flour to make it soft and pliable. After kneading, press the dough into a 9 × 5 × 3-inch bread pan. Let rise in a warm place for 1 hour until doubled in volume. Punch down and let it rise again for 45 minutes to 1 hour, or until the dough looks soft and fluffy. Brush with the egg white and bake in an oven preheated to 350°F. for 30 minutes, or until golden brown. Remove from the pan and let cool before serving.

Serving size = ¹⁄₁₀ loaf
130 calories
0.3 grams total fat
0.1 grams saturated fat
0 milligrams cholesterol

CORN BREAD

YIELD: 1 9 × 5-INCH LOAF (10 SERVINGS)   BY MARK HALL

Adding jalapeño chilies and corn to this quick bread will give it a Southwestern flair.

1⅔ cups whole wheat pastry flour
1 cup cornmeal
2 tablespoons baking powder
1 tablespoon sugar
½ teaspoon salt

1 cup water
1 egg white
¼ cup fresh corn kernels or
   chopped jalapeño chili peppers
   (optional)

Preheat the oven to 400°F. Mix all of the dry ingredients together. In a separate bowl, combine the water and egg white. Fold the dry ingredients, and the corn or chili peppers if they are being used, into the wet ones. Be careful not to overmix or it will not rise. Pour the batter into a nonstick 9 × 5 × 3-inch bread pan. Bake for 20 to 25 minutes until golden brown.

RYE BREAD

YIELD: 2 1½-POUND LOAVES (56 SERVINGS)   BY ALICE WATERS

2 tablespoons dry yeast
½ cup water
2 cups sparkling hard cider or
   beer

1¼ pounds unbleached
   all-purpose flour
¾ pound rye flour
1 tablespoon salt

Soften 2 tablespoons yeast in ½ cup warm water in a large mixing bowl and stir in 2 cups sparkling hard cider or beer. Mix 1¼ pounds all-purpose flour with ¾ pound rye flour and salt. Whisk the flour into the liquid, a cup at a time, until the dough is too thick to continue. Stir in the remaining flour, a cup at a time, until the dough comes together in a solid, sticky mass. Turn the dough onto a floured surface and begin kneading. Use a gentler motion than in kneading a white-bread dough, so that the dough stretches less. The dough will probably remain sticky throughout the kneading, but do not add more flour. After 3 to 4 minutes the dough will have a limp, silky elasticity. Put the dough in a container that allows for triple expansion, cover, and refrigerate overnight.

Allow 3 to 4 hours for the dough to come to room temperature. Work out all air from the dough, then shape it into 1-pound balls or baguettes. Let the dough rise to slightly less than double in bulk, as the bread is better dense than light. Bake in a preheated 400°F. oven for 35 to 40 minutes, until the loaves are a deep ruddy brown.

Serving size = 1 slice
67 calories
0.2 grams total fat
trace saturated fat
124 milligrams cholesterol

PEASANT BREAD

YIELD: 4 ROUND 1-POUND LOAVES (64 SERVINGS)   BY ALICE WATERS

3 cups water
½ cup sourdough starter
½ pound whole-wheat flour
2 tablespoons and 1 teaspoon
  active dry yeast

1½ pounds unbleached
  all-purpose flour
¼ pound barley flour
¼ pound rye flour
4 teaspoons salt

Prepare the "sponge" the night before baking. Mix 3 cups water, ½ cup sourdough starter, and ½ pound whole-wheat flour thoroughly with a whisk and leave it, covered, at room temperature overnight.

The next day, add 2 tablespoons and 1 teaspoon yeast to the sponge and stir. Let the yeast dissolve. Mix 1½ pounds unbleached all-purpose flour with the ¼ pound barley flour, ¼ pound rye flour, and 4 teaspoons salt. When the yeast has dissolved, whisk the flour in, a cup at a time, until the dough is smooth and too thick to whisk. Incorporate the rest of the flour, a cup at a time, with a wooden paddle. When the dough forms a shaggy mass, turn it onto a floured surface and knead for 5 to 10 minutes, until it is smooth and elastic. Leave it in a container, covered, until it doubles in bulk, between 1 and 1½ hours.

Divide the dough into four equal parts and work the air from each portion, one at a time. Form each portion into a ball and place on baking sheets lined with bakers' parchment. Cover the loaves lightly and let them rise until double in bulk. Slash the tops, spray lightly with water, and bake in a preheated 400°F. oven for 40 to 45 minutes. The loaves are done when they are an even dark-brown color and make a hard hollow sound when rapped.

Serving size = 1 slice (¹⁄₁₆ loaf)
63 calories
0.2 grams total fat
trace saturated fat
0 milligrams cholesterol

GARLIC BREAD

YIELD: ½ LOAF (8 SERVINGS)   BY OLIVE MCFARLANE

1½ tablespoons freshly minced
  garlic
¾ cup hot water
2 packets Butter Buds
½ loaf French bread (4 ounces)

6 tablespoons chopped and seeded
  fresh tomato (optional)
Pinch each freshly chopped
  rosemary and oregano or basil
  (optional)

Preheat the oven to 350°F.

Bring the garlic and water to a boil. Simmer for 5 to 10 minutes. Turn off the heat and whisk in the Butter Buds. Pour or spoon the garlic stock over the sliced bread. If desired, distribute tomato and herbs over the bread. Wrap the bread in foil and then bake for about 10 minutes. Open the foil and broil for about 1 minute more until the desired warmth or crispness.

Serving size = ½ ounce bread
57 calories
0.6 grams total fat
0.1 grams saturated fat
1 milligram cholesterol

OAT BRAN HUSHPUPPIES

YIELD: 35 (10 TO 11 SERVINGS)   BY FATHER ROBERT ROYALL

Instead of being fried, as hushpuppies traditionally are, these are to be baked on a nonstick cookie sheet or one that has been lightly sprayed with vegetable oil. To reduce the amount of oil used, wipe off some of the oil.

2½ cups oat bran
1 tablespoon baking powder
¼ cup honey

¼ cup nonfat skim milk
2 egg whites
¼ cup freshly minced onions

Preheat the oven to 375°F. Mix the oat bran and baking powder in a large bowl and set aside. In a smaller bowl, stir the honey into the milk, then add with the egg whites to the oat bran mix. Stir until just combined. Fold in the onions.

Wet your hands and lightly shape about 1 tablespoon batter into a 1-inch ball and place on a nonstick cookie sheet or one that was lightly sprayed with vegetable oil. Continue this until the sheet is full. Bake for 25 to 35 minutes until crispy brown. Be careful not to overcook. The hushpuppies should be soft on the inside. Eat them soon after removing from the oven.

VARIATION: Substitute ¼ cup of raisins for the onions.

Serving size = 3 each
100 calories
1.3 grams total fat
0.3 grams saturated fat
trace cholesterol

Raisin variation:
Serving size = 3 each
108 calories
1.3 grams total fat
0.3 grams saturated fat
trace cholesterol

WILD MUSHROOM PIZZA

MAKES 1 12-INCH MEDIUM THICK CRUSTED PIZZA   BY PAMELA MORGAN

Use the best mushrooms you can find for this elegant pizza.

Dough:

1 package active dry yeast
1 cup warm tap water
1 pinch of sugar
3 to 3½ cups all-purpose flour
1 teaspoon salt
Cornmeal

4 to 5 fresh basil leaves, torn
½ teaspoon each dried oregano and dried thyme or 4 to 5 sprigs each of thyme and oregano
Freshly ground black pepper

Topping:

1 cup Marinara Sauce (p. 515)
1 pound wild mushrooms, thinly sliced

Preheat the oven to 450°F. Empty the package of yeast into the warm water with the sugar and stir until the yeast granules dissolve. Let this sit for 10 to 15 minutes until a thin layer of bubbles forms over the water.

Combine 3 cups of flour and the salt in your food processor or bowl. Add the yeast-water mixture and process continuously until a ball is formed. Knead for 10 minutes by hand or follow your processor's instructions. If the dough sticks to your fingers easily, gradually add more flour as you continue kneading until it no longer sticks.

Transfer the dough to a bowl that has been lightly rubbed with oil. Place the bowl in a warm, dry place, cover lightly and let the dough rise for 30 to 60 minutes until doubled in bulk, then punch it down to release the air. Take the dough out of the bowl and knead for 1 minute more. The dough is now ready to be shaped.

Stretch the dough with your fingertips to form a circle. It should be flat in the middle and thicker around the edges. Sprinkle cornmeal over a pizza stone or heavy baking pan and then transfer the dough to the stone or pan.

Spread the tomato sauce evenly over the uncooked dough. Arrange the mushrooms (raw, or braised for 1 minute in a small amount of the marinara sauce) over the tomato sauce. Sprinkle the herbs on top and bake for 10 to 15 minutes, until the crust has browned.

⅙ pan = 290 calories
1.1 grams total fat
0.1 grams saturated fat
0 milligrams cholesterol

VARIATIONS: For a *zucchini-mushroom* pizza, slice one 8-ounce zucchini and then grill until cooked and lightly browned. Arrange this over the mushrooms. Add the herbs and bake as above.

For an *eggplant-mushroom* pizza, slice one medium eggplant (approximately *¾ pound*) into ¼-inch slices. Use ½ teaspoon of salt to sprinkle over the eggplant and let it sit for about 1 hour on paper towels. Rinse off the salt and then grill until cooked. Arrange the eggplant over the marinara sauce with some of the wild mushrooms and the herbs. Bake as above. If you must pay close attention to your salt intake, you may omit salting the eggplant, which is done to remove the excess moisture.

PIZZA PROVENÇAL

MAKES 1 12-INCH MEDIUM THICK-CRUSTED PIZZA   BY PAMELA MORGAN

A delicious pizza for onion lovers. The sweet taste of caramelized onions in combination with the tomatoes and peppers is wonderfully pleasing.

3 cups Onion Confit with
    Croutons (page 428)
Wild Mushroom Pizza Dough
    (page 522)
2 heads garlic
4 plum tomatoes
1 red bell pepper, roasted and
    julienned
1 yellow bell pepper, roasted and
    julienned

4 to 5 fresh basil leaves, torn
½ teaspoon each dried oregano
    and dried thyme or 4 to 5
    sprigs each of thyme and
    oregano
4 to 5 sprigs fresh rosemary or 1
    teaspoon dried

Prepare the Onion Confit with Croutons as per page 428 with two slight variations. First, omit the baguettes for the croutons. Second, to help caramelize the onions, add 2 tablespoons of sugar to the onions at the start of cooking. Be sure that most of the liquid has evaporated from the onions before using for the pizza.

Prepare the dough as per the Wild Mushroom Pizza on page 522 and lay out on a pizza stone or pan.

To roast the garlic, separate the cloves and place in a nonstick pan with ¼ cup of water. Cover the pan with foil and bake for 40 to 60 minutes at 450°F. until very soft. Let the garlic cool until it is easy to handle.

Slice each tomato into eight segments and arrange over the dough. Distribute the onions over the tomatoes, and then the mixed peppers over the onions. Squeeze the softened garlic from each clove onto the pizza. Sprinkle with herbs and bake for 10 to 15 minutes at 450°F., until the crust has browned.

⅙ pan = 374 calories
1.5 grams total fat
0.2 grams saturated fat
0 milligrams cholesterol

BREAKFAST FOODS

Breakfast is full of delicious options: warm, satisfying hot cereals, crunchy cold cereals, pancakes, waffles, and more.

If you're always in a hurry in the morning, you can make hot cereal in a thermos the night before just by pouring boiling water over the cereal. Whether cooked or uncooked, these cereals are high-fiber and high in protein, and they'll make a real difference in how you feel through the morning.

Pancakes and waffles are also a wonderful treat, and you'll find they're just as delicious spread with unsweetened jam or applesauce as with butter and syrup. Try them topped with fresh fruit or berries with some nonfat yogurt.

The number of nationally available commercial cereals, both hot and cold, that fit this program's guidelines are too numerous to mention. Look for those cereals containing less than 1 gram of fat per serving. Wheatena and Nabisco's Cream of Wheat or Rice are examples of hot cereals. Some of Kellogg's Nutri-Grain cereals and Post's Raisin Bran are examples of cold cereals. Read labels. You may have already chosen a suitable one.

Of course, you can also make a delicious breakfast from any of the breads in the "Breads and Pizza" section. Enjoy some slices, toasted or untoasted, with your favorite spread or unsweetened jam.

OATMEAL WITH RAISINS AND CINNAMON

YIELD: 4 CUPS (4 SERVINGS)   BY MARY CARROLL

A favorite that is particularly warming during winter.

8 cups boiling water
2 sticks cinnamon, left whole
1/2 cup raisins
3 tablespoons orange juice
   concentrate

2 cups rolled oats
Freshly grated nutmeg for garnish

Place all ingredients in a heavy saucepan and bring to a boil. Lower heat and simmer for 20 minutes, or until all the water is absorbed. Serve with a dusting of nutmeg.

Serving size = 1 cup
229 calories
2.7 grams total fat
0.5 grams saturated fat
0 milligrams cholesterol

GRANOLA

YIELD: 3 CUPS (3 SERVINGS)   BY MARY CARROLL

This recipe can easily be doubled and you can substitute other dried fruit such as apples, figs, apricots, figs and pineapple for the dates and raisins.

2 cups rolled oats
¼ cup oat bran
¼ cup rye flakes
2 tablespoons soy flakes
¼ cup apple juice
1 teaspoon vanilla extract

1 teaspoon ground cinnamon
½ teaspoon freshly grated
* nutmeg*
¼ cup chopped and pitted dates
¼ cup raisins

Preheat the oven to 300°F.

Mix together all ingredients except for the dates and raisins. Toss well to coat evenly with the apple juice. Spread on a nonstick baking sheet. Bake until evenly golden brown in color, stirring every 30 minutes, for about 1½ to 2 hours. After the granola is cooled, remove from the baking sheet and toss in the dates and raisins. Store in airtight containers in a cool place.

Serving size = 1 cup
347 calories
4.6 grams total fat
0.8 grams saturated fat
0 milligrams cholesterol

MILLET CEREAL WITH RAISINS

YIELD: 4 CUPS (4 SERVINGS)   BY MARY CARROLL

This is an interesting change of pace for hot cereal lovers.

1 cup hulled millet
1½ cups water
1½ cups apple juice
½ tablespoon apple juice
   concentrate

¼ cup raisins
½ teaspoon ground cinnamon
½ teaspoon freshly grated
   nutmeg
1 tablespoon fresh lemon juice

Rinse the millet in warm water and drain. Place in a pot with water, juice, juice concentrate and raisins. Heat to boiling, then lower heat and simmer for 10 minutes, stirring occasionally to prevent burning. Remove from the heat, add cinnamon, nutmeg, and lemon juice. Cover and let sit for 45 minutes. Serve hot as is, or with a dollop of yogurt.

Serving size = 1 cup
172 calories
1.1 grams total fat
0.3 grams saturated fat
0 milligrams cholesterol

BUCKWHEAT PANCAKES

YIELD: 12 3-INCH PANCAKES (4 SERVINGS)   BY VICTOR KARPENKO

Top the pancakes with fresh fruit, unsweetened preserves, applesauce, or nonfat yogurt.

½ cup nonfat yogurt
½ cup nonfat milk
1 teaspoon vanilla extract
¼ cup buckwheat flour
½ cup rolled oats

¼ teaspoon baking soda
¼ teaspoon baking powder
1 egg white
1 tablespoon apple juice
   concentrate

Mix the yogurt and milk with the vanilla. In a separate bowl, combine the buckwheat flour and rolled oats with the baking soda and powder. Fold all of these ingredients together. Beat the egg white until it is stiff, then gently fold into the other ingredients.

Pour onto a very hot nonstick skillet or one that has been lightly coated with vegetable oil spray. Turn the pancakes when the edges have browned and bubbles have formed on the top. Cook another minute or so until done.

Serving size = 3 pancakes
103 calories
0.8 grams total fat
0.2 grams saturated fat
1 milligram cholesterol

WAFFLES

YIELD: 13 4-INCH WAFFLES (6 TO 7 SERVINGS)   BY MARY CARROLL

These waffles are delicious topped with fresh fruit.

¼ cup water	¼ teaspoon ground cinnamon
¼ cup nutritional yeast	⅛ teaspoon freshly grated
1 cup sifted light rye flour	nutmeg
1½ cups sifted whole wheat	2 to 2½ cups water
pastry flour	6 egg whites
3 teaspoons baking powder	2 teaspoons cream of tartar

Gradually add the ¼ cup of water to the yeast to make a thick paste. Sift the dry ingredients and spices together. While stirring, gradually add the water and the yeast-water mixture until you get a cake batter consistency. Beat vigorously for several minutes. Beat the egg whites and cream of tartar until the whites are stiff and will form a peak. Gently fold the whites into the batter. Do not stir or beat. Use a nonstick waffle iron to bake to your taste.

Serving size = 2 waffles
178 calories
0.8 grams total fat
trace saturated fat
0 milligrams cholesterol

APPLE-CINNAMON OAT BRAN MUFFINS

YIELD: 12 MUFFINS (12 SERVINGS)   BY DR. ANDREW WEIL

The muffins are fairly high in calories secondary to the apple juice concentrate. You can dilute the juice concentrate with water to reduce the number of calories per muffin. If you decide to add water, remember to keep the same volume of liquid for the recipe (approximately 1½ cups).

1½ cups whole wheat pastry flour	*2½ teaspoons baking soda*
1½ cups unbleached all-purpose flour	*1¼ cups oat bran*
1 teaspoon ground cinnamon	*2 large cooking apples, such as Rome beauty or Granny Smith*
½ teaspoon freshly grated nutmeg	*12-ounce container apple juice concentrate, thawed*

Preheat the oven to 325°F.

Sift together the flours with the cinnamon, nutmeg, and baking soda. Add the oat bran. Then peel, core, and coarsely chop the apples. Toss the chopped apples with the oat bran mixture.

Mix in the apple juice concentrate, then fill the juice container ⅓ full with water (about ½ cup). Add this and mix just enough to moisten.

Spoon the batter into nonstick or lightly oil-sprayed muffin tins and bake for 25 minutes.

VARIATION: Add ½ cup raisins, dates, or other dried fruit with the apples.

Serving size = 1 muffin
204 calories
1.2 grams fat
trace saturated fat
0 milligrams cholesterol

DESSERTS

Desserts are definitely allowed on this diet! The ones you'll find here are based on fruit and grains, and most are only minimally sweetened. You'll be amazed at how many irresistible combinations of fruit, spices, wine, and fruit concentrates there are. It's easy to make a simple plate of fruit into a special dessert, just by adding a little something unexpected—sweet muscat wine to melon or lime juice to mangos. No extra sweetening is required. Dishes like the Rice Pudding (page 536) and the Lemon Semolina Pudding (page 535) are somewhat heavier than the fruit dishes, but also high in protein, and provide you with amino acids that may be lacking in the rest of the meal. You can also enjoy leftover grain desserts for breakfast.

In addition to the desserts here, remember that an unadorned piece of fresh fruit picked at the height of its season makes as good a dessert as anything.

APPLE AND APPLE CIDER SHERBET
(AN ADAPTATION OF A LINDA GUENZEL RECIPE)

YIELD: 6 SERVINGS   BY ALICE WATERS

12 to 15 apples, pippins or
  Granny Smiths
2 bottles sparkling apple cider
¹/₄ teaspoon ground cinnamon or
  3 cinnamon sticks
3 vanilla beans, cut and scraped
¹/₄ to ¹/₂ cup lemon juice

A clove or nutmeg for a musty,
  autumnal flavor (optional)
Zest of 1 to 2 lemons
³/₄ cup sugar per quart of apple
  puree
Pinch salt

Core the apples and cut them into twelfths into a bowl of acidulated water (about 3 tablespoons lemon juice per cup of water); do not peel. Drain them and stew them in a large saucepan with 2 cups of the sparkling cider, the cinnamon, and the vanilla beans. Bring to a boil and cook for approximately 10 minutes, or until the apples are quite soft. Puree the apples in a very fine sieve, using a wooden pestle to force the mixture through the holes. Discard the peels.

Combine the apple puree, the rest of the apple cider, the lemon juice and the zest, the sugar, and the salt. The puree should still be hot so that the sugar will dissolve. The amounts of lemon and cider will vary depending on the tartness of the apples.

Let the mixture cool well and adjust for flavor before freezing. Freeze according to the directions for your ice-cream freezer.

After freezing, store the sherbet in a covered container. This sherbet is best served the same day it is made; ice crystals begin to form after one day.

Serving size = 1 serving
324 calories
1.2 grams total fat
0.2 grams saturated fat
0 milligrams cholesterol

PEARS WITH BLACK CHERRY SAUCE

YIELD: 6 PEARS (6 SERVINGS)   BY CAROL CONNELL

This is an exquisitely elegant dessert—very simple to make and quite pleasing to the eye and palate.

6 large pears
1 ½ cups black cherry juice
2 tablespoons arrowroot

¼ cup cold water
Whole mint leaves for garnish

Place the pears in a pot with the stem-end upward. Add the cherry juice to the bottom of the pot. Cover and steam the pears in the juice until almost soft, about 20 minutes. Remove the pears from the juice.

Dilute the arrowroot in the cold water. Add to the juice, reheat, and stir until thick and clear. Ladle the sauce over the pears. Garnish with whole mint leaves.

VARIATION: Serve the pear halves fanned over a slice of angel food cake that has been covered with some black cherry sauce or fruit preserves. Then top with a dollop of Whipped "Cream" (page 542).

Serving size = 1 pear
109 calories
0.5 grams total fat
0.1 grams saturated fat
0 milligrams cholesterol

BALSAMIC STRAWBERRIES

YIELD: 4 CUPS (4 SERVINGS)   BY MOLLIE KATZEN

A traditional Italian way to serve fresh berries is simply to let them sit and macerate for a few hours with a small amount of sugar, then to drizzle in a little vinegar just before serving. Perfectly ripe berries taste exquisite prepared this way. It is also a magical way to salvage imperfect berries, especially those that may have been picked too soon and would otherwise suffer the fate of being considered boring and disappointing.

Balsamic vinegar is a special aged variety made in Modena, Italy. It is deep reddish brown and has a full-bodied, slightly sweet flavor that sets it apart from other vinegars. In recent years it has become widely popular and increasingly available in the United States. It can be found in specialty or gourmet shops, as well as in some grocery stores, either with the other vinegars or in the gourmet department. If you can't get balsamic vinegar, substitute another variety. If not exactly transcendent, the result will still be good.

The strawberries can be sliced and sugared up to a day in advance. The vinegar should be applied within 30 minutes of serving.

2 pints (1 quart) strawberries   1 tablespoon balsamic vinegar
4 to 6 teaspoons sugar

Clean the strawberries by wiping them with a damp paper towel. (If they are washed directly in water, they will absorb it and their flavor will become dilute.)

Hull the strawberries and halve or slice them, depending on their size. Place them in a shallow pan (a 10-inch glass pie pan works well) and sprinkle with sugar.

Cover tightly with plastic wrap and let sit for at least several hours, stirring them or shaking the pan every now and then. (If they are going to sit for much longer than 3 or 4 hours, cover and refrigerate them, but allow them to return to room temperature before serving.)

Sprinkle on the vinegar within a half hour of serving and serve in small individual bowls.

Serving size = 1 cup
65 calories
0.6 grams total fat
trace saturated fat
0 milligrams cholesterol

MELON WITH GINGER LEMON SYRUP

YIELD: 2 CUPS (4 SERVINGS)   BY MARK HALL

*Any sweet melon can be used such as canteloupe, honeydew, or watermelon.
The light taste of ginger gives it an unexpected lift.*

1 inch-long slice gingerroot,
  grated or shredded
1 1/2 tablespoons sugar
1 1/2 teaspoons lemon juice
1/2 cup plus 2 tablespoons water

1 1/2 teaspoons arrowroot
2 cups sliced sweet melon
1 1/2 teaspoons mint or Italian
  parsley for garnish

Add the ginger, sugar, and lemon juice to the 1/2 cup water in a saucepan
and bring to a boil. Let cook for a few minutes. Dilute the arrowroot in 2
tablespoons of cold water. Stir into the liquid after it has simmered for a
while. When it starts to thicken, turn off the heat. Let it cool. Divide the
melon slices into 4 bowls, drizzle the syrup over each portion, garnish with
mint or parsley, and serve.

Serving size = 1/2 cup
51 calories
0.2 grams total fat
0.2 grams saturated fat
0 milligrams cholesterol

MANGO COMPOTE

YIELD: 2 CUPS (4 SERVINGS)   BY ALICE WATERS

5 large ripe mangoes
About 2 teaspoons lime juice

2 cups sauterne

Peel the mangoes and slice them from the stones in about 1/8-inch slices.
Put them in a shallow dish and sprinkle with 2 teaspoons lime juice. Pour
2 cups sauterne over the mangoes, cover, and refrigerate for 2 to 3 hours.
Remove from the refrigerator 1 hour before serving and taste for lime juice.
There should be a hint of lime flavor; add more juice if necessary.

Serving size = 1/2 cup
249 calories
0.8 grams total fat
0.1 grams saturated fat
0 milligrams cholesterol

BERRY SORBET

YIELD: 3 CUPS (6 SERVINGS)   BY MARY CARROLL

This can be prepared in an ice-cream maker or in your freezer.

5 ½ cups fresh raspberries
Mint leaves for garnish
1 cup fresh blueberries
1 cup orange sections
2 peaches, peeled

1 tablespoon orange juice
  concentrate
¼ cup apple juice concentrate
1 teaspoon vanilla extract

Reserve 1 ½ cups of the raspberries and the mint leaves. Puree the other ingredients in a blender or food processor until smooth. Transfer the ingredients to your ice-cream maker or to an ice tray. Prepare as per your ice-cream maker instructions or freeze the pureed fruit and immediately before serving, puree it in the blender or food processor. Transfer to serving cups and garnish with the mint and fresh raspberries.

Serving size = ½ cup
99 calories
0.7 grams total fat
trace saturated fat
0 milligrams cholesterol

BAKED BANANAS

YIELD: 3 BANANAS (6 SERVINGS)   BY MARK HALL

This dessert is very sweet. Serve it with a dollop of yogurt or Whipped "Cream" (page 542).

3 large bananas
½ cup brown sugar
2 tablespoons rum

2 tablespoons fresh lime or lemon
  juice

Preheat the oven to 375°F. Peel the bananas and cut them in half lengthwise. Place them in a flat baking dish. In a saucepan, combine the brown sugar, rum and juice. Heat until it thickens, then pour over the bananas. Bake for 15 minutes, basting periodically. Let cool and serve.

Serving size = ½ banana
136 calories
0.3 grams total fat
0.1 grams saturated fat
0 milligrams cholesterol

POACHED PEARS

YIELD: 2 PEARS (4 SERVINGS)   BY MARK HALL

The key to this simple, elegant dessert is cooking the pears until they have softened but are still firm.

1 cup sweet white wine (such as Rhine)	*¼ cup apple juice concentrate*
¾ cup water	*1 teaspoon vanilla extract*
	2 pears, peeled and cored

Heat the wine, water, apple juice concentrate, and vanilla to near boiling. Lower the flame before adding the pears. Cover and simmer for 5 to 7 minutes in the hot liquid or until the pears are soft. Take care not to overcook the pears, or they well turn mushy and fall apart. Cool and serve.

Serving size = ½ pear + juice
112 calories
0.4 grams total fat
0.1 grams saturated fat
0 milligrams cholesterol

LEMON SEMOLINA PUDDING

YIELD: 2¼ CUPS (4 SERVINGS)   BY MARK HALL

Even though it uses semolina, this dessert is very light and has the delightful tartness of lemon.

2¼ cups water	*3 tablespoons apple juice concentrate*
½ cup semolina	
¼ cup fresh lemon juice	*1 tablespoon lemon zest*
2 teaspoons honey	*Fresh mint leaves for garnish*
2 teaspoons sugar	

Bring the water to a boil and gradually whisk in the semolina, stirring to prevent lumps from forming. Let cook about 2 minutes. Turn off the heat. Whisk in the lemon juice, honey, sugar, juice concentrate, and zest. Cool. Serve garnished with mint leaves.

Serving size = ½ cup
71 calories
0.3 grams total fat
trace saturated fat
0 milligrams cholesterol

RICE PUDDING

YIELD: 3 CUPS (6 SERVINGS)   BY JOE AND ANITA CECENA

1 cup short-grain white rice
3 cups nonfat milk
2 cinnamon sticks
½ teaspoon vanilla extract
¼ cup apple juice concentrate, 2
* tablespoons honey, or 10*
* packets sugar substitute*

8- or 10-ounce can crushed or
* diced pineapple, drained*
½ cup raisins
Ground cinnamon for garnish

Pour the rice into a large pan and add the nonfat milk. Cover and bring to a boil. Reduce the heat and simmer 20 to 25 minutes. Stir frequently throughout the cooking until the rice grains plump up. Then add the cinnamon sticks, vanilla, and apple juice concentrate or honey, if using. Continue stirring to prevent the rice from sticking and burning. When the mixture is thick, stir in the sugar substitute, if using, the pineapple, and raisins. Remove the cinnamon sticks and pour the rice pudding into a serving dish. Dust with cinnamon.

Serving size = ½ cup
223 calories
0.5 grams total fat
0.2 grams saturated fat
2 milligrams cholesterol

PEACH BREAD PUDDING

YIELD: 8 CUPS (16 SERVINGS)   BY PHYLLIS GINSBERG

The peaches and Amaretto give a decidely nontraditional twist to this wonderfully old-fashioned dessert.

6 medium peaches
2 cups skim milk
1/2 teaspoon salt
1 pound loaf of stale sourdough
   bread
1 teaspoon Amaretto

1/4 teaspoon freshly grated
   nutmeg
1/2 cup apple juice concentrate
Juice of 1/2 lemon
6 egg whites, beaten

Blanch, peel, pit, and then dice the peaches. Set aside.

In a large bowl, mix together the skim milk and salt. Tear the bread into 1-inch cubes. Mash the bread into the milk and let soak for 15 minutes.

While soaking, use another bowl to combine the Amaretto, nutmeg, apple juice concentrate, lemon juice, and peaches. Add the beaten egg whites. Add to the bread mixture and toss gently.

Pour into a nonstick an 8- or 9-inch square pan. Bake in a preheated oven at 350°F. for 45 minutes, or until set and browned on top. Serve warm.

Serving size = 1/2 cup
122 calories
1.3 grams total fat
0.3 grams saturated fat
1 milligram cholesterol

PEAR COBBLER

YIELD: 7 1/2 × 12-INCH BAKING PAN (16 SERVINGS)   BY IRENE WHITE

The Grape-Nuts soften to give the crust of this cobbler a surprisingly light crunch.

2 tablespoons brandy
1/2 cup raisins
4 1/4 cups water
1/4 cup apple juice concentrate

1 cinnamon stick
6 Bosc pears
3 to 4 cloves
2 tablespoons agar flakes

The Crust:

2 cups Grape-Nuts
½ cup apple juice concentrate

Meringue:

8 egg whites
1 teaspoon cream of tartar
2 packets sugar substitute
2 teaspoons vanilla

Preheat the oven to 350°F. Put the brandy and raisins into a saucepan with 1½ cups of water. Bring this to a boil. Remove this from the heat and let soak until they are called for in the recipe.

Combine 2¾ cups of water, the juice concentrate, and cinnamon stick in a large saucepan. Bring this to a boil and lower the heat. Halve, core, and peel the pears and place them in the water. Bring to a gentle boil, cover, and continue cooking for 20 minutes. Do not let the pears become mushy. Remove from the heat and add the cloves to the poaching liquid. Refrigerate.

To form the crust, mix the Grape-Nuts and apple juice concentrate. Pat this into the bottom of a 7½ × 12-inch Pyrex dish. Bake for 10 minutes. Let the crust cool before filling with the fruit.

Drain the liquid from the pears into a saucepan. Then drain the liquid from the soaked raisins and add this to the pear "juice" until you have 3 cups of combined liquid. Add the agar flakes and slowly heat until the agar is dissolved. Dice the pears and place the pieces along with the raisins over the crust. Pour the warm liquid over the fruit and let this cool and set in the refrigerator.

To prepare the meringue, whip the egg whites until frothy. Add the cream of tartar and continue whipping the whites until they are stiff but not dry. Add the sugar substitute and the vanilla. Beat until firm. Spread this over the cooled cobbler. Bake for 10 to 12 minutes in a preheated 400°F. oven, or until nicely browned.

Serving size = ¹⁄₁₆ of pan
135 calories
0.3 grams total fat
trace saturated fat
0 milligrams cholesterol

GLAZED FRUIT TART

YIELD: 12-INCH TART (12 SERVINGS)   BY BARBARA MUSSER

This is ablaze with color. The glaze holds this cornucopia of fruit together.

2 cups Grape-Nuts
1/4 cup apple juice concentrate
2 tablespoons arrowroot
2 cups strawberry-apple juice

3 peaches, sliced
1 pint strawberries, halved
3 kiwis, sliced
30 green seedless grapes, halved

Preheat the oven to 400°F. Mix together the cereal and apple juice concentrate. Pat this into a 12-inch nonstick pie pan and bake for 5 to 10 minutes until browned. Let cool before filling.

Gradually add the arrowroot to 1/2 cup juice. Stir as the arrowroot is added to get a mixture that is lump-free. Pour into a saucepan with the rest of the juice. Heat over medium heat, stirring constantly. The liquid will become cloudy, then crystal-like and will then start to boil. Boil for 3 minutes. It should become thicker than honey. Set aside to cool.

Arrange the fruit in an interesting pattern over the cooled pie crust. Pour a thin layer of the fruit juice glaze over it. Refrigerater for at least 30 minutes before serving.

Serving size = 1/12 tart pan
146 calories
0.5 grams total fat
trace saturated fat
0 milligrams cholesterol

APPLE STRUDEL

YIELD: 18 × 5-INCH LOAF (10 SERVINGS)   BY DONNA NICOLETTI

Much of the commercially available phyllo does contain oil, but oil-free varieties are available. This recipe proves that you do not need fat for a beautiful crust.

10 18 × 12-inch sheets of oil-free
   phyllo
1/4 cup honey
1/4 cup water
5 cups thinly sliced apples
2 tablespoons apple juice

1 1/2 ounces raisins
1/2 teaspoon ground cinnamon
1 tablespoon vanilla extract or the
   seeds of 1/2 vanilla bean and 1
   tablespoon water
1 egg white

Keep the phyllo dough covered with a clean, damp cloth until you are ready to work with it. It dries out very quickly.

Mix together the honey and water, then set aside. Peel, core, and slice the apples. Sauté the apples with the apple juice, raisins, cinnamon, and vanilla until they begin to soften. Remove from the heat and let cool. When the apples are cool you can begin to assemble the phyllo.

Preheat the oven to 325°F. Lay a phyllo sheet down with the short end of the rectangle in front of you. Brush liberally with the honey water. Lay the next sheet down directly on top of the first sheet and brush it as before. Repeat this procedure with the remaining 8 layers.

Spread the apple mixture evenly in the center of the phyllo. Leave a 1½-inch border around the phyllo rectangle. Starting at the short end, roll up the phyllo like a jelly roll. Have a nonstick or vegetable oil-sprayed baking sheet ready. Quickly pick up the roll and transfer it to the baking sheet. Twist the ends of the phyllo to prevent the filling from seeping out. Brush the top of the roll with the egg white.

Bake for approximately 30 minutes, or until golden brown. Let cool before cutting.

Serving size = ⅒ roll
111 calories
0.2 grams total fat
trace saturated fat
0 milligrams cholesterol

CARROT CAKE

YIELD: 10 SLICES (10 SERVINGS)   BY MARK HALL

Here's a perfect snacking cake.

1 teaspoon ground cinnamon	*1½ teaspoons baking powder*
1 teaspoon ground allspice	*1 teaspoon baking soda*
½ teaspoon freshly grated nutmeg	*1 cup grated carrots*
¼ teaspoon ground cloves	*1 cup raisins or other dried fruit*
1½ cups whole wheat pastry flour	*¾ cup honey*
⅓ cup wheat bran	*1½ cups water*

Preheat the oven to 350°F. Combine all the dry ingredients and mix well. In a separate bowl combine the liquid ingredients. Fold the dry ingredients into the wet ones and mix well. Do not overbeat or mix. Pour into a nonstick 9 × 5 × 3-inch loaf pan. Bake for 1 hour and 15 minutes, or until a toothpick comes out clean.

Serving size = 1 slice
191 calories
0.6 grams total fat
trace saturated fat
0 milligrams cholesterol

MOLASSES CAKE

YIELD: 8 × 8 × 2-INCH CAKE (9 SERVINGS)   BY DON VAUPEL

Molasses and raisins make this an especially luscious dessert.

$1/2$ cup molasses
$2/3$ cup hot water
$1/2$ cup seedless raisins
$1/2$ teaspoon salt
$1/2$ teaspoon ground cinnamon

$1/2$ teaspoon ground cloves
$1/2$ teaspoon baking soda
$1^3/4$ cups unbleached all-purpose
  flour

Preheat the oven to 350°F. Combine the molasses, hot water, and raisins. Bring to a boil and let boil for 5 minutes. Cool to room temperature. In a separate bowl, sift the remaining ingredients together. Stir this into the cooled molasses mixture until smooth.

Pour into a nonstick 8 × 8 × 2-inch baking pan or one that has been sprayed with vegetable oil. Bake for 45 minutes, cool, and serve.

Serving size = $1/9$ pan
151 calories
0.3 grams total fat
trace saturated fat
0 milligrams cholesterol

BANANA BREAD

YIELD: 9 × 5 × 3-INCH LOAF (10 SERVINGS)   BY MARK HALL

This quick bread is perfect for snacks, even breakfast.

2 cups unbleached all-purpose
  flour
1/2 cup whole wheat flour
1 tablespoon baking powder
1/4 teaspoon baking soda
4 very ripe bananas, mashed

1/2 cup apple juice concentrate
2 teaspoons vanilla extract
1/2 cup raisins
3 egg whites
2/3 cup water

Preheat the oven to 350°F. Mix all dry ingredients together. In a separate bowl, combine all the wet ingredients. Fold the dry ingredients into the wet ones. Do not overmix or the bread will not rise. Pour the batter into a 9 × 5 × 3-inch nonstick loaf pan or one that's been sprayed with vegetable oil. Bake for 1 hour. Cool, slice, and serve.

Serving size = 1 slice (1/10 pan)
204 calories
0.7 grams total fat
0.1 grams saturated fat
0 milligrams cholesterol

WHIPPED "CREAM"

YIELD: 1 1/2 CUPS (12 SERVINGS)   BY SHIRLEY BROWN

There is no cream in this but it will still make a light stiff topping if you can get one of the high-speed hand mixers such as the Bamix or Kitchen Mate that can beat air into the milk. Compare the amount of calories and fat in this to that of regular whipped cream. Be sure to use nonfat milk that is very well chilled.

1/2 cup nonfat milk
1/2 teaspoon rum extract
1/2 teaspoon apple juice
  concentrate

1 tablespoon superfine sugar

Whip the milk with a hand mixer until peaks form, about 20 to 30 seconds. Add the flavorings and sugar, then whip for a few moments more. Serve immediately.

Serving size = 2 tablespoons
8 calories
.03 grams total fat
0.03 grams saturated fat
trace cholesterol

"Regular" whipped cream:
Serving size = 2 tablespoons
50 calories
5.4 grams total fat
3.3 grams saturated fat
20 milligrams cholesterol

"Better put a strong fence around the top of the cliff
Than an ambulance down in the valley."

—Joseph Malins

■

"In nature there are neither rewards nor punishments;
there are only consequences."

—Robert B. Ingersoll

■

"Nothing in life is to be feared. It is only to be
understood."

—Marie Curie

Epilogue

"I Have Hope"

"I'm Hank Ginsberg, and I'm sixty-three years old. I have been an investment banker and an investor in a number of different companies.

"I first realized I had a heart problem in 1970. I went to a movie with a friend of mine, who was a physician. As we were walking up a hill together, I started feeling short of breath and some pressure in my chest. I'd been having these symptoms for about six months, but I'd ignored them. I didn't want to believe that I might have a heart problem. But this time, I was with a doctor. He knew something was wrong, even if I didn't want to face it. The doctor took me to his office and did some tests. Soon after, I went for an angiogram.

"The angiogram showed that I had some moderate blockages, about 50 percent, in several arteries. Naturally, I was upset and disturbed. The doctor said he didn't think it was necessary to have bypass surgery yet, but if I didn't change my lifestyle then my blockages would continue to worsen and he'd need to operate.

"He told me to go on a diet, lose weight, and get away from stress—but he didn't tell me how. I got scared enough then to do something. Although I was only forty-four at the time, I decided to retire. The doctor scared me.

"Even though I stopped doing business, I had a lot of friends and former business associates who would call and bring me deals or ask for advice. It seemed I just couldn't get away from the stress.

"My wife (Phyllis) and I were living in a big house in Beverly Hills—the whole bit—and I just sold it and decided to hell with it. I just wanted to get away from everyone and everything that gave me stress. So we decided to move out of the country, to London. It was a major decision, all because of the heart problem.

"I did change my lifestyle to some degree, although nothing like I'm doing now on Dr. Ornish's program. Back then, I don't think that the medical profession knew enough about what we had to do. My doctor didn't tell me to stay away from meat. All he told me was to eat less of the same foods that I had been eating.

"Mainly, I focused on losing weight. I've lost weight many times but I always gained it back because I didn't really change my life-style. I'd go back to my same eating habits. That must have happened at least twenty times in my adult life.

"My father died at fifty-nine with heart problems, and he had it at least for ten years before that. Four of his brothers died in their early fifties. So I figured my angiogram was a signal, a warning, and it was. But I guess I didn't do enough. Recently I got angry at myself that I had such a good warning nineteen years ago and didn't make bigger lifestyle changes then. But Dr. Ornish's research hadn't been done yet.

"I was fine the first three years in London. I didn't do very much work, just enough to make a good living without overdoing it. I worked with the stock market and I put a deal together once a year or so. But then I got bored. I needed the stimulation and excitement of the creative part of what I used to do.

"So we moved back to the U.S. and I went back to doing what I had been. But I was involved with some people that made it a little more stressful.

"Then I had some real serious chest pain and went back to a

couple of doctors. I ended up in the hospital with a dangerously high blood pressure of 250/150, and that was another signal. And everyone said that I had to get away from this sort of stress, so I quit working again. My doctor prescribed some diuretics to control my blood pressure and a drug to lower my cholesterol. I took them for many years, but the cholesterol-lowering drug damaged my liver, so I stopped taking it.

"I was scared, but I didn't know what to do except to run away again. It's what I always did in the past when things got too stressful. Our kids were all in college, so Phyllis and I decided to take a year off. It was our twenty-fifth wedding anniversary. We started traveling around the world.

"We did that for a few years, traveling, staying somewhere as long as we were having fun. And it was a very nice life.

"We moved back to California. Soon after, I started to have more pain. So I had another angiogram. It showed that the disease had gotten worse since the last one. Again, they told me the same thing: lose weight, reduce stress—but they didn't tell me how. Telling me to do it wasn't enough.

"It still wasn't serious enough for an operation, so I felt that I was all right. So I lost weight again and I went through the same process.

"Two years later, I had more chest pain again, and I had another angiogram. This time, the coronary artery blockages were much worse, and the doctor said I needed to have bypass surgery.

"I had a lot of denial. I went in without fear because I wasn't really accepting what was happening to me. At some deep level, I really didn't believe it. When the doctor told me I needed bypass surgery, I said to Phyllis, 'Well, I guess he knows best.' Phyllis said we should get some more opinions, but I said, 'These are professionals. They know.' I just accepted whatever the doctors said.

"But I didn't really understand what was happening. It wasn't until many years later, when Dr. Ornish sat down with me and showed me a diagram of where my blockages were—'This is 95 percent blocked, this one is 86 percent blocked, this is 100 percent blocked'—did it finally sink in how sick my heart really was. When he asked me, 'Were you aware of how serious your heart disease is?' I replied, 'Of course.' But I really wasn't aware. I really didn't let it register. I didn't *want* to accept it. I blocked it out. It's hard to face the truth. I guess we put up a lot of walls to protect ourselves.

"So I had the surgery. It was a terrible experience. Most people don't realize how traumatic and painful bypass surgery is. I remember waking up and I couldn't breathe. I just felt awful. And I almost gave up. I mean, I just felt my life would never be the same. I didn't know what I would be able to do and what I wasn't going to be able to do.

"After I went home from the hospital, my doctor said I could have three ounces of fish, or chicken, or beef a day. But when he said three ounces—then I'd slip little by little by little and I would just eat more. 'Is this three ounces or five ounces? Is it three times a week or five times a week—is it really that important? I'm really doing so well, etc.' Then I'd slip a little bit more and say, 'Well. . . .' and cheat, which is something that I've done with every diet, all my life. And I feel more deprived if I have a little of something and I can't have more than if I don't have it at all.

"The Reversal Diet works better because there is no fish, chicken, or beef. So you can't kid yourself or fool yourself as to what is allowed and what isn't. You don't have to judge if what you're having is enough or too much. The guidelines are clear. It's easier to stay on the diet for that reason.

"Instead of worrying about how much meat I can eat, I found it easier to make the food interesting that I *am* allowed to eat. You can make it *very* tasty. You can have good food. To this day, I still feel very strongly that interesting food is important to me since it's one of the real pleasures I have. It would be very hard for me to stay on a diet if I had to eat bland, uninteresting food. But the Reversal Diet can be very exciting.

"I make the food interesting by trying to be creative. You can use all the spices. With any food, no matter what you have, the real flavor comes from the spices that you use. It doesn't come from the fat; it comes from how you prepare it.

"We like ethnic foods: Chinese food, Mexican food, Italian food, Indian food. We go out for it, and we make it at home. We take recipes from regular cookbooks and modify them to fit Dr. Ornish's guidelines to cut out most of the fat. And nine times out of ten, the food comes out as tasty as the original recipe—sometimes better!

"Food is still a very important part of my life, and I don't feel like I'm missing anything—except the chest pain I used to have. I don't have to choose between tasty food that's going to kill me or healthful food that tastes bad. If it isn't tasty I feel deprived. I get angry. But I don't feel deprived if the food is delicious. High-fat food can taste bad, and low-fat food can taste great. It all depends on how you make it. The recipes in this book are terrific.

"And I'm eating now as much or more than I ever used to eat before. I lost about thirty-five pounds during the first six months, and I've kept it off for over two years now. And I eat a lot of food. On every other diet, I'd gain the weight back. I used to starve myself to lose the weight. But then after that I'd get famished and overeat. On Dr. Ornish's diet, I don't have to count calories. He doesn't say you can't eat. It's *what* you eat.

"Anyway, after my bypass I bought one company and was the chairman of two others. I tried not to work as hard as I had been, but it was pretty stressful.

"About two and a half years after my bypass, I started having some more chest pain. The doctors told me I needed a third angiogram. It showed that my bypasses had closed—*all* of them. Every one of the six bypasses. And they were ready to do another operation. As a matter of fact, three doctors told me that I had to go back, to have more bypass surgery. They felt that I was in really big trouble.

"When I found out that all of my bypasses closed up, I think I was still going through my denial period. I didn't fully feel the impact. But everyone was telling me I *had* to do something.

"So I had an angioplasty. Six months later, the arteries closed up again! It didn't sink in because I wasn't getting as much pain as before. At that point, though, I realized that I couldn't kid myself any longer.

"At first, I sort of gave up to some degree. I remember my surgeon telling me, 'Go home, take care of your insurance, and don't expect to live to be an older person.' I became very depressed.

"When you're told that there's not much you can do, you give up. There were times when I said, 'Well, whatever happens, happens.' You don't feel that there is something that you can do to help yourself. So I started getting involved again in a lot of different business deals—at least those were exciting and rewarding. I felt I was doing *something*.

"I was discouraged that the lifestyle changes I'd made during the previous several years weren't enough: First my bypasses clogged up, then my angioplasty clogged up. Then I learned about Dr. Ornish's program—which had more comprehensive lifestyle changes than I'd been making—and that it might work. His research was beginning to prove that changing my lifestyle could make a big difference even if I had bad genes.

"OK, so I started out with a couple of strikes. Most of the men in my family died of heart attacks at relatively young ages. But there was still a lot I could do. I couldn't change my genes, but I could change my lifestyle.

"I realized it was up to me to do something for myself. So I entered Dr. Ornish's program. And for the first time, I realized that I was in control of my life. To the degree that I'm the one causing the problem, then I'm the one who can do something to help me— and maybe others by my example. And here was my opportunity. I felt empowered, not blamed.

"It was a powerful realization. Before that, I would deny it—it was too hard to acknowledge it, even to myself. It's painful to face the truth: that you're really killing yourself. To look at yourself square in the eye and say, 'You still have an opportunity not to kill yourself.' To admit what you're doing to yourself is very painful, so I guess that's why I denied the truth for so many years. But when you're finally in enough pain, as I was, then it's less painful to acknowledge the truth than to keep going the way you have been. You can't deny it any more.

"But until I learned that there was something I could do about it, then it was hard to face what I was doing to myself. Because if you don't have something you can do to help yourself, then the denial serves a function. Why face a bad situation if you can't do anything about it?

"So when Dr. Ornish told me that there was a lot that I *could* do about it, I really believed, for the first time since I found out that I had heart disease, that *I* was in control. *I* could do something about it. Which then allowed me to face what I was doing and to make different choices.

"Once I found out that there was something I could do to help myself, it helped the depression, too. That goes away when you realize you're in control. You realize that it's *you,* it's not the outside world, it's not other people that are doing it to you. Once you understand what it is that you're doing, you can't deny it any more. Then you can't get away from the truth.

"It finally sunk in. I was the one hurting myself. I faced it. And I decided to do something about it. That, I think, was the key.

"I began to really believe in it. The people I saw there, everybody was feeling so much better. It wasn't just me. And I didn't even know about the results of the testing at that point. But just looking at the people, seeing how they were changing, seeing what they were now able to do, and seeing how I felt—I believed my own eyes and my own experience.

"Then *I* started feeling so much better. And when I saw the angiograms getting better—not only mine, but also everyone else's results—then it confirmed it even more. Each one made the belief even stronger. The scientific data can help other people to have that confidence, too.

"I don't know if anybody at this point can say, stress reduction is more important, diet is more important, exercise is more important—it's not that meaningful. Because as long as you're doing it all, it doesn't matter what is more important. All that matters to me is that it works.

"Twenty years ago, when I first found out I had a heart problem, they didn't have this information. Dr. Ornish's research convinced me, logically, that heart disease can be reversed. 'These are the people who have done it, these are the reasons, and this is what has happened to their test results. There has been improvement.' If he had done his research twenty years ago, there's no question that I would have followed his program then. And I probably wouldn't have needed a bypass or angioplasty.

"You can't escape the truth of that. I reduced the fat in my diet from 40 percent to 30 percent. And I got worse. I made other changes, but it wasn't enough. I kept getting worse. Now, I'm getting better.

"I feel better physically. I lost a lot of weight. I started exercising. I was never in shape, ever, since I was fifteen years old. Never have I been able to do a lot of exercise. And now I'm capable of doing it. I mean, now I walk up some of the biggest hills in San Francisco without any problems. Before I used to get chest pain just looking at them.

"I feel better emotionally. I have hope, which I didn't have before. And it feels good to have that. Before, I said, 'Well, I have so many years, whatever it is, I sort of accept it.' Now, I really believe that I can live to an old age. I look at my new grandson, who was born just three months ago, and I'm expecting to dance at his wedding one day. That's a very good feeling.

"My relationship with Phyllis has improved a lot. I've been married for forty years and I'm finally learning how to communicate with my wife—and that's very valuable. I still feel like I have a ways to go to improve my communication skills. Because you fall back into old habits all the time. But there's no question that it is much better.

"My wife and I love each other, we have a good relationship, but I used to blow up quite frequently and lose my cool over stupid little things. I think that probably affected my health, too—these violent eruptions due to things that are, when I sit down and look back at them, not really that important. Now I have learned how to communicate better, how to express myself in ways other than blowing up.

"I still feel like I've got a ways to go, but things don't get to me in the same way that they used to. It's much better. I'm not so explosive. I'm not even sure why. I'm aware that it doesn't just improve 100 percent; it improves in degrees.

"My heart disease, which was getting worse every year despite the bypass surgery and angioplasty, now is getting better! The angiogram after less than a year on Dr. Ornish's program showed that my coronary artery blockages were actually beginning to reverse, and the PET scan showed that my heart is getting more blood flow.

"I think it's important that people realize that *they* are in control of their lives. That it's up to them. And there is information around, scientific information, proof, about the mind and body, which a lot of people, including me, didn't accept for a long, long time. Now I do.

"Some of my friends are also investment bankers and very busy people. When they find out what I've been doing, sometimes they say, 'I don't have time for that. I've got deals to do.'

"You don't have to give up making deals—as long as you make some time to take care of yourself. You can make appointments to exercise and do stress management like you make appointments to meet with someone. So I tell them to decide what's important to them: if life is more important or if the deal is more important. It's your choice, as long as you face it realistically. You're in control.

"When you realize that you're in control and you're doing it to yourself—no one else is doing it to you and you can't blame anybody—then it's up to you to decide what's important. Get the facts. Once you've got the facts and if you're an intelligent human being, then it's hard to go back to doing what you did before.

"It surprised me that I've been able to follow [The Opening Your Heart Program] and not cheat. It's very hard to change patterns. But I finally did it. And if I can, then other people can, too."

The Preventive Medicine Research Institute (PMRI) is a nonprofit, tax-exempt public foundation. PMRI, Dr. Ornish, and his colleagues will be offering a variety of resources and educational opportunities.

For information, please write:
PMRI
1001 Bridgeway, Box 305
Sausalito, CA 94965

Appendix
Nutrient Analysis of Common Foods

Food	Unit	Weight (g)	Cal	CHO (g)	Prot (g)	Fat (g)	Sat Fat (g)	Mono Fat (g)	Poly Fat (g)	Chol (mg)	Na (mg)
Almonds: dried, shelled, slivered (not packed)	1 tbsp	7	43	1.4	1.3	3.9	0.3	2.7	0.7	0	tr
Anchovy: 1-4" flat	1 whole	4	5	0	0.8	0.3	0.1	0.1	0.1	5	32
Angel food cake: see Cake											
Apple: raw with skin	1 whole	150	80	20.0	0.3	0.8	0	0	0.8	0	1
Apple: raw, pared, ¼" slices or diced pieces	1 cup	110	59	15.5	0.2	0.3	0	0	0.3	0	1
Apple butter	1 tbsp	18	33	8.2	0.1	0.1	0	0	0.1	0	tr
Apple juice: canned or bottled	1 cup	248	117	29.5	0.2	0	0	0	0	0	2
Applesauce: canned, sweetened	1 cup	255	232	60.7	0.5	0.3	0	0	0.3	0	5
Apricots: raw	3 whole	114	55	13.7	1.1	0.2	0	0	0.2	0	1
Apricot nectar: canned or bottled	1 cup	251	143	36.6	0.8	0.3	0	0	0.3	0	tr
Artichoke: frozen, cooked, bud or globe	1 whole	300	52	11.9	3.4	0.2	0	0	0.2	0	36
Asparagus: canned spears, ½" diameter	4 spears	80	17	2.7	1.9	0.3	0	0	0.3	0	189
Asparagus: canned, cut spears, low sodium	1 cup	235	47	7.3	6.1	0.7	0	0	0.7	0	7
Avocado: California, raw, 3½" diameter (unpeeled)	1 whole	284	369	12.9	4.7	36.7	7.3	16.5	4.8	0	9
Avocado: California, raw, pureed, mashed, or sieved	1 tbsp	14	25	0.9	0.3	2.4	0.5	1.1	0.3	0	1
Bacon: Canadian, cooked, 3⅜ × ³/₁₆"	1 oz	28	78	0.1	7.7	5.0	1.7	1.9	0.4	25	726
Bacon: cooked (approximately 20 slices/lb raw)	2 slices	15	86	0.5	3.8	7.8	2.7	3.4	0.8	11	153
Bacon bits: with coconut oil	1 tsp	3	15	0.9	1.3	0.6	0.6	0	0	0	115
Bacon bits: with soy oil	1 tsp	3	14	0.9	1.4	0.6	0.1	0.2	0.2	0	115
Bagel: water	1 whole	73	212	41.1	7.9	1.3	0.2	0.2	0.3	0	120
Baking powder: double acting	1 tsp	3	3	0.7	0	0	0	0	0	0	290
Baking powder: low sodium	1 tsp	4	7	1.8	0	0	0	0	0	0	tr
Baking soda	¼ tsp	4	0	0	0	0	0	0	0	0	345
Banana, raw, medium	1 whole	175	101	26.4	1.3	0.2	0	0	0.2	0	1

Appendix
Nutrient Analysis of Common Foods (Continued)

Food	Unit	Weight (g)	Cal	CHO (g)	Prot (g)	Fat (g)	Sat Fat (g)	Mono Fat (g)	Poly Fat (g)	Chol (mg)	Na (mg)
Barbecue sauce: commercial (corn oil)	1 tbsp	16	14	1.3	0.2	1.1	0.1	0.3	0.6	0	127
Beans: garbanzos or chick-peas	1 cup	185	248	42.1	14.1	3.3	1.0	0.3	2.0	0	18
Beans: pork and beans in tomato sauce, canned	1 cup	255	311	48.5	15.6	6.6	2.4	2.8	0.6	6	1,181
Beans: kidney	1 cup	185	218	39.6	14.4	0.9	0.3	0.1	0.6	0	6
Beans: lentils	1 cup	200	212	38.6	15.6	0	0	0	0	0	4
Beans: lima, frozen, cooked	1 cup	170	168	32.5	10.2	0.2	0	0	0.1	0	172
Beans: lima, canned	1 cup	170	163	31.1	9.2	0.5	0.2	0	0.3	0	401
Beans: lima, canned, low sodium	1 cup	170	162	30.1	9.9	0.5	0.1	0	0.2	0	7
Beans: pinto, calico, red Mexican	1 cup	185	218	39.6	14.4	0.9	0.3	0.1	0.6	0	6
Beans: mung, sprouts, cooked and drained	1 cup	125	35	6.5	4.0	0.3	0	0	0.3	0	5
Beans: mung, sprouts, uncooked	1 cup	105	37	6.9	4.0	0.2	0	0	0	0	5
Beans: green, snap, fresh, frozen, cooked	1 cup	130	34	7.8	2.1	0.1	0	0	0.1	0	3
Beans: green, snap, canned	1 cup	135	32	7.0	1.9	0.3	0	0	0	0	319
Beans: green, snap, canned, low sodium	1 cup	135	30	6.5	2.0	0.1	0	0	0.1	0	3
Beans: white, Great Northern, navy, cooked	1 cup	180	212	38.2	14.0	1.1	0.3	0.1	0.7	0	13
Beans: yellow or wax, frozen, cooked	1 cup	125	28	5.8	1.8	0.3	0	0	0.3	0	4
Beans: yellow or wax, canned	1 cup	135	32	7.0	1.9	0.4	0	0	0.4	0	319
Beans: yellow or wax, canned, low sodium	1 cup	135	28	6.3	1.6	0.1	0	0	0.1	0	3

This information is current as of this printing. Check the manufacturer's label for updated analysis.

A dash (—) indicates that data are not available. Trace (tr) indicates that a very small amount of the constituent is present.

Abbreviations used in this table are: tbsp = tablespoon; tsp = teaspoon; oz = ounce; lb = pound; gm = gram; mg = milligrams; " = inches; Cal = calories; CHO = carbohydrate; Prot = protein; Sat Fat = saturated fat; Mono Fat = monounsaturated fat; Poly Fat = polyunsaturated fat; Chol = cholesterol; Na = Sodium.

Appendix
Nutrient Analysis of Common Foods

Food	Unit	Weight (g)	Cal	CHO (g)	Prot (g)	Fat (g)	Sat Fat (g)	Mono Fat (g)	Poly Fat (g)	Chol (mg)	Na (mg)
Beef: dried, chipped, uncooked	1 oz	28	58	0	9.7	1.8	0.8	0.8	0	26	1,219
Beef: <6% fat; flank, round (lean only)	1 oz	28	53	0	8.9	1.7	0.9	0.8	0.1	26	19
Beef: 10% fat; chuck, filet mignon, New York strip, porterhouse, T-bone, tenderloin, ground round, choice grade (lean only)	1 oz	28	61	0	8.5	2.7	1.3	1.1	0.1	26	19
Beef: 15% fat; club, rib eye roast (lean only)	1 oz	28	74	0	8.1	4.4	2.2	2.0	0.2	27	18
Beef: 20% fat; ground chuck	1 oz	28	82	0	7.7	5.5	2.9	2.6	0.2	27	16
Beef: 25% fat; ground beef (hamburger), chuck, steak, pot roast (lean and fat)	1 oz	28	93	0	7.4	6.8	3.4	3.1	0.3	27	16
Beef: > 30% fat; brisket, rib eye steak, standing rib roast, spareribs (lean and fat)	1 oz	28	110	0	6.5	9.1	4.8	4.4	0.3	27	15
Beef: corned	1 oz	28	110	0	6.5	9.1	4.8	4.4	0.3	27	264
Beef tongue: medium-fat, cooked, 3 × 2 × 1/8"	1 slice	20	49	0.1	4.3	3.3	1.8	2.0	0.1	18	12
Beef: kidney, cooked, 1/2 × 1/2 × 1/4"	1 oz	140	353	1.1	46.2	16.8	6.6	2.5	2.7	1,126	354
Beef: liver	1 oz	28	40	1.5	5.7	1.1	0.4	0.2	0.2	86	39
Beef tallow: suet	1 tbsp	14	120	0	0.2	13.2	6.8	5.9	0.6	11	0
Beer: regular	12 oz	360	151	13.7	1.1	0	0	0	0	0	25
Beets: red, canned, diced, sliced, or whole	1 cup	170	63	15.0	1.7	0.2	0	0	0.2	0	401
Beets: red, canned, diced, sliced, or whole, low sodium	1 cup	170	63	14.8	1.5	0.2	0	0	0.2	0	78
Biscuit: made with shortening	1 whole	28	103	12.8	2.1	4.8	—	—	—	—	175
Blackberries: raw (also boysenberries, dewberries)	1 cup	144	84	18.6	1.7	1.3	0.3	0.3	0.7	0	1
Bologna: 1 slice	1 oz	28	86	0.3	3.4	8.3	3.4	4.0	0.3	52	287
Bouillon cube: all kinds (1 tsp instant bouillon)	1 cube	4	5	0.2	0.8	0.1	0.1	0	0	0	960
Braunschweiger (liver sausage)	1 oz	28	90	0.7	4.2	9.2	3.1	4.4	1.2	—	287

Appendix
Nutrient Analysis of Common Foods (Continued)

Food	Unit	Weight (g)	Cal	CHO (g)	Prot (g)	Fat (g)	Sat Fat (g)	Mono Fat (g)	Poly Fat (g)	Chol (mg)	Na (mg)
Bread: cracked wheat	1 slice	25	66	13.0	2.2	0.6	0.1	0.2	0.2	0	132
Bread: English muffin	1 whole	57	133	25.5	4.4	1.4	0.4	0.6	0.4	0	263
Bread: French, enriched, 2½ × 2 × ½"	1 slice	15	44	8.3	1.4	0.5	0.1	0.2	0.1	0	87
Bread: pita, pocket	1 large	52	145	30.0	5.0	1.0	0.3	0.4	0.2	0	86
Bread: pumpernickel (dark rye)	1 slice	32	79	17.0	2.9	0.4	0.1	0.2	0.1	0	182
Bread: raisin	1 slice	25	66	13.4	1.7	0.7	0.1	0.3	0.2	0	91
Bread: rye (light)	1 slice	25	61	13.0	2.3	0.3	0.1	0.2	0.1	0	139
Bread: white, enriched	1 slice	25	68	12.6	2.2	0.8	0.2	0.4	0.2	0	127
Bread: whole wheat, firm crumb	1 slice	25	61	11.9	2.6	0.8	0.1	0.3	0.2	0	132
Bread: white, low sodium	1 slice	28	76	14.1	2.4	0.9	0.2	0.4	0.2	0	3
Broccoli: medium stalk, fresh, cooked, and drained	1 stalk	180	47	8.1	5.6	0.5	0	0	0.5	0	18
Brussels sprouts: frozen, cooked, and drained	1 cup	155	51	10.1	5.0	0.3	0	0	0.3	0	22
Butter: 1 pat	1 tsp	5	36	0	0	4.1	2.5	1.2	0.2	12	49
Buttermilk: made from skim milk	1 cup	245	88	12.5	8.8	0.2	0.1	0.1	0	2	319
Buttermilk: made from low-fat milk	1 cup	245	99	11.7	8.1	2.2	1.3	0.6	0.1	9	257
Cabbage: common or Chinese; shredded, cooked, and drained	1 cup	145	29	6.2	1.6	0.3	0	0	0.3	0	20
Cabbage: common or Chinese varieties, raw, shredded	1 cup	90	22	4.9	1.2	0.2	0	0	0.2	0	18
Cake: angel food, 1/12 of 10" tube cake	1 slice	60	161	36.1	4.3	0.1	0.1	0	0.1	0	170
Cake: coffee cake (mix), 2⅝ × 2¾ × 1¼"	1 slice	72	232	37.7	4.5	6.9	2.0	3.2	1.3	35	310
Cake: cream cheese, without crust or topping	1 slice	85	368	25.7	7.6	26.8	6.0	6.0	1.0	163	173
Cake: devil's food (frozen), ⅛ of 7½" cake	1 slice	85	323	47.3	3.7	15.0	7.7	5.4	0.7	37	357
Cake: devil's food cupcake with icing (mix), 2½" diameter	1 whole	35	119	20.4	1.5	4.3	1.8	2.1	0.4	17	92

558

Appendix
Nutrient Analysis of Common Foods (Continued)

Food	Unit	Weight (g)	Cal	CHO (g)	Prot (g)	Fat (g)	Sat Fat (g)	Mono Fat (g)	Poly Fat (g)	Chol (mg)	Na (mg)
Cake: gingerbread (mix), 2¾ × 2¾ × 1⅜"	1 slice	63	174	32.2	2.0	4.3	1.1	2.1	1.0	0.6	192
Cake: marble with white icing (mix), 1/12 of layer cake	1 slice	87	288	53.9	3.8	7.6	4.8	2.1	0.7	40	225
Cake: yellow with chocolate icing (mix), 1/12 of layer cake	1 slice	92	310	53.0	3.8	10.4	4.6	5.5	0.9	44	209
Candy: candy corn, approximately 72 pieces	¼ cup	50	182	44.8	0	1.0	0.3	0.5	0.2	0	106
Candy*: chocolate, bittersweet	1 oz	28	135	13.3	2.2	11.3	6.3	4.2	0.2	5	1
Candy*: chocolate, sweet	1 oz	28	150	16.4	1.2	10.0	5.6	3.7	0.2	5	9
Candy: chocolate covered mint, 1⅜ × ⅜"	1 small	11	45	8.9	0.2	1.2	0.4	0.7	0.1	0.6	20
Candy: chocolate covered raisins	1 cup	190	808	134.0	10.3	32.5	18.1	11.8	0.7	19	122
Candy: chocolate covered vanilla cream	1 piece	13	56	9.1	0.5	2.2	0.8	1.0	0.1	2	24
Candy: fudge, plain, 1 cubic inch	1 piece	21	84	15.8	0.6	2.6	0.9	1.2	0.4	1	44
Candy: gum drops, 1 large or 8 small	1 large	10	34	8.7	0	0.1	0	0	0.1	0	4
Candy: jellybeans	10 pieces	28	104	26.4	0	0.1	0	0	0.5	0	3
Candy: M & M® type	¼ cup	49	230	35.8	2.6	9.7	5.4	3.5	0.2	3	36
Candy: peanut brittle, 2½ × 2½ × ⅓" piece	1 oz	28	119	23.0	1.6	2.9	0.6	1.3	0.9	0	9
Candy: chocolate-flavored roll (Tootsie Roll®) 1 × ½"	1 piece	7	28	5.8	0.2	0.6	0.2	0.3	0.1	1	14
Candy bar*: chocolate coated almonds, or peanut bar (Mr. Goodbar®)	1 oz	28	161	11.2	3.5	12.4	2.1	8.2	1.6	—	17
Candy bar*: chocolate coated with coconut center (Mound®)	1 oz	28	124	20.4	0.8	5.0	2.9	1.9	0	3	56
Candy bar*: fudge, peanut, caramel (O'Henry®, Snicker®, Rally®, Baby Ruth®)	1 oz	28	130	16.6	2.7	6.5	1.8	3.5	1.0	3	36
Candy bar*: Hershey Krackel® or Nestlés Crunch®	1 oz	28	144	15.0	2.3	8.3	4.4	3.1	0.6	3	35

Appendix
Nutrient Analysis of Common Foods (Continued)

Food	Unit	Weight (g)	Cal	CHO (g)	Prot (g)	Fat (g)	Sat Fat (g)	Mono Fat (g)	Poly Fat (g)	Chol (mg)	Na (mg)
Candy bar*: milk chocolate bar or 7 chocolate kisses	1 oz	28	147	16.1	2.2	9.2	5.1	3.3	0.2	5	27
Cantaloupe: 5" diameter	1 whole	91	159	39.8	3.7	0.5	0	0	0.5	0	64
Cantaloupe: cubed or diced, approximately 20/cup	1 cup	160	48	12.0	1.1	0.2	0	0	0.2	0	19
Carbonated beverage: Coca-Cola®	12 oz	369	144	37.2	0	0	0	0	0	0	30
Carbonated beverage: ginger ale	12 oz	366	108	28.8	0	0	0	0	0	0	—
Carbonated beverage: Sprite®	12 oz	366	143	36.0	0	0	0	0	0	0	63
Carbonated beverage: Sprite® without sugar	12 oz	366	5	0	0	0	0	0	0	0	63
Carbonated beverage: Fresca®	12 oz	366	3	0	0	0	0	0	0	0	86
Carbonated beverage: Tab®	12 oz	366	1	0.1	0	0	0	0	0	0	45
Carrot: raw, approximately 1⅛ × 7½"	1 whole	81	30	7.0	0.8	0.1	0	0	0.1	0	34
Carrots: fresh, cooked, sliced	1 cup	155	48	11.0	1.4	0.3	0	0	0.3	0	51
Carrots: canned solids, sliced	1 cup	155	47	10.4	1.2	0.5	0	0	0.5	0	366
Carrots: canned solids, sliced, low sodium	1 cup	155	39	8.7	1.2	0.2	0	0	0.2	0	60
Cashew: roasted in oil, unsalted (14 large, 18 medium, or 26 small)	1 oz	28	159	8.3	4.9	12.8	2.6	7.3	2.1	0	4
Catfish: freshwater, raw	1 oz	28	29	0	5.0	1.0	0.2	0.3	0.3	—	17
Cauliflower: frozen, cooked, approximately 7 florets	1 cup	180	32	5.9	3.4	0.4	0	0	0.4	0	18
Caviar: sturgeon, granular	1 tbsp	16	42	0.5	4.3	2.4	0.6	0.7	1.0	48	352
Celery: green, raw, 8 × 1½" stalk	1 stalk	40	7	1.6	0.4	0	0	0	0	0	50
Cereal: bran, unprocessed, 1.17 cup	1 oz	28	91	12.3	3.9	0.4	0.2	0.2	0.7	0	2
Cereal: bran buds	1 cup	60	144	44.6	7.6	1.8	0.3	0.3	1.1	0	493
Cereal: 40% bran flakes	1 cup	35	106	28.2	3.6	0.6	0.1	0.1	0.3	0	207

*The weight of candy bars often changes. The analysis here is given for 1 ounce and can be calculated for the total unit (1 piece of candy)

Appendix
Nutrient Analysis of Common Foods

Food	Unit	Weight (g)	Cal	CHO (g)	Prot (g)	Fat (g)	Sat Fat (g)	Mono Fat (g)	Poly Fat (g)	Chol (mg)	Na (mg)
Cereal: Cheerios® or puffed oats	1 cup	25	99	18.8	3.0	1.4	0.3	0.5	0.6	0	317
Cereal: corn flakes	1 cup	25	97	21.3	2.0	0.1	0	0	0.1	0	251
Cereal: corn grits, enriched, cooked without salt	1 cup	245	125	27.0	2.9	0.2	0	0	0.1	0	2
Cereal: cream of rice, cooked without salt	1 cup	245	123	27.4	2.0	0	0	0	0	0	2
Cereal: cream of wheat, cooked without salt	1 cup	240	180	40.6	5.3	1.0	0.2	0.1	0.5	0	2
Cereal: farina, enriched, regular, cooked without salt	1 cup	245	103	21.3	3.2	0.5	0.1	0	0.2	0	4
Cereal: farina, enriched, quick-cooking, cooked with salt	1 cup	245	105	21.8	3.2	0.5	0.1	0	0.2	0	466
Cereal: farina, enriched, instant-cooking, cooked without salt	1 cup	245	135	27.9	4.2	0.5	0.1	0	0.2	0	13
Cereal: granola, without coconut or other saturated fat	¼ cup	28	139	16.9	2.9	6.7	5.1	0	0.6	0	30
Cereal: granola, cooked (¼ cup dry = ½ cup cooked)	½ cup	120	100	21.0	3.0	1.0	0.2	0.4	0.4	0	30
Cereal: Grape-Nuts®	1 cup	110	430	92.8	11.0	0.7	0	0	0.7	0	814
Cereal: oatmeal, cooked without salt	1 cup	240	132	23.3	4.8	2.4	0.4	0.8	1.0	0	2
Cereal: puffed rice	1 cup	15	60	13.4	0.9	0.1	0	0	0.1	0	0
Cereal: puffed wheat	1 cup	15	54	11.8	2.3	0.2	0	0	0.2	0	1
Cereal: raisin bran	1 cup	50	144	39.7	4.2	0.7	0.1	0.1	0.4	0	212
Cereal: Rice Krispies®	1 cup	30	117	26.3	1.8	0.1	0	0	0.1	0	283
Cereal: Spoon Size Shredded Wheat®, approximately 50 biscuits per cup	1 cup	50	180	40.0	5.0	1.3	0.2	0.2	0.7	0	2
Cereal: Shredded Wheat® biscuit, 3¾ × 2¼ × 1"	1 whole	25	90	20.0	2.5	0.6	0.1	0.1	0.3	0	1
Cereal: sugar-coated corn flakes	1 cup	40	154	36.5	1.8	0.1	0	0	0.1	0	267
Cereal: Wheat Chex®	⅓ cup	28	110	23.0	2.0	1.0	0.9	0.1	0	0	198

Appendix
Nutrient Analysis of Common Foods (Continued)

Food	Unit	Weight (g)	Cal	CHO (g)	Prot (g)	Fat (g)	Sat Fat (g)	Mono Fat (g)	Poly Fat (g)	Chol (mg)	Na (mg)
Cereal: wheat germ	1 tbsp	6	23	3.0	1.8	0.7	0.1	0.1	0.4	0	1
Cereal: Wheaties® or Total®	1 cup	30	104	24.2	3.1	0.7	0.1	0.1	0.4	0	310
Cheese: American	1 oz	28	106	0.5	6.3	8.9	5.6	2.5	0.3	27	406
Cheese: blue	1 oz	28	100	0.7	6.1	8.2	5.3	2.2	0.2	21	396
Cheese: brick	1 oz	28	105	0.8	6.6	8.4	5.3	2.4	0.2	27	159
Cheese: brie	1 oz	28	95	0.1	5.9	7.9	—	—	—	28	178
Cheese: camembert	1 oz	28	85	0.1	5.6	6.9	4.3	2.0	0.2	20	239
Cheese: cheddar	1 oz	28	114	0.4	7.1	9.4	6.0	2.7	0.3	30	176
Cheese: colby	1 oz	28	112	0.4	6.7	9.1	5.7	2.6	0.3	27	171
Cheese: cottage, creamed (4% fat)	¼ cup	53	54	1.4	6.6	2.4	1.5	0.7	0.1	8	212
Cheese: cottage, low-fat (2% fat)	¼ cup	57	51	2.1	7.8	1.1	0.7	0.3	0	5	230
Cheese: cottage, dry curd	¼ cup	36	31	0.7	6.3	0.2	0.1	0	0	3	5
Cheese: cream cheese, 2 tbsp	1 oz	28	99	0.8	2.1	9.9	6.2	2.8	0.4	31	84
Cheese: edam	1 oz	28	101	0.4	7.1	7.9	5.0	2.3	0.2	25	274
Cheese: feta	1 oz	28	75	1.2	4.0	6.0	4.2	1.3	0.2	25	316
Cheese: gouda	1 oz	28	101	0.6	7.1	7.8	5.0	2.2	0.2	32	232
Cheese: gruyère	1 oz	28	117	0.1	8.5	9.2	5.4	2.9	0.5	31	95
Cheese: monterey	1 oz	28	106	0.2	6.9	8.6	—	—	—	—	152
Cheese: mozzarella, part-skim, low-moisture	1 oz	28	79	0.9	7.8	4.9	3.1	1.4	0.1	15	150
Cheese: mozzarella, whole milk	1 oz	28	80	0.6	5.5	6.1	3.7	1.9	0.2	22	106
Cheese: muenster	1 oz	28	104	0.3	6.6	8.5	5.4	2.5	0.2	27	178
Cheese: neufchatel	1 oz	28	74	0.8	2.8	6.6	4.2	1.9	0.2	22	113
Cheese: parmesan, grated	1 tbsp	5	23	0.2	2.1	1.5	1.0	0.4	0	4	93
Cheese: provolone	1 oz	28	100	0.6	7.3	7.6	4.8	2.1	0.2	20	248

Appendix
Nutrient Analysis of Common Foods (Continued)

Food	Unit	Weight (g)	Cal	CHO (g)	Prot (g)	Fat (g)	Sat Fat (g)	Mono Fat (g)	Poly Fat (g)	Chol (mg)	Na (mg)
Cheese: ricotta, whole milk (13% fat)	¼ cup	62	108	1.9	7.0	8.1	5.2	2.3	0.2	32	52
Cheese: ricotta, part skim milk (8% fat)	¼ cup	62	86	3.2	7.1	4.9	3.1	1.4	0.2	19	77
Cheese: romano	1 oz	28	110	1.0	9.0	7.6	—	—	—	29	340
Cheese: roquefort	1 oz	28	105	0.6	6.1	8.7	5.5	2.4	0.4	26	513
Cheese: Swiss	1 oz	28	95	0.6	7.0	7.1	4.6	2.0	0.2	24	388
Cheese: Velveeta® (cheese spread)	1 oz	28	82	2.5	4.7	6.0	3.8	1.8	0.2	16	381
Cheese: 1% butterfat (Countdown®)	1 oz	28	40	3.6	6.6	0.3	0.2	0.1	0	1	409
Cheese: 4–8% butterfat, processed (Breeze®, Chef's Delight®, Country Club®, Mellow Age®, Tasty®, Lite-Line®, low-fat DI-ET®)	1 oz	28	50	2.8	5.8	1.7	1.1	0.5	0	10	428
Cheese: 5% butterfat, natural (St. Otho)	1 oz	28	49	3.1	9.1	1.1	0.8	0.3	0	10	—
Cheese: 19–32% polyunsaturated fat (Golden®, Image®, Cheez-ola®, Dorman®, Nutrend®, Scandic®, Unique®)	1 oz	28	98	1.1	6.2	7.5	1.5	1.4	4.1	4	330
Cheese: 23% polyunsaturated fat, low sodium (Cheez-ola®)	1 oz	28	90	0.6	6.8	6.3	0.8	1.5	3.6	1	156
Cherries: raw, sweet, unpitted	10 whole	75	47	11.7	0.9	0.2	0	0	0.2	0	1
Cherries: canned, sweet, syrup-packed, pitted	1 cup	257	208	52.7	2.3	0.5	0	0	0.5	0	3
Chicken: gizzard, all classes, cooked, chopped	1 cup	145	215	1.0	39.2	4.8	1.4	1.8	1.2	283	83
Chicken: light meat, no skin	1 oz	28	51	0	9.2	1.4	0.4	0.7	0.3	22	18
Chicken: dark meat, no skin	1 oz	28	52	0	8.3	1.8	0.5	0.6	0.4	26	24
Chicken: dark and light meat, with skin	1 oz	28	70	0	7.7	4.2	1.2	1.4	1.0	25	—
Chicken fat	1 tbsp	14	126	0	0	14.0	4.6	6.4	2.5	9	0
Chicken liver: cooked, whole, 2 × 2 × ⅝"	1 liver	25	41	0.2	6.6	1.1	0.4	0.3	0.2	158	13

Appendix
Nutrient Analysis of Common Foods *(Continued)*

Food	Unit	Weight (g)	Cal	CHO (g)	Prot (g)	Fat (g)	Sat Fat (g)	Mono Fat (g)	Poly Fat (g)	Chol (mg)	Na (mg)
Chick-peas: see *Beans*											
Chocolate: bitter or baking	1 oz	28	143	8.2	3.0	15.0	8.4	5.6	0.3	0	1
Chocolate syrup (or topping): fudge type	2 tbsp	38	124	20.3	1.9	5.1	2.6	1.9	0.2	0	33
Clams: canned solids (chopped or minced)	1 cup	160	143	3.0	25.3	2.4	0.7	0.4	0.9	101	192
Cocoa: dry powder, medium fat, plain	1 tbsp	5	14	2.8	0.9	1.0	0.6	0.4	0	0	tr
Cocoa mix: 1 oz package	1 pkg	28	102	20.1	5.3	0.8	0.6	0.3	0	2	149
Coconut: shredded, fresh, meat only	1 cup	80	277	7.5	2.8	28.2	25.0	1.7	0.5	0	18
Cookie: commercial, chocolate chip, 2¼ × ⅜"	1 cookie	11	50	7.3	0.6	2.2	0.7	0.8	0.5	5	42
Cookie: commercial, fig bar, 1⅝ × 1⅝"	1 cookie	14	50	10.6	0.6	0.8	0.2	0.4	0.2	0	35
Cookie: commercial, gingersnap, 2 × ¼"	1 cookie	7	29	5.6	0.4	0.6	0.2	0.3	0.1	0	40
Cookie: commercial, macaroon, 2¾ × ¼"	1 cookie	19	91	12.5	1.0	4.4	1.9	0.2	0.1	0	7
Cookie: commercial, marshmallow, chocolate-coated, 1¾ × ¾"	1 cookie	13	53	9.4	0.5	1.7	0.9	0.9	0	4	27
Cookie: commercial, oatmeal with raisins, 2⅝ × ¼"	1 cookie	13	59	9.6	0.8	2.0	0.5	1.0	0.5	4	21
Cookie: commercial, peanut butter sandwich, 1¾ × ½"	1 cookie	12	58	8.2	1.2	2.4	0.6	1.2	0.6	5	21
Cookie: commercial, sandwich, round, 1¾ × ⅜"	1 cookie	10	50	6.9	0.5	2.3	0.6	1.1	0.5	5	48
Cookie: commercial, vanilla wafer, 1¾ × ¼"	1 wafer	4	19	2.9	0.2	0.6	0.2	0.3	0.2	1	10
Cookie: prepared mix, brownies, 1¾ × 1¾ × ⅞"	1 piece	20	86	12.6	1.0	4.0	0.8	1.5	1.3	17	33
Cordial: apricot brandy, benedictine, anisette, crème de menthe, or curaçao	4 tsp	20	66	6.3	0	0	0	0	0	0	0
Corn: canned, whole kernel	1 cup	165	139	32.7	4.3	1.3	0.4	0.1	0.7	0	389
Corn: canned, whole kernel, low sodium	1 cup	165	152	29.7	4.1	1.2	0.4	0.1	0.7	0	3

Appendix
Nutrient Analysis of Common Foods *(Continued)*

Food	Unit	Weight (g)	Cal	CHO (g)	Prot (g)	Fat (g)	Sat Fat (g)	Mono Fat (g)	Poly Fat (g)	Chol (mg)	Na (mg)
Corn: canned, cream style, low sodium	1 cup	256	210	47.4	6.7	2.8	0.8	0.3	1.7	0	5
Corn chips: 1½ oz package = 1¼ cups or 60 chips	1¼ cup	43	239	22.7	2.9	15.8	3.8	7.9	3.8	0	240
Corn meal: white and yellow, enriched, degermed	1 cup	138	502	108.2	10.9	1.7	0.5	0.2	1.0	0	1
Corned beef: see *Beef*											
Cornstarch: not packed	1 tbsp	8	29	7.0	0	0	0	0	0	0	tr
Cottage cheese: see *Cheese*											
Crab: fresh, cooked, not packed	1 cup	125	106	0.6	21.6	1.3	0.2	0.2	0.4	125	263
Crab: canned solids, packed	1 cup	160	149	1.8	27.8	2.6	0.4	0.5	0.9	162	1,600
Crackers: animal	10 whole	26	112	20.8	1.7	2.4	0.6	1.2	0.5	16	79
Cracker: graham, chocolate-coated, 2½ × 2 × ¼"	1 whole	13	62	8.8	0.7	3.1	0.9	1.9	0.2	7	53
Crackers: graham, sugar honey, 2 squares, 2½" each	2 whole	14	58	10.8	1.0	1.6	0.4	0.8	0.4	1	72
Cracker: matzo	1 whole	30	118	26.1	3.2	0.3	0	0	0.1	0	10
Crackers: melba toast	3 whole	12	60	9.0	2.0	2.0	0.8	0.9	0.2	0.6	2
Crackers: melba toast, low sodium	3 whole	12	60	9.0	2.0	2.0	0.8	0.9	0.2	0.6	1
Crackers: saltines, single crackers	4 whole	11	48	8.0	1.0	1.3	0.3	0.6	0.3	1	123
Crackers: sandwich, cheese and peanut butter (1 oz pack)	4 whole	28	139	15.9	4.3	6.8	1.8	3.1	1.6	6	281
Crackers: Triscuit®	1 whole	4	21	3.0	0.4	0.8	0.4	0.4	0.1	0	20
Cranberries: raw, chopped	1 cup	110	51	11.9	0.4	0.8	0	0	0.8	0	2
Cranberry juice: cocktail, sweetened	1 cup	253	164	41.7	0.3	0.3	0	0	0.3	0	3
Cranberry sauce: sweetened, canned	1 cup	277	404	103.9	0.3	0.6	0	0	0.6	0	3
Cream: fluid, half and half (11.7% fat)	1 tbsp	15	20	0.7	0.5	1.7	1.1	0.5	0.1	6	6
Cream: fluid, light (20.6% fat)	1 tbsp	15	29	0.6	0.4	2.9	1.8	0.8	0.1	10	6

565

Appendix
Nutrient Analysis of Common Foods *(Continued)*

Food	Unit	Weight (g)	Cal	CHO (g)	Prot (g)	Fat (g)	Sat Fat (g)	Mono Fat (g)	Poly Fat (g)	Chol (mg)	Na (mg)
Cream: fluid, light, whipping (31.3% fat), approximately 2 cups whipped	1 cup	239	699	7.1	5.2	73.9	46.2	21.7	2.1	265	82
Cream: fluid, heavy or whipping (37.6% fat), approximately 2 cups whipped	1 cup	238	821	6.6	4.9	88.1	54.8	25.4	3.3	326	89
Cream: sour	1 tbsp	14	31	0.6	0.5	3.0	1.9	0.9	0.1	6	8
Cream: sour, imitation (IMO®, Wonder®)	1 tbsp	15	26	0.7	0.5	2.4	2.0	0.3	0.1	1	7
Creamer: nondairy, powder, containing saturated fat (Creamora® and Coffee-Mate®)	1 tbsp	6	33	3.3	0.3	2.1	2.1	0	0	0	12
Creamer: nondairy, liquid, containing saturated fat (Coffee Rich®)	1 tbsp	15	20	1.7	0.2	1.5	1.4	0	0	0	12
Creamer: nondairy, liquid, containing polyunsaturated fat (Poly Perx® and Mocha Mix®)	1 tbsp	15	20	1.8	0.1	1.5	0.2	0.7	0.6	0	1
Cucumbers: raw, pared, whole, 2⅛ × 8¼"	1 whole	280	39	9.0	1.7	0.3	0	0	0.3	0	17
Dates: hydrated, without pits	10 whole	80	219	58.3	1.8	0.4	0	0	0.4	0	1
Dessert topping: frozen, semisolid (Cool Whip®)	1 tbsp	4	13	0.9	0.1	1.0	0.9	0.1	0	0	1
Dessert topping: nondairy, pressurized	1 tbsp	4	11	0.6	0	0.9	0.8	0.1	0	0	2
Doughnut: cake type, plain, 1½ × ¾"	1 whole	14	55	7.2	0.6	2.6	0.7	1.3	0.5	7	70
Doughnut: yeast leavened, plain, 3¾ × 1¼"	1 whole	42	176	16.0	2.7	11.3	2.8	5.6	2.5	12	99
Duck: flesh only, raw, domesticated	1 oz	28	47	0	6.1	2.3	0.5	1.1	0.3	21	21
Duck: flesh and skin, raw, domesticated	1 oz	28	92	0	4.5	8.1	1.9	4.1	0.9	—	21
Eclair: custard filling with chocolate, 5 × 2 × 1¾"	1 whole	100	239	23.2	6.2	13.6	4.4	6.2	2.1	145	82
Egg: chicken, fresh, medium	1 whole	50	79	0.6	6.1	5.6	1.7	2.2	0.7	274	69
Egg: chicken, white, fresh	1 white	33	16	0.4	3.4	tr	0	0	0	0	50
Egg: chicken, yolk, fresh	1 yolk	17	63	0	2.8	5.6	1.7	2.2	0.7	272	8

Appendix
Nutrient Analysis of Common Foods (Continued)

Food	Unit	Weight (g)	Cal	CHO (g)	Prot (g)	Fat (g)	Sat Fat (g)	Mono Fat (g)	Poly Fat (g)	Chol (mg)	Na (mg)
Eggnog: commercial	1 cup	254	342	34.4	9.7	19.0	11.3	5.7	0.9	149	138
Egg substitute: Egg Beaters®, 1 egg equivalent	¼ cup	60	40	3.0	7.0	0	0	0	0	0	130
Egg substitute: Second Nature®, 1 egg equivalent	3 tbsp	47	35	0.5	4.7	1.6	0.3	0.6	0.8	0	79
Egg substitute: Lucern®, 1 egg equivalent	¼ cup	60	50	2.0	6.0	2.0	—	—	—	tr	—
Eggplant: cooked, diced	1 cup	200	38	8.2	2.0	0.4	0	0	0.4	0	2
English muffin: see Bread											
Fig: raw, whole, 1½" diameter	1 small	40	32	8.1	0.5	0.1	0	0	0.1	0	1
Fish: see Catfish, Haddock, Halibut, Herring, Snapper, Flounder, Sole											
Fish sticks: breaded, cooked, frozen, 4 × 1 × ½"	1 oz	28	50	1.0	4.7	2.5	0.7	1.0	0.7	17	20
Flounder: raw	1 oz	28	22	0	4.7	0.2	0	0	0.1	14	22
Flour: white, all purpose, enriched, unsifted	1 cup	125	455	95.1	13.1	1.3	0.3	0.1	0.8	0	3
Flour: white, self-rising, enriched, unsifted	1 cup	125	440	92.8	11.6	1.3	0.4	0.1	0.8	0	1,349
Flour: whole wheat	1 cup	120	400	85.2	16.0	2.4	0.7	0.2	1.4	0	4
Frankfurter: 5 × ¾"	1 whole	45	139	0.8	5.6	12.4	4.7	5.9	0.8	27	495
Frosting mix: prepared	1 tbsp	15	61	13.2	0.3	1.5	0.4	0.8	0.1	0	9
Frosting: ready to spread (with animal or vegetable shortening)	1 tbsp	15	55	10.8	0.1	1.6	0.5	0.9	0.2	0	9
Fruit cocktail: canned, solids and liquid, water-packed	1 cup	245	91	23.8	1.0	0.2	0	0	0.2	0	12
Garbanzos: see Beans											
Gelatin: dry, unflavored, 1 envelope	1 pkg	7	23	0	6.0	0	0	0	0	0	0
Gelatin: sweetened dessert powder (JELL-O®), prepared with water, plain	½ cup	120	71	16.9	1.8	0	0	0	0	0	61
Gelatin: low calorie, prepared with water	½ cup	120	8	0	2.0	0	0	0	0	0	8

Appendix
Nutrient Analysis of Common Foods *(Continued)*

Food	Unit	Weight (g)	Cal	CHO (g)	Prot (g)	Fat (g)	Sat Fat (g)	Mono Fat (g)	Poly Fat (g)	Chol (mg)	Na (mg)
Gin: see *Liquor*											
Gizzard: chicken, all classes, cooked, chopped	¼ cup	36	54	0.3	9.8	1.2	0.4	0.5	0.3	71	21
Goose: flesh only, raw	1 oz	28	45	0	6.3	2.0	0.5	0.9	0.2	—	24
Grapes: raw, seedless (Thompson)	10 grapes	50	34	8.7	0.3	0.2	0	0	0.2	0	2
Grape juice: frozen concentrate, sweetened, diluted	1 cup	250	133	33.3	0.5	0	0	0	0	0	3
Grapefruit: all varieties	1 whole	400	80	20.8	1.0	0.2	0	0	0.2	0	2
Grapefruit juice: unsweetened, frozen concentrate, diluted	1 cup	247	101	24.2	1.2	0.2	0	0	0.2	0	2
Greens, collard: frozen: cooked	1 cup	170	51	9.5	4.9	0.7	0	0	0.7	0	27
Haddock: raw	1 oz	28	29	0	6.6	0.1	0	0	0.1	17	17
Halibut: Atlantic or Pacific, broiled	1 oz	28	28	0	5.9	0.3	0.1	0	0.1	14	15
Ham: see *Pork*											
Hamburger: see *Beef*											
Herring: canned, solids and liquid, plain	1 oz	28	59	0	5.6	3.1	0.7	1.6	0.5	24	—
Honey: strained	1 tbsp	21	64	17.3	0.1	0	0	0	0	0	1
Honeydew: 7 × 2″ wedge, ¹⁄₁₀ of melon	1 slice	226	49	11.5	1.2	0.4	0	0	0.4	0	18
Horseradish: prepared	1 tbsp	15	6	1.4	0.2	0	0	0	0	0	14
Ice cream: rich, approximately 16% fat, hardened	1 cup	148	349	32.0	4.1	23.7	14.7	6.8	0.9	88	108
Ice cream: regular, approximately 10% fat, hardened	1 cup	133	269	31.7	4.8	14.3	8.9	4.1	0.5	59	116
Ice cream bar: chocolate-covered (Eskimo Pie)	1 bar	85	270	22.0	2.9	19.1	14.7	2.8	0.5	35	—
Ice cream sandwich: 3 oz size	1 whole	85	238	35.8	4.3	8.5	4.0	2.2	0.4	34	1
Ice cream cone	1 cone	3	11	2.3	0.3	0.1	0	0.1	0	0	—
Ice milk: 5.1% fat, soft serve	1 cup	175	223	38.4	8.0	4.6	2.9	1.3	0.2	13	163
Ice milk: 5.1% fat, hardened	1 cup	131	184	29.0	5.2	5.6	3.5	1.6	0.2	18	105

Appendix
Nutrient Analysis of Common Foods (Continued)

Food	Unit	Weight (g)	Cal	CHO (g)	Prot (g)	Fat (g)	Sat Fat (g)	Mono Fat (g)	Poly Fat (g)	Chol (mg)	Na (mg)
Instant breakfast: dry powder, all flavors except eggnog	1¼ oz	36	130	23.4	7.2	0.9	0.5	0.3	0.1	4	tr
Jelly: sweetened	1 tbsp	18	49	12.7	0	0	0	0	0	0	3
Knockwurst link: 4 × 1⅛"	1 link	68	165	1.5	9.6	18.5	6.8	8.8	1.8	42	748
Ladyfingers	1 whole	11	40	7.1	0.9	0.9	0.3	0.4	0.1	39	8
Lamb: <7% fat, chop, leg, roast, sirloin chop (lean only)	1 oz	28	53	0	8.2	2.0	0.9	0.8	0.1	28	15
Lamb: 10% fat, shank, shoulder (lean only)	1 oz	28	58	0	7.6	2.8	1.4	1.2	0.2	28	15
Lamb: 20% fat, leg, roast, sirloin chop (lean and fat)	1 oz	28	79	0	7.2	5.4	2.8	2.4	0.4	28	14
Lamb: 30% fat, breast, chop, rib (lean and fat)	1 oz	28	96	0	6.2	7.7	3.6	3.1	0.4	28	14
Lard	1 tbsp	13	117	0	0	12.8	5.1	5.7	1.5	12	0
Lemon: raw, 1 wedge (⅛ of 2⅛" lemon)	1 slice	18	3	1.0	0.1	0	0	0	0	0	0
Lemon juice: canned, unsweetened	1 tbsp	15	4	1.2	0.1	tr	0	0	tr	0	tr
Lemonade: concentrate, frozen, diluted	1 cup	248	88	22.9	0.2	0	0	0	0	0	0
Lentils: see Beans											
Lettuce: raw, crisp head varieties, chopped or shredded	1 cup	55	7	1.6	0.5	0.1	0	0	0.1	0	5
Liquor: gin, rum, vodka, whiskey	1 oz	28	70	0	0	0	0	0	0	0	0
Liver: see Beef or Chicken											
Lobster: northern, cooked, ½" cubes	1 cup	145	138	0.4	27.1	1.5	0.2	0.2	0.5	123	305
Luncheon meal: see Salami, Bologna, Braunschweiger, Sausage, Turkey											
Macadamia nuts: 15 whole nuts	1 oz	28	196	4.5	2.2	20.3	3.1	16.3	0.6	0	—
Macaroni: enriched, cooked, hot	1 cup	140	155	32.2	4.8	0.6	0	0.3	0.3	0	1

Appendix
Nutrient Analysis of Common Foods *(Continued)*

Food	Unit	Weight (g)	Cal	CHO (g)	Prot (g)	Fat (g)	Sat Fat (g)	Mono Fat (g)	Poly Fat (g)	Chol (mg)	Na (mg)
Mackerel: canned, solids and liquids	¼ cup	35	64	0	7.5	3.5	0.9	1.3	0.8	33	148
Mango: raw	1 whole	300	152	38.8	1.6	0.9	0	0	0.9	0	16
Margarine: P/S > 3.1 (Promise® soft, Parkay® soft safflower, Hains® soft, Saffola® soft)	1 tbsp	14	102	0.1	0.1	11.5	1.5	3.5	6.3	0	140
Margarine: P/S 2.6 to 3.0 (Mrs. Filbert's® soft corn oil, Promise® stick, Parkay® liquid squeeze)	1 tbsp	14	102	0.1	0.1	11.5	1.7	4.6	4.9	0	140
Margarine: P/S 2.0 to 2.5 (Fleischmann's® soft, Chiffon® soft, Parkay® corn oil soft)	1 tbsp	14	102	0.1	0.1	11.5	2.1	4.1	5.0	0	110
Margarine: P/S 1.6 to 1.9 (Fleischmann's® stick, Chiffon® stick, Meadow Gold® stick)	1 tbsp	14	102	0.1	0.1	11.5	2.1	5.0	3.6	0	110
Margarine: P/S 1.0 to 1.5 (Mazola® stick, Parkay® corn oil stick, Imperial® stick)	1 tbsp	14	100	0.1	0.1	11.3	2.0	5.1	4.0	0	115
Margarine: low sodium, P/S 1.7 (Fleischmann's®, Mazola®)	1 tbsp	14	100	0.1	0.1	11.2	2.1	5.0	3.6	0	tr
Margarine: P/S < 0.5, all vegetable fat (Kraft® all purpose stick, Swift® all purpose stick)	1 tbsp	14	102	0.1	0.1	11.5	2.2	7.5	1.5	0	140
Margarine: P/S < 0.5, vegetable and animal or all animal (Gaylord® stick, Meadowlake® stick)	1 tbsp	14	102	0.1	0.1	11.5	4.7	5.6	1.0	0	140
Margarine: P/S 2.4, (diet tub Fleischmann's® soft, Imperial® soft)	1 tbsp	14	50	0.1	0	5.6	1.0	2.1	2.4	0	135
Mellorine	1 cup	131	244	30.8	5.9	11.1	9.5	0.6	0.2	18	105
Milk: skim (less than 1% fat)	1 cup	245	86	11.9	8.4	0.4	0.3	0.1	0	4	126
Milk: low fat (1% to 2% fat)	1 cup	244	102	11.7	8.0	2.6	1.6	0.8	0.1	10	123
Milk: whole (3.3% fat)	1 cup	244	150	11.4	8.0	8.2	5.1	2.4	0.3	33	120

Appendix
Nutrient Analysis of Common Foods (*Continued*)

Food	Unit	Weight (g)	Cal	CHO (g)	Prot (g)	Fat (g)	Sat Fat (g)	Mono Fat (g)	Poly Fat (g)	Chol (mg)	Na (mg)
Milk: canned, evaporated, whole	1 cup	252	338	25.3	17.2	19.1	11.6	5.9	0.6	74	267
Milk: canned, evaporated, skim	1 cup	256	200	29.0	19.4	0.6	0.4	0.2	0	10	294
Milk: nonfat, dry powder, approximately 1 cup reconstituted	⅓ cup	23	81	11.8	8.0	0.2	0.1	0	0	4	124
Milk: canned, condensed, sweetened	1 cup	306	982	166.2	24.2	26.6	16.8	7.4	1.0	104	389
Milk: chocolate drink, fluid, commercial, made with whole milk	1 cup	250	213	27.5	8.5	8.5	5.3	2.5	0.3	30	118
Milk: low sodium (whole)	1 cup	244	149	10.9	7.6	8.4	5.3	2.4	0.3	33	6
Milkshake: chocolate	11 oz	311	369	65.9	9.5	8.4	5.2	2.4	0.3	33	346
Milkshake: vanilla	11 oz	313	350	55.6	12.1	9.5	5.9	2.7	0.4	37	299
Molasses: light	1 tbsp	21	52	13.3	0	0	0	0	0	0	3
Mushrooms: raw, sliced, chopped, or diced	1 cup	70	20	3.1	1.9	0.2	0	0	0.2	0	11
Mustard: prepared, yellow	1 tsp	5	4	0.3	0.2	0.2	0	0	0.2	0	63
Nectarine: raw, 2½" diameter	1 whole	150	88	23.6	0.8					0	8
Noodles: egg, enriched, cooked	1 cup	160	200	37.3	6.6	2.4	0.8	1.1	0.2	50	3
Noodles: chow mein, canned	1 cup	45	220	26.1	5.9	10.6	2.8	4.3	2.9	5	—
Oil: coconut	1 tbsp	14	120	0	0	13.6	11.7	0.8	0.2	0	0
Oil: cod liver	1 tbsp	14	120	0	0	13.6	2.4	7.0	3.5	—	0
Oil: corn	1 tbsp	14	120	0	0	13.6	1.7	3.4	7.9	0	0
Oil: cottonseed	1 tbsp	14	120	0	0	13.6	3.6	2.6	6.9	0	0
Oil: olive	1 tbsp	14	119	0	0	13.5	1.9	9.8	1.2	0	0
Oil: palm kernel	1 tbsp	14	120	0	0	13.6	11.1	1.6	0.2	0	0
Oil: peanut	1 tbsp	14	119	0	0	13.5	2.6	6.2	4.1	0	0
Oil: safflower	1 tbsp	14	120	0	0	13.6	1.3	1.7	10.0	0	0

Appendix
Nutrient Analysis of Common Foods (Continued)

Food	Unit	Weight (g)	Cal	CHO (g)	Prot (g)	Fat (g)	Sat Fat (g)	Mono Fat (g)	Poly Fat (g)	Chol (mg)	Na (mg)
Oil: soybean	1 tbsp	14	120	0	0	13.6	2.0	3.1	7.8	0	0
Oil: soybean-cottonseed blend	1 tbsp	14	120	0	0	13.6	2.2	3.1	7.7	0	0
Oil: sunflower	1 tbsp	14	120	0	0	13.6	1.4	2.8	8.7	0	0
Okra: frozen, cooked, cuts	1 cup	185	70	16.3	4.1	0.2	0	0	0.2	0	4
Olives: ripe, whole, extra large	10 whole	55	61	1.2	0.5	6.5	0.7	5.0	0.5	0	385
Olives: green, whole, large	10 whole	46	45	0.5	0.5	4.9	0.5	3.7	0.3	0	926
Onions: green, raw, 4⅛ × ⅝"	2 med	30	14	3.2	0.3	0.1	0	0	0.1	0	2
Onions: mature, raw, chopped	1 cup	170	65	14.8	2.6	0.2	0	0	0.2	0	17
Onions: mature, cooked, whole or sliced	1 cup	210	61	13.7	2.5	0.2	0	0	0.2	0	15
Orange: Florida, medium, 2¹¹/₁₆" diameter	1 whole	204	71	18.1	1.1	0.3	0	0	0.3	0	2
Orange juice: concentrate, frozen, unsweetened, diluted	1 cup	249	122	28.9	1.7	0.2	0	0	0.2	0	2
Oysters: canned, 18 to 27 medium or 27 to 44 small	12 oz	340	224	11.6	28.6	6.1	1.8	0.7	2.0	170	248
Oysters: raw, 13 to 19 medium or 19 to 31 small	1 cup	240	158	8.2	20.2	4.3	1.2	0.5	1.4	120	175
Pancake: made from mix, 6 × ½"	1 cake	73	164	23.7	5.3	5.3	—	—	—	—	412
Peach: raw, pared, 2¾" diameter, approximately 2½ per lb	1 whole	175	51	12.9	0.8	0.1	0	0	0.1	0	1
Peaches: canned, syrup packed, halves, slices, or chunks	1 cup	256	200	51.5	1.0	0.3	0	0	0.3	0	5
Peanut butter	1 cup	258	1,520	48.5	65.0	130.5	27.1	60.7	39.0	0	1,561
Peanuts: roasted, salted, 10 Virginia, 20 Spanish, or 1 tbsp chopped	10 nuts	9	53	1.7	2.3	4.5	0.8	2.1	1.3	0	38
Pear: raw, Bartletts, 2½ × 3½"	1 whole	180	100	25.1	1.1	0.7	0	0	0.7	0	3
Pear: canned, syrup-packed, with 1⅔ tbsp liquid	1 half	76	58	14.9	0.2	0.2	0	0	0.2	0	1
Pear nectar: canned	1 cup	250	130	33.0	0.8	0.5	0	0	0.5	0	3

Appendix
Nutrient Analysis of Common Foods (Continued)

Food	Unit	Weight (g)	Cal	CHO (g)	Prot (g)	Fat (g)	Sat Fat (g)	Mono Fat (g)	Poly Fat (g)	Chol (mg)	Na (mg)
Peas: cow or black-eyed, canned, cooked	1 cup	255	179	31.6	12.8	0.8	0.2	0	0.3	0	602
Peas: green, immature, canned solids	1 cup	170	150	28.6	8.0	0.7	0	0.4	0.7	0	401
Peas: green, immature, canned solids, low sodium	1 cup	170	122	22.1	7.5	0.7	0	0.4	0.7	0	5
Pecans: chopped or pieces	1 tbsp	7	51	1.1	0.7	5.2	0.5	3.1	1.3	0	tr
Pepper: immature, green, raw, 3¾ × 3"	1 whole	200	36	7.9	2.0	0.3	0	0	0.3	0	21
Pepper: jalapeño, canned	1 whole	18	5	1.1	0.2	0	0	0	0	0	72
Pepper: jalapeño, fresh	1 whole	18	7	1.6	0.2	0	0	0	0	0	5
Pheasant: flesh only, raw	1 oz	28	46	0	6.7	1.9	0.5	0.8	0.2	—	
Pickle: dill or sour, large, 4 × 1¾"	1 whole	135	15	3.0	0.9	0.3	0	0	0.3	0	1,928
Pickle: dill or sour, 3¾ × 1¼", low sodium	1 whole	65	7	1.4	0.5	0.1	0	0	0.1	0	4
Pickles: fresh, sweetened (bread and butter), 1½ × ¼"	2 slices	15	11	2.7	0.1	0	0	0	0	0	101
Pickle: sweet, gherkins, large, 3 × 1"	1 whole	35	51	12.8	0.2	0.1	0	0	0.1	0	500
Pickle relish: finely chopped, sweet	1 tbsp	15	21	5.1	0.1	0.1	0	0	0.1	0	107
Pie: frozen, baked, apple, 8" diameter	1 pie	550	1,386	219.0	10.6	54.8	13.6	27.3	12.2	0	1,168
Pie: frozen, baked, cherry, 8" diameter	1 pie	580	1,690	257.4	12.5	70.0	17.4	34.8	15.6	0	1,333
Pie: mix, baked, coconut custard (eggs and milk), 8" diameter	1 pie	797	1,618	231.9	34.3	63.0	27.1	31.1	8.0	837	1,873
Pineapple: raw, diced pieces	1 cup	155	81	21.2	0.6	0.3	0	0	0.3	0	2
Pineapple: canned, syrup-packed, chunk, tidbit, or crushed	1 cup	255	189	49.5	0.8	0.3	0	0	0.3	0	3
Pineapple: canned, water-packed, tidbits	1 cup	246	96	25.1	0.7	0.2	0	0	0.2	0	2
Pineapple: in its own juice (no sugar added), 4 slices with juice or 1 cup with juice	1 cup	227	140	35.0	1.0	1.0	0	0	1.0	0	2

Appendix
Nutrient Analysis of Common Foods *(Continued)*

Food	Unit	Weight (g)	Cal	CHO (g)	Prot (g)	Fat (g)	Sat Fat (g)	Mono Fat (g)	Poly Fat (g)	Chol (mg)	Na (mg)
Pineapple juice: canned, unsweetened	1 cup	250	138	33.8	1.0	0.3	0	0	0.3	0	3
Plum: hybrid, fresh, 2⅛" diameter	1 whole	70	32	8.1	0.3	0.1	0	0	0.1	0	1
Plums: canned, served with 2¾ tbsp syrup	3 whole	140	110	28.7	0.5	0.1	0	0	0.1	0	1
Popcorn: no salt or fat added to popped corn	1 cup	6	23	4.6	0.8	0.3	0	0.1	0.2	0	tr
Pork: fresh, 10% fat, ham or picnic ham (lean only)	1 oz	28	61	0	8.4	2.8	0.9	1.2	0.3	25	18
Pork: fresh, 13–20% fat, Boston butt roast, chop, loin, shoulder (lean only)	1 oz	28	71	0	8.0	3.9	1.6	2.1	0.5	25	20
Pork: fresh, 23–30% fat, Boston butt, ground pork, ham, loin picnic, shoulder (lean and fat)	1 oz	28	103	0	6.6	8.3	2.9	3.8	0.9	25	16
Pork: spareribs, 37% fat (lean and fat)	1 oz	28	125	0	5.9	11.0	3.8	5.1	1.2	25	10
Pork: cured, 7–10% fat, ham or picnic ham (lean only)	1 oz	28	56	0	7.6	2.7	0.9	1.1	0.2	25	273
Pork: cured, 13–20% fat, Boston butt, shoulder (lean only)	1 oz	28	75	0	6.9	5.1	1.8	2.4	0.6	25	247
Pork: cured, 23–30% fat, ham, picnic, shoulder (lean and fat)	1 oz	28	93	0	6.4	7.2	2.5	3.4	0.8	25	230
Pork: deviled ham, canned	¼ cup	56	198	0	7.8	18.2	6.4	8.5	2.0	35	703
Potato chips	10 chips	20	114	10.0	1.1	8.0	2.0	1.7	4.0	0	200
Potatoes: fresh, boiled, diced, or sliced	1 cup	155	101	22.5	2.9	0.2	0	0	0.2	0	3
Potato: fresh, baked in skin, 2⅓ × 4¾"	1 whole	202	145	32.8	4.0	0.2	0	0	0.2	0	6
Potato: frozen, french fried, 4" strips (oven-heated)	10 strips	78	172	26.3	2.8	6.6	1.6	1.4	3.3	0	3
Potato, sweet: fresh, baked, 5 × 2"	1 whole	146	161	37.0	2.4	0.6	0	0	0.6	0	14
Potatoes, sweet: pieces, canned in syrup	1 cup	200	216	49.8	4.0	0.4	0	0	0.4	0	96
Pretzels: extruded type, rods, 7½ × ½"	1 whole	14	55	10.6	1.4	0.6	0.2	0.4	0.1	0	235

Appendix
Nutrient Analysis of Common Foods (Continued)

Food	Unit	Weight (g)	Cal	CHO (g)	Prot (g)	Fat (g)	Sat Fat (g)	Mono Fat (g)	Poly Fat (g)	Chol (mg)	Na (mg)
Pretzels: twisted type, rings (3), 1⅞ × 1¾ × ¼"	10 whole	30	117	22.8	2.9	1.4	0.3	0.8	0.2	0	504
Prunes: dried, uncooked, without pits	10 whole	102	260	68.7	2.1	0.6	0	0	0.6	0	8
Prunes: dried, cooked, no added sugar	1 cup	250	253	66.7	2.1	0.6	0	0	0.6	0	9
Prune juice: canned or bottled	1 cup	256	197	48.6	1.0	0.3	0	0	0.3	0	5
Pudding mix: chocolate, regular, prepared with whole milk	1 cup	260	322	59.3	8.8	7.8	4.3	2.6	0.2	36	335
Pudding mix: chocolate, instant, prepared with whole milk	1 cup	260	325	63.4	7.8	6.5	3.6	2.2	0.3	36	322
Pudding mix: low calorie, dry form, 1 package (all kinds)	4 oz	128	100	24.0	0	0	0	0	0	0	280
Pumpkin: canned	1 cup	245	81	19.4	2.5	0.7	0	0	0.7	0	5
Quail: flesh and skin, raw	1 oz	28	48	0	7.2	2.0	0.5	0.9	0.5	—	11
Raisins: natural, seedless, uncooked, whole, not packed	1 tbsp	9	26	7.0	0.2	tr	0	0	tr	0	2
Raspberries: raw, red	1 cup	123	70	16.7	1.5	0.6	0	0	0.6	0	1
Rhubarb: frozen, sweetened	1 cup	270	381	97.2	1.4	0.3	0	0	0.3	0	5
Rice: brown, cooked without salt	1 cup	195	232	49.7	4.9	1.2	0.3	0.3	0.6	0	5
Rice: white, enriched, cooked without salt	1 cup	205	221	49.6	4.1	0.4	0.1	0.1	0.1	0	5
Roll: hard, enriched	1 roll	25	78	14.9	2.5	0.8	0.2	0.4	0.2	0	157
Roll: soft, enriched, brown and serve, or Parker House	1 roll	28	83	14.8	2.3	1.6	0.4	0.7	0.4	0	142
Roll: enriched, hotdog (6 × 2") or hamburger (3½ × 1½")	1 whole	40	119	21.2	3.3	2.2	0.5	1.1	0.5	0	202
Rum: see Liquor											
Salad dressing: blue or roquefort	1 tbsp	15	76	1.1	0.7	8.0	1.6	1.8	3.8	10	164

Appendix

Nutrient Analysis of Common Foods *(Continued)*

Food	Unit	Weight (g)	Cal	CHO (g)	Prot (g)	Fat (g)	Sat Fat (g)	Mono Fat (g)	Poly Fat (g)	Chol (mg)	Na (mg)
Salad dressing: blue or roquefort, low calorie	1 tbsp	16	12	0.7	0.5	0.9	0.5	0.3	0	1	177
Salad dressing: French	1 tbsp	16	66	2.8	0.1	6.2	1.1	1.3	3.2	0	219
Salad dressing: French, low calorie	1 tbsp	16	15	2.5	0.1	0.7	0.1	0.1	0.4	0	126
Salad dressing: Italian	1 tbsp	15	83	1.0	tr	9.0	1.5	1.9	4.6	0	314
Salad dressing: Italian, low calorie	1 tbsp	15	8	0.4	tr	0.7	0.1	0.2	0.4	0	118
Salad dressing: mayonnaise	1 tbsp	15	101	0.3	0.2	11.2	2.0	2.4	5.5	9	84
Salad dressing: mayonnaise, low sodium	1 tbsp	14	99	0.3	0.2	11.0	2.0	2.4	5.5	9	2
Salad dressing: mayonnaise type (Miracle Whip®)	1 tbsp	15	65	2.2	0.2	6.3	1.1	1.4	3.1	7	88
Salad dressing: mayonnaise type, low calorie	1 tbsp	16	22	0.8	0.2	2.0	0.4	0.4	1.0	0	19
Salad dressing: Russian	1 tbsp	15	74	1.6	0.2	7.6	1.4	1.7	3.9	7	130
Salad dressing: Thousand Island	1 tbsp	16	80	2.5	0.1	8.0	1.4	1.7	3.9	7	112
Salad dressing: Thousand Island, low calorie	1 tbsp	15	27	2.3	0.1	2.1	0.4	0.5	1.1	0	105
Salami: cooked, 4½" diameter slice	1 oz	28	73	0.4	5.0	5.8	2.1	2.7	0.6	15	297
Salmon: fresh, broiled or baked, no added fat	1 oz	28	48	0	7.7	1.6	0.5	0.8	0.1	10	33
Salmon: canned, drained, pink	1 oz	28	49	0	5.7	1.9	0.2	0.3	1.0	10	135
Salmon: smoked (Lox)	1 oz	28	50	0	6.1	2.6	0.5	0.8	0.1	10	135
Salt: table	1 tsp	6	0	0	0	0	0	0	0	0	2,196
Salt pork	1 oz	28	219	0	1.1	24.0	8.5	11.3	2.7	20	340
Sandwich spread: with chopped pickle	1 tbsp	15	58	2.4	0.1	5.5	1.1	1.4	3.1	8	96
Sandwich spread: low calorie	1 tbsp	15	17	1.2	0.2	1.4	0.3	0.3	0.8	0	94
Sardine: canned in oil, 3 × 1 × ½"	1 whole	12	24	0	2.9	1.3	0.4	0.4	0.4	17	99
Sauerkraut: canned, solids and liquid	1 cup	235	42	9.4	2.4	0.5	0	0	0.5	0	1,755
Sausage, Polish: 5⅝ × 1"	1 link	76	231	0.9	11.9	19.6	6.9	9.1	1.7	47	836
Sausage, pork: 4 × ⅞" (uncooked)	1 link	13	49	0	2.4	4.2	1.5	2.0	0.5	8	125

Appendix
Nutrient Analysis of Common Foods *(Continued)*

Food	Unit	Weight (g)	Cal	CHO (g)	Prot (g)	Fat (g)	Sat Fat (g)	Mono Fat (g)	Poly Fat (g)	Chol (mg)	Na (mg)
Sausage, Vienna: canned, 2 × ⅞" diameter	1 whole	16	56	0	2.2	5.2	1.8	2.5	0.6	10	157
Scallops: fresh, cooked, steamed	1 oz	28	32	—	6.6	0.3	0	0	0.1	15	75
Sesame seeds: dry, hulled	1 tbsp	8	47	1.4	1.5	4.4	0.6	1.6	1.8	0	—
Sherbet: orange	1 cup	193	270	58.7	2.2	3.8	2.4	1.1	0.1	14	88
Shortening: animal	1 tbsp	13	111	0	0	12.5	6.3	5.5	0.8	10	0
Shortening: animal-vegetable	1 tbsp	13	111	0	0	12.5	5.6	5.5	1.1	6	0
Shortening: vegetable	1 tbsp	13	111	0	0	12.5	3.3	5.8	3.5	0	0
Shrimp: 4½ oz can drained	1 cup	128	148	0.8	31.0	1.5	0.2	0.2	0.6	192	—
Shrimp: canned, approximately 2" long (small)	10 whole	17	20	0.1	4.1	0.2	0	0	0.1	26	81
Shrimp: fresh, cooked, 8 shrimp, each 3¼" long	2 oz	58	67	0.4	14.0	0.7	0.1	0.1	0.3	87	19
Snapper: red or gray, raw	1 oz	28	26	0	5.6	0.3	0.1	0.1	0.1	—	22
Sole: raw	1 oz	28	22	0	4.7	0.2	0	0	0.1	—	22
Soup: canned, bean with pork, prepared with equal volume of water	1 cup	250	170	21.8	8.0	6.0	1.5	2.2	1.8	4	1,008
Soup: canned, beef broth, prepared with equal volume of water	1 cup	240	31	2.6	5.0	0	0	0	0	0	782
Soup: canned, cream of celery, prepared with equal volume of water	1 cup	240	86	8.9	1.7	5.5	1.4	1.2	2.4	7	955
Soup: canned, cream of chicken, prepared with equal volume of water	1 cup	240	94	7.9	2.9	5.8	2.0	3.2	1.4	8	970
Soup: canned, cream of mushroom, prepared with equal volume of water	1 cup	240	132	10.1	2.4	9.4	2.5	1.8	4.4	6	955
Soup: canned, chicken noodle, prepared with equal volume of water	1 cup	240	67	7.9	3.4	2.4	0.6	1.0	0.5	6	979

Appendix
Nutrient Analysis of Common Foods (*Continued*)

Food	Unit	Weight (g)	Cal	CHO (g)	Prot (g)	Fat (g)	Sat Fat (g)	Mono Fat (g)	Poly Fat (g)	Chol (mg)	Na (mg)
Soup: canned, clam chowder, Manhattan style, prepared with equal volume of water	1 cup	245	78	12.3	2.2	2.2	0.4	0.4	1.3	6	938
Soup: canned, minestrone, prepared with equal volume of water	1 cup	245	105	14.2	4.9	2.7	0.6	0.7	1.2	2	995
Soup: canned, onion, prepared with equal volume of water	1 cup	240	65	5.3	5.3	2.4	0.8	1.0	0.6	6	1,051
Soup: canned, split pea, prepared with equal volume of water	1 cup	245	145	20.6	8.6	3.2	1.0	1.5	0.3	6	941
Soup: canned, tomato, prepared with equal volume of water	1 cup	245	88	15.7	2.0	2.0	0.4	0.4	0.9	2	970
Soup: canned, vegetable beef, prepared with equal volume of water	1 cup	245	89	9.6	5.3	3.4	0.8	0.9	1.6	6	1,046
Soup: canned, vegetarian vegetable, prepared with equal volume of water	1 cup	245	80	13.2	2.2	2.2	0.5	0.6	0.9	2	838
Soup: dehydrated, onion, 1 package	1½ oz	43	150	23.2	6.0	4.6	1.0	2.0	1.0	0	2,871
Sour cream: see *Cream*											
Soy sauce	1 tbsp	18	12	1.7	1.0	0.2	0	0	0.2	0	1,319
Soybeans: mature seeds, cooked	1 cup	180	234	19.4	19.8	10.3	1.5	2.1	5.3	0	4
Soybean curd (tofu): 2½ × 2¾ × 1"	1 piece	120	86	2.9	9.4	5.0	0.8	1.0	2.6	0	8
Soybean seeds: sprouted, raw	1 cup	105	48	5.6	6.5	1.5	0.5	0.1	0.9	0	—
Soybean seeds: sprouted, cooked	1 cup	125	48	4.6	6.6	1.8	0.5	0.2	1.1	0	—
Spaghetti: enriched, cooked without salt	1 cup	140	155	32.2	4.8	0.6	0	0	0.6	0	1
Spaghetti with meat balls and tomato sauce: canned, rings	1 cup	250	258	28.5	12.3	10.3	2.2	3.3	3.9	39	1,220

Appendix
Nutrient Analysis of Common Foods (Continued)

Food	Unit	Weight (g)	Cal	CHO (g)	Prot (g)	Fat (g)	Sat Fat (g)	Mono Fat (g)	Poly Fat (g)	Chol (mg)	Na (mg)
Spinach: frozen, cooked	1 cup	205	47	7.6	6.2	0.6	0	0	0.6	0	107
Spinach: canned, low sodium	1 cup	205	53	8.2	6.6	1.0	0.3	0.1	0.6	0	66
Squash, summer: fresh, cooked, sliced	1 cup	180	25	5.6	1.6	0.2	0	0	0.2	0	2
Squash, winter: frozen, cooked	1 cup	240	91	22.1	2.9	0.7	0	0	0.7	0	2
Steak: see Beef											
Stew: beef and vegetable, canned	1 cup	245	194	17.4	14.2	7.6	3.2	3.1	0.2	36	1,007
Strawberries: fresh, whole	1 cup	149	55	12.5	1.0	0.7	0	0	0.7	0	1
Sugar: brown, packed	1 cup	220	821	212.1	0	0	0	0	0	0	66
Sugar: granulated	1 tbsp	12	46	11.9	0	0	0	0	0	0	tr
Sugar: powdered (confectioners'), unsifted	1 tbsp	8	31	8.0	0	0	0	0	0	0	tr
Sunflower seed kernels: dry, hulled	1 tbsp	9	51	1.8	2.2	4.3	0.5	0.9	2.7	0	3
Sweet roll: Danish pastry, without nuts or fruit, 4½ × 1"	1 whole	65	274	29.6	4.8	15.3	4.5	7.1	2.8	17	238
Sweetbreads (thymus), beef	1 oz	28	90	0	7.3	6.6	—	—	—	132	99
Syrup: cane and maple	1 tbsp	20	50	12.8	0	0	0	0	0	0	tr
Taco shell: fried tortilla	1 whole	30	146	19.7	2.6	5.6	1.5	2.3	1.5	0	tr
Tangerine: large, 2½" diameter	1 whole	136	46	11.7	0.8	0.2	0	0	0.2	0	2
Tapioca: dry	1 tbsp	10	33	8.2	0.1	tr	0	0	tr	0	tr
Tartar sauce	1 tbsp	14	76	0.6	0.2	8.3	1.0	2.1	4.1	7	102
Tofu: see Soybean curd											
Tomatoes: canned, solids and liquid	1 cup	241	51	10.4	2.4	0.5	0	0	0.5	0	313
Tomatoes: fresh, raw, 3 × 2⅛" high (tomato = 6 slices)	1 whole	200	40	8.6	2.0	0.4	0	0	0.4	0	5
Tomatoes: fresh, cooked	1 cup	241	63	13.3	3.1	0.5	0	0	0.5	0	10

Appendix
Nutrient Analysis of Common Foods (Continued)

Food	Unit	Weight (g)	Cal	CHO (g)	Prot (g)	Fat (g)	Sat Fat (g)	Mono Fat (g)	Poly Fat (g)	Chol (mg)	Na (mg)
Tomatoes: canned, solids and liquid, low sodium	1 cup	241	48	10.1	2.4	0.5	0	0	0.5	0	7
Tomato catsup: canned or bottled	1 cup	273	289	69.3	5.5	1.1	0	0	1.1	0	2,845
Tomato chili sauce: bottled	1 cup	273	284	67.7	6.8	0.8	0	0	0.8	0	3,653
Tomato juice: canned or bottled	1 cup	243	46	10.4	2.2	0.2	0	0	0.2	0	486
Tomato juice: canned or bottled, low sodium	1 cup	242	46	10.4	1.9	0.2	0	0	0.2	0	7
Tomato paste: canned	1 cup	262	215	48.7	8.9	1.0	0.3	0.1	0.6	0	100
Tomato paste: low sodium	1 cup	262	215	48.7	8.9	1.0	0.3	0.1	0.6	0	40
Tomato sauce	1 cup	240	80	18.0	3.0	0	0	0	0	0	882
Tomato sauce: low sodium	1 cup	240	80	18.0	3.0	0	0	0	0	0	13
Tortilla: corn, 6" diameter	1 whole	30	70	13.4	1.6	0.6	0	0	0	0	tr
Tortilla: flour	1 whole	30	108	22.4	2.9	1.2	0.6	0.8	0.3	0	120
Tuna: water-packed, canned, chunk style, solids and liquid, low sodium	6½ oz	184	234	0	51.5	1.5	0.4	0.3	0.4	115	75
Tuna: oil-packed, canned (drained), 1 cup	4½ oz	127	295	0	46.1	10.9	3.6	2.8	2.9	104	1,280
Turkey: light meat, without skin	1 oz	28	45	0	9.3	0.7	0.2	0.2	0.2	22	23
Turkey: dark meat, without skin	1 oz	28	48	0	8.5	1.5	0.4	0.4	0.4	29	28
Turkey: light and dark with skin	1 oz	28	63	0	9.0	2.9	0.8	1.0	0.8	30	—
Turkey bologna or franks	1 oz	28	71	2.1	3.5	5.4	2.4	2.1	0.9	37	336
Turkey ham	1 oz	28	40	0.5	5.5	1.5	0.4	0.4	0.4	28	280
Turkey pastrami	1 oz	28	34	0.8	5.2	1.6	0.4	0.4	0.4	29	525
Turkey salami: with skin	1 oz	28	50	0.5	4.6	3.6	0.8	1.0	0.8	26	454
Turnip greens: frozen, chopped, cooked	1 cup	165	38	6.4	4.1	0.5	0	0	0.5	0	28
Turnips: fresh, cooked, cubes	1 cup	155	36	7.6	1.2	0.3	0	0	0.3	0	53

Appendix
Nutrient Analysis of Common Foods *(Continued)*

Food	Unit	Weight (g)	Cal	CHO (g)	Prot (g)	Fat (g)	Sat Fat (g)	Mono Fat (g)	Poly Fat (g)	Chol (mg)	Na (mg)
Veal: <6% fat, breast riblet, cutlet, leg, loin, rump, shank, shoulder steak (lean only)	1 oz	28	40	0	5.7	1.7	0.9	0.8	0.1	28	16
Veal: 10% fat, cutlet, leg, rump, shank, shoulder, steak (lean and fat)	1 oz	28	61	0	8.2	3.0	1.4	1.3	0.2	28	13
Veal: 15% fat, loin (lean and fat)	1 oz	28	67	0	7.5	3.8	1.8	1.6	0.2	29	13
Veal: 20% fat, rib (lean and fat)	1 oz	28	86	0	7.4	6.0	3.2	2.9	0.3	29	14
Veal: 25% fat, breast riblet (lean and fat)	1 oz	28	89	0	4.7	7.7	3.6	3.1	0.4	29	14
Vodka: see *Liquor*											
Vinegar: cider	1 cup	240	34	14.2	0	0	0	0	0	0	2
Waffle: made from mix, 7 × 5/8"	1 waffle	75	206	27.2	6.6	8.0	—	—	3.1	—	515
Walnuts: English, chopped pieces	1 tbsp	8	49	1.2	1.1	4.8	0.5	0.7	3.1	0	tr
Water chestnuts	4 nuts	25	20	4.8	0.4	0.1	0	0	0.1	0	5
Watermelon: diced pieces	1 cup	160	42	10.2	0.8	0.3	0	0	0.3	0	2
Watermelon: 10 × 1" wedge, or 4" arc × 8" radius	1 slice	926	111	27.3	2.1	0.9	0	0	0.9	0	4
Whiskey: see *Liquor*											
Weiner: 5 × 3/4"	1 whole	45	139	0.8	5.6	12.4	4.7	5.9	0.8	27	495
Wine: dessert (port, madeira, sweet sherry)	1 oz	30	41	2.3	0	0	0	0	0	0	1
Wine: table (burgundy, rosé, white, dry sherry)	1 oz	29	25	1.2	0	0	0	0	0	0	1
Worcestershire sauce	1 tbsp	15	6	1.4	0.1	0	0	0	0	0	267
Yeast: bakers, dry package, scant tbsp	¼ oz	7	20	2.7	2.6	0.1	0	0	0.1	0	4
Yogurt: skim, home recipe	1 cup	227	127	17.4	13.0	0.4	0.3	0.1	0	4	174
Yogurt: plain, low fat	1 cup	227	144	16.0	11.9	3.5	2.3	1.0	0.1	14	159
Yogurt: whole milk	1 cup	227	139	10.6	7.9	7.4	4.8	2.0	0.2	29	105
Yogurt: with fruit (1–2% fat)	1 cup	227	225	42.3	9.0	2.6	1.7	0.7	0.1	10	121
Yogurt: frozen (2% fat)	1 cup	227	244	48.0	6.0	3.0	1.9	0.7	0.1	10	121

"No one but the author is interested in a long list of references stuck onto the end of an article like barnacles on a ship's bottom."

—Editor, *New England Journal of Medicine,* 1964

■

"There is an accuracy that defeats itself by the overemphasis of details. I often say that one must permit oneself, and quite advisedly and deliberately, a certain margin of misstatement."

—Benjamin Cardozo [1870–1938]

■

"First have something to say, second say it, third stop when you have said it, and finally give it an accurate title."

—John Shaw Billings [1838–1913]

Selected
References

INTRODUCTION

Sontag S. *Illness as Metaphor.* New York: Farrar, Straus, 1978.

Wagner J. *The Search for Signs of Intelligent Life in the Universe.* New York: Harper and Row, 1986.

1. "WHY DON'T YOU DO SOMETHING MORE CONVENTIONAL?"

Achterberg J. *Imagery in Healing.* Boston: New Science Library, 1985.

Armstrong ML, Warner Ed, Connor WE. "Regression of coronary atheromatosis in rhesus monkeys." *Circ Res.* 1970;27:59.

Arntzenius AC. "Regression of atherosclerosis." Presented at the Second International Conference on Preventive Cardiology, Washington, D.C., June 1989.

Arntzenius AC, Kromhout D, Barth JD, et al. "Diet, lipoproteins, and the progression of coronary atherosclerosis." *N Engl J Med.* 1985;312:805–11.

Barndt R. Blankenhorn DH, Crawford DW, et al. "Regression and progression of early femoral atherosclerosis in treated hyperlipoproteinemic patients." *Ann Int Med.* 1977;86:139–46.

Bassler TJ. " 'Regression' of atheroma." *Western J Med.* 1980;132:474–75.

Basta LL, Williams C, Kioschos JM. "Regression of atherosclerotic stenosing lesions of the renal arteries and spontaneous cure of systemic hypertension through control of hyperlipidemia." *Amer J Med.* 1976;61:420–23.

Benson H: "Systemic hypertension and the relaxation response." *N Engl J Med.* 1977;296:1152–56.

Blankenhorn DH, Johnson RL, El Zein HA, et al. "Dietary fat influences human coronary lesion formation." *Circulation.* 1988;78(suppl II):11.

Blankenhorn DH, Johnson RL, Mack WJ, et al. "The influence of diet on the appearance of new lesions in human coronary arteries." *JAMA.* 1990;263:1646–52.

Blankenhorn DH, Kramsch DM. "Reversal of atherosis and sclerosis. The two components of atherosclerosis." *Circulation.* 1989;79:1–15.

Blankenhorn DH, Nessim SA, Johnson RL, et al. "Beneficial effects of combined colestipol-niacin therapy on coronary atherosclerosis and coronary venous bypass grafts." *JAMA.* 1987;257:3233–40.

Bond MG, Adams MR, Bullock BC. "Complicating factors in evaluating coronary artery atherosclerosis." *Artery.* 1981;9:21–29.

Brand RJ, Paffenbarger RS, Sholtz RI, et al. "Work activity and fatal heart attack studied by multiple logistic risk analysis." *Am J Epidemiol.* 1979;110:52–62.

Brown BG, Bolson EL, Dodge HT. "Arteriographic assessment of coronary atherosclerosis. Review of current methods, their limitations, and clinical applications." *Arteriosclerosis.* 1982;2:2–15.

Brown BG, Lin JT, Schaefer SM, et al. "Niacin or lovastatin, combined with colestipol, regress coronary atherosclerosis and prevent clinical events in men with elevated apolipoprotein B." *Circulation* 1989;80(4):II-266.

Brunzell JD, Austin MA. "Plasma triglyceride levels and coronary disease," *N Engl J Med.* 1989;320:1273–74.

Cousins N. *The Healing Heart.* New York: Avon Books, 1983.

Daoud AS, et al. "Regression of advanced atherosclerosis in swine." *Arch Pathol Lab Med.* 1976;100:372.

Demer LL, Kirkeeide RL, Haynie MP, Wallschlaeger EA, Holmes RL, Elson BM, Ornish DM, Gould KL. "Feasibility of following progression or regression of coronary artery stenosis by positron emission tomography during dipyridamole-hand grip stress." Presented at the American Heart Association 60th Scientific Sessions, Anaheim, 1987.

DePalma RG, Klein L. Bellon EM, et al. "Regression of atherosclerotic plaques in rhesus monkeys." *Arch Surg.* 1980;115:1268.

Dimsdale JE, Herd JA. "Variability of plasma lipids in response to emotional arousal." *Psychosomatic Medicine.* 1982;44:413–30.

Duffield RGM et al. "Treatment of hyperlipidemia retards progression of symptomatic femoral atherosclerosis." *Lancet.* 1983;2:639.

Eliot RS. "Lessons learned and future directions." *Am Heart J.* 1988;116:682–86.

Eliot RS and Breo DL. *Is It Worth Dying For?* New York: Bantam Books, 1986.

Farrar DJ, Green HD, Wagner WD, et al. "Reduction in pulse wave velocity and improvement of aortic distensibility accompanying regression of atherosclerosis in the rhesus monkey." *Circ Res.* 1980; 47:425.

Friedman M, Thoresen CE, Gill JJ, et al. "Feasibility of altering Type A behavior pattern after myocardial infarction." *Circulation.* 1982;66:83–91.

Froelicher V, Jensen D, Genter F, et al. "A randomized trial of exercise training in patients with coronary heart disease." *JAMA.* 1984;252(10):1291–97.

Froelicher V, Jensen D, Sullivan M. "A randomized trial of the effects of exercise training after coronary artery bypass surgery." *Arch Intern Med.* 1985 145(4):689–92.

Glagov S, Weisenberg E, Zarins CK, et al. "Compensatory enlargement of human atherosclerotic coronary arteries." *N Engl J Med.* 1987;316:1371–75.

Gould KL, Kirkeeide RL, Ornish DM, et al. "Improvement of stenosis geometry by quantitative coronary arteriography after adequate cholesterol lowering in man." *Circulation.* 1989;80(4):II-102.

Hackett TP, Rosenbaum JF. "Emotion, psychiatric disorders, and the heart." In: Braunwald, E, ed. *Heart Disease.* Philadelphia: W.B. Saunders, 1980: 1923–43.

Haft JI. "Role of blood platelets in coronary artery disease." *Amer J Cardiol.* 1979; 43:1197–1206.

Harvey W. *Exercitatio de motu cordis et sanguinis.* Cited in Eastwood MR, Trevelyan H. "Stress and coronary heart disease." *J Psychosom Res.* 1971;15:289–92.

Hjermann I, Velve Byre K, et al. "Effect of diet and smoking intervention on the incidence of coronary heart disease." *Lancet.* 1981;1303–10.

Kannel WB. "Contribution of the Framingham study to preventive cardiology: the Bishop lecture." *JACC.* 1990;15:206–11.

Kaplan JR, Manuck SB, Clarkson TB, et al. "Social stress and atherosclerosis in normocholesterolemic monkeys." *Science.* 1983;220(4598):733–35.

Kempner W. "Treatment of hypertensive vascular disease with rice diet." *Arch Intern Med.* 1974;133(5):758–90.

Kramer JR, Kitazume H, Proudfit WL, Matsuda Y, Williams GW, & Sones FM: "Progression and regression of coronary atherosclerosis: Relation to risk factors." *Am Heart J.* 1983;105:134–44.

Kramsch DM, Aspen AJ, Abramowitz BM et al. "Reduction of coronary atherosclerosis by moderate conditioning exercise in monkeys on an atherogenic diet." *NEJM.* 1981;305:1483–89.

Lawrence RS et al. *Report of the U.S. Preventive Services Task Force: Guide to Clinical Preventive Services.* U.S. Department of Health and Human Services, Public Health Service, Washington, D.C., Government Printing Office, 1989.

Lazare A. "Shame and humiliation in the medical encounter." *Arch Int Med.* 1987;147:1653–58.

Leon AS, Connett J, Jacobs DR, & Rauramaa R. "Leisure-time physical activity levels and risk of coronary heart disease and death: The Multiple Risk Factor Intervention Trial." *JAMA.* 1987;258:2388–95.

Levy RI, Brensike JF, Epstein SE, et al. "The influence of changes in lipid values induced by cholestyramine and diet on progression of coronary artery disease: results of the NHLBI Type II Coronary Intervention Study." *Circulation.* 1984;69:325–37.

Malinow MR. "Atherosclerosis: regression in nonhuman primates." *Circ Res.* 1980;46:311.

Malinow MR. "Regression of atherosclerosis in humans: fact or myth?" *Circulation.* 1981;64:1–3.

Moncada S, Vane JR. "Arachidonic acid metabolites and the interactions between platelets and blood vessel walls." *N Engl J Med.* 1979; 300:1142–47.

Morrison LM and Schjeide OA. *Arteriosclerosis: Prevention, Treatment, and Regression.* Springfield, Ill.: C.C. Thomas, 1984.

"Multiple Risk factor intervention trial." *JAMA.* 1982;248:1465–77.

Nash DT et al. "Regression of coronary artery lesions during lipid lowering therapy, demonstrated by scheduled serial arteriography." *Int J. Cardiol.* 1983;3: 257–60.

Nerem RM, Levesque MJ, Cornhill JF, et al. "Social environment as a factor in diet-induced atherosclerosis." *Science.* 1980;208:1475.

Oliva PB. "Pathophysiology of acute myocardial infarction, 1981." *Ann Intern Med.* 1981; 94:236–50.

Ornish DM. "Mind/heart interactions: for better and for worse." *Health Values.* 1978;2:266–69.

Ornish DM. *Stress, Diet, & Your Heart.* New York: Holt, Rinehart and Winston, 1982; New American Library (Signet Books), 1983.

Ornish DM. "Stress and coronary heart disease: new concepts." In *For Your Health,* ed. Carlson RJ and Newman B. New York: C.V. Mosby, 1987.

Ornish DM, Brown SE, Scherwitz LW, et al. "Can lifestyle changes reverse coronary atherosclerosis?" Presented at the Second International Conference on Preventive Cardiology and the 29th Annual Meeting of the American Heart Association Council on Epidemiology, Washington, D.C., 1989.

Ornish DM, Brown SE, Scherwitz LW, et al. "Can lifestyle changes reverse coronary heart disease? The Lifestyle Heart Trial." *Lancet* (in press).

Ornish DM, Gotto AM, Miller RR, et al. "Effects of a vegetarian diet and selected yoga techniques in the treatment of coronary heart disease." *Clinical Research.* 1979;27:720A.

Ornish DM, Scherwitz LW, Brown SE, et al. "Adherence to lifestyle changes and reversal of coronary atherosclerosis." *Circulation.* 1989;80(4):II-57.

Ornish DM, Scherwitz LW, Brown SE, et al. "Can lifestyle changes reverse atherosclerosis?" *Circulation.* 1988;78(4):II-11.

Ornish DM, Scherwitz LW, Brown SE, et al. "Effects of lifestyle changes on lipids, lipoproteins, and apolipoproteins." Presented at the Society of Behavioral Medicine's 9th Annual Scientific Session, Boston, 1988.

Ornish DM, Scherwitz LW, Brown SE, et al. "The Lifestyle Heart Trial: design, methods, and selected baseline results." *Clinical Trials* (in press).

Ornish DM, Scherwitz LW, Doody RS, et al. "Effects of stress management training and dietary changes in treating ischemic heart disease." *JAMA.* 1983; 249:54–59.

Ornish DM, Scherwitz LW, Doody RS, et al. "Effects of stress management training and dietary changes in treating ischemic heart disease." Presented at the 31st Annual Scientific Session of the American College of Cardiology, Atlanta, 1982.

Patel C, Marmot MG, Terry DJ, Carruthers M, Hunt B, & Patel M. "Trial of relaxation in reducing coronary risk: Four-year follow-up." *Br Med J.* 1985;290: 1103–1106.

Roth D, Kostuk WJ. "Noninvasive and invasive demonstration of spontaneous regression of coronary artery disease." *Circulation.* 1980;62:888–96.

Sacks FM, Castelli WP, Donner A, Kass EH. "Plasma lipids and lipoproteins in vegetarians and controls." *N Engl J Med.* 19751 292:1148–51.

Sacks FM, Ornish DM, Rosner B, et al. "Consumption of coffee and fatty acids predict blood pressure levels in vegetarians." Presented at the American Heart Association 56th Scientific Sessions, Dallas, 1983.

Sacks FM, Ornish DM, Rosner B, McLanahan S, Castelli WP, and Kass EH. "Dietary predictors of blood pressure and plasma lipoproteins in lactovegetarians." *JAMA.* 1985;254:1337–41.

Scherwitz L, Graham LE, Ornish DM. "Self-involvement and the risk factors for coronary heart disease." *Advances.* 1985;2:6–18.

Scherwitz LW, Ornish DM, Brown SE, et al. "The effects of lifestyle changes on psychosocial risk factors." Presented at the Society of Behavioral Medicine's 10th Annual Scientific Session, San Francisco, 1989.

Schiffer F, Hartley LH, Schulman CL, Abelmann WH. "Evidence for emotionally induced coronary arterial spasm in patients with angina pectoris." *Br Heart J.* 1980;44:62–66.

Schuler G, Schlierf G, Wirth A, et al. "Low-fat diet and regular, supervised physical exercise in patients with symptomatic coronary artery disease: reduction of stress-induced myocardial ischemia." *Circulation.* 1988;77(1):172–81.

Seravalli EP. "The dying patient, the physician, and the fear of death." *N Engl J Med.* 1988;319:1728–30.

Shekelle RB, Shyrock AM, Paul O, et al. "Diet, serum cholesterol, and death from coronary heart disease: The Western Electric Study." *N Engl J Med.* 1981; 304:65–70.

Siegel B. *Love, Medicine, and Miracles.* New York: Harper & Row, 1986.

Simonton C and Simonton SM. *Getting Well Again.* New York: Bantam, 1982.

Small DM. "Progression and regression of atherosclerotic lesions." *Arteriosclerosis.* 1988;8(2):103–29.

Stuart MJ, Gerrard JM, White JG. "Effects of cholesterol on production of thromboxane B_2 by platelets in vitro." *N Engl J Med.* 1980; 302:6–10.

"The lipid research clinics' coronary primary prevention trial results." *JAMA.* 1984;251:351–64.

Wissler RW. "Evidence for regression of advanced atherosclerotic plaques." *Artery.* 1979;5:398.

Zelis R, Mason DT, Braunwald EG, Levy RI. "Effects of hyperlipoproteinemias and their treatment on the peripheral circulation." *JCI.* 1970;49:1007.

Zmuda A, Dembinska-Kiec A, Chytkowski A, Gryglewski RJ. "Experimental atherosclerosis in rabbits." *Prostaglandins.* 1977; 14:1035–43.

3. "YES, THAT'S TRUE, BUT WHAT IS THE CAUSE?"

Adams MR, Kaplan JR, Koritnik DR, et al. "Erectile failure in cynomolgus monkeys with atherosclerosis of the arteries supplying the penis." *J Urol.* 1984;-131(3),571–73.

Arnold G, Kaiser C, Fischer R. "Myofibrillar degeneration—a common type of myocardial lesion and its selective identification by a modified luxol fast blue stain." *Pathol Res Pract.* 1985;180(4):405–15.

Arntzenius AC. "Can atherogenesis be slowed, stopped, or reversed? Human studies." Presented at the 2nd International Conference on Preventive Cardiology, June 19, 1989, Washington, D.C.

Ascher EK, Stauffer JC, Gaasch WH. "Coronary artery spasm, cardiac arrest, transient electrocardiographic Q waves and stunned myocardium in cocaine-associated acute myocardial infarction." *Am J Cardiol.* 1988;61(11):939–41.

Benfante R, Reed D. "Is elevated serum cholesterol a risk factor for coronary heart disease in the elderly?" *JAMA.* 1990;263:393–96.

Benson H, McCallie DP. "Angina pectoris and the placebo effect." *N Engl J Med.* 1979;300:1424–29.

Berenson GS, Srinivasan SR, Nicklas TA, Webber LS. "Cardiovascular risk factors in children and early prevention of heart disease." *Clin Chem.* 1988;34(8B):B115–22.

Brensike JF, Levy RI, et al. "Effects of therapy with cholestyramine on progression of coronary arteriosclerosis: results of the NHLBI Type II coronary intervention study." *Circulation.* 1984;69:313–24.

Brett AS. "Treating hypercholesterolemia: how should practicing physicians interpret the published data for patients?" *N Engl J Med.* 1989;321:676–80.

Brodsky MA, Sato DA, Iseri LT, et al. Ventricular tachyarrhythmia associated with psychological stress. The role of the sympathetic nervous system." *JAMA.* 1987;257(15):2064–67.

Burke GL, Cresanta JL, Shear CL, et al. "Cardiovascular risk factors and their modification in children." *Cardiol-Clin.* 1986;4(1):33–46.

Clarkson TB, Kaplan JR, Adams MR, Manuck SB. "Psychosocial influences on the pathogenesis of atherosclerosis among nonhuman primates." *Circulation.* 1987;76(1 Pt 2):I29–40.

Cleeman JI, Lenfant C. "New guidelines for the treatment of high blood cholesterol in adults from the National Cholesterol Education Program." *Circulation.* 1987;76:960–62.

Croft JB, Cresanta JL, Webber LS, et al. "Cardiovascular risk in parents of children with extreme lipoprotein cholesterol levels: the Bogalusa Heart Study." *South Med J.* 1988;81(3):341–49, 353.

Cutler JA, MacMahon SW, Furberg CD. "Controlled clinical trials of drug treatment for hypertension." *Hypertension.* 1989;13(suppl I):I-36–I-44.

Deanfield JE, Selwyn AP. "Character and causes of transient myocardial ischemia during daily life. Implications for treatment of patients with coronary disease." *Am J Med.* 1986;80(4C):18–24.

Deanfield JE, Shea M, Kensett M, et al. "Silent myocardial ischaemia due to mental stress." *Lancet.* 1984;2(8410):1001–1005.

Feldman RL. "Coronary thrombosis, coronary spasm, and coronary arthero-sclerosis and speculation on the link between unstable angina and acute myocardial infarction." *Am J Cardiol.* 1987;59:1187–98.

Ferguson T. "A conversation with Ken Pelletier." *Medical Self-Care.* 1979; 5:3–9.

Goldstein JL, Brown MS. "Cholesterol and cardiovascular disease: regulation of low-density lipoprotein receptors: implications for pathogenesis and therapy of hypercholesterolemia and atherosclerosis." *Circulation.* 1987;76:504–507.

Gotto AM Jr., Bierman EL, Connor WE, et al. "Recommendations for treat-ment of hyperlipidemia in adults: a joint statement of the Nutrition Committee and the Council on Arteriosclerosis." *Circulation.* 1984;69:1065A–1090A.

Graboys TB. "Celtics fever: playoff-induced ventricular arrhythmia [letter]." *N Engl J Med.* 1981;305(8):467–68.

Graboys TB, Headley A, Lown B, et al. "Results of a second-opinions program for coronary artery bypass graft surgery." *JAMA.* 1987;258(12):1611–14.

Harrison DG, Armstrong ML, Freiman PC, et al. "Restoration of endothe-lium-dependent relaxation by dietary treatment of atherosclerosis." *J Clin Investig.* 1987;80(6),1808–11.

Hennekens CH et al. "Final report on the aspirin component of the ongoing physicians' health study." *N Engl J Med.* 1989;321:129–35.

Kaplan JR, Manuck SB, Clarkson TB, et al. "Social status, environment, and atherosclerosis in cynomolgus monkeys." *Arteriosclerosis.* 1982;2(5):359–68.

Kaplan NM. "Misdiagnosis of systemic hypertension and recommendations for improvement." *Am J Cardiol.* 1987;60:1383–85.

Keys AB. *Seven Countries: A Multivariate Analysis of Death and Coronary Heart Disease.* Cambridge, Mass.: Harvard University Press, 1980.

Langford HG. "Nonpharmacological therapy of hypertension. Commentary on diet and blood pressure." *Hypertension.* 1989;13:I98–102.

Lapin BA, Cherkovich GM, Iakovleva LA. [The experimental production of cardiovascular diseases in monkeys]. "Eksperimental'noe vosproizvedenie na obez'ianakh zabolevanii serdechno-sosudistoi sistemy." *Vestn Akad Med Nauk SSSR.* 1966;21(4):73–81.

Leaf A. "Management of hypercholesterolemia." *N Engl J Med.* 1989;321: 680–83.

Liang B, Verrier RL, Melman J, Lown B. "Correlation between circulating catecholamine levels and ventricular vulnerability during psychological stress in conscious dogs." *Proc Soc Exp Biol Med.* 1979;161(3):266–69.

Lown B. "Neural and psychologic factors in sudden death." *Verh Dtsch Ges Herz Kreislaufforsch,* 1980;46:28–37.

Lown B. "Sudden cardiac death: biobehavioral perspective." *Circulation.* 1987;76(1 Pt 2):I186–96.

Lown B, DeSilva RA, Reich P, Murawski BJ. "Psychophysiologic factors in sudden cardiac death." *Am J Psychiatry.* 1980;137(11):1325–35.

Lown B. "Higher nervous activity and sudden cardiac death." *Bull Mem Acad R Med Belg.* 1980;135(8):487–505.

Manuck SB, Kaplan JR, Clarkson TB. "Social instability and coronary artery atherosclerosis in cynomolgus monkeys." *Neurosci Biobehav Rev.* 1983;7(4):485–91.

Manuck SB, Kaplan JR, Adams MR, Clarkson TB. "Effects of stress and the sympathetic nervous system on coronary artery atherosclerosis in the cynomologus macaque." *Am Heart J.* 1988;116(1 Pt 2), 328–33.

Marzilli M, Goldstein S, Trivella MG, et al. "Some clinical considerations regarding the relation of coronary vasospasm to coronary artherosclerosis: a hypothetical pathogenesis." *Am J Cardiol.* 1980;45(4):882–86.

Maseri A. "Louis F. Bishop lecture. Role of coronary artery spasm in symptomatic and silent myocardial ischemia." *J Am Coll Cardiol.* 1987;9(2):249–62.

Maseri A, Chierchia S. "Coronary artery spasm: demonstration, definition, diagnosis, and consequences." *Prog Cardiovasc Dis.* 1982;25(3):169–92.

Maseri A, L'Abbate A, Chierchia S, et al. "Significance of spasm in the pathogenesis of ischemic heart disease." *Am J Cardiol.* 1979;44(5):788–92.

Morley JE, Korenman SG, Kaiser FE, et al. "Relationship of penile brachial pressure index to myocardial infarction and cerebrovascular accidents in older men." *Am J Med.* 1988;84:445–48.

Multiple Risk Factor Intervention Trial Research Group. "Mortality rates after 10.5 years for participants in the Multiple Risk Factor Intervention Trial." *JAMA.* 1990;263:1795–1801.

Phillips DP, Smith DG. "Postponement of death until symbolically meaningful occasions." *JAMA.* 1990;263:1947–51.

Rozanski A, Bairey N, et al. "Mental stress and the induction of silent myocardial ischemia in patients with coronary artery disease." *N Engl J Med.* 1988;318:1005–12.

Samuels MA. "Neurogenic heart disease: a unifying hypothesis." *Am J Cardiol.* 1987;60(18):15J–19J.

Schachne JS, Roberts BH, Thompson PD. "Coronary-artery spasms and myocardial infarction associated with cocaine use [letter]." *N Engl J Med.* 1984;310(25):1665–66.

Schnall PL, Pieper C, Schwartz JE, et al. "The relationship between 'job strain,' workplace diastolic blood pressure, and left ventricular mass index." *JAMA.* 1990;263:1929–35.

Selwyn AP, Shea MJ, Deanfield JE, et al. "Clinical problems in coronary disease are caused by wide variety of ischemic episodes that affect patients out of hospital." *Am J Med.* 1985;79(3A):12–17.

Sempos C, Fulwood R, Haines C, et al. "The prevalence of high blood cholesterol levels among adults in the United States." *JAMA.* 1989;262(1):45–52.

Shepherd RFJ, Vanhoutte PM. "Mechanisms of coronary artery spasm." *Cardio.* May 1987, p. 46–48.

Sibai AM, Haroutune KA, Alam S. "Wartime determinants of arteriographically confirmed coronary artery disease in Beirut." *Am J Epid.* 1989;130:623–31.

Skinner JE, Beder SD, Entman ML. "Psychological stress activates phosphorylase in the heart of the conscious pig without increasing heart rate and blood pressure." *Proc Natl Acad Sci USA.* 1983;80(14):4513–17.

Skinner JE, Lie JT, Entman ML. "Modification of ventricular fibrillation latency following coronary artery occlusion in the conscious pig." *Circulation.* 1975;51(4):656–67.

Strandberg T, Naukkarinen V, Salomaa, et al. "Factors related to increased incidence of coronary heart disease by multifactorial prevention measures." *JAMA.* 1985;254:2097. Also presented at the Second International Conference on Preventive Cardiology, June 1989, Washington, D.C.

Stuart EM, Caudill M, Leserman J, Borrington C, Friedman R, Benson-H. "Nonpharmacologic treatment of hypertension: a multiple-risk-factor approach." *J. Cardiovasc Nurs.* 1987;1(4):1–14.

Tazelaar HD, Karch SB, Stephens BG, Billingham ME. "Cocaine and the heart." *Hum Pathol.* 1987;18(2):195–99.

Tomoike H, Egashira K, Yamamoto Y, Nakamura M. "Enhanced responsiveness of smooth muscle, impaired endothelium-dependent relaxation and the genesis of coronary spasm." *Am J Cardiol.* 1989;63(10):33E–39E.

Varnauskas E and the European Coronary Surgery Study Group. "Twelve year follow-up of survival in the randomized European coronary surgery study." *N Engl J Med.* 1988;319:332–37.

Verrier RL, Lown B. "Autonomic nervous system and malignant cardiac arrhythmias." *Res Publ Assoc Res Nerv Ment Dis.* 1981;59:273–91.

Verrier RL, Lown B. "Behavioral stress and cardiac arrhythmias." *Annu Rev Physiol.* 1984;46:155–76.

Verrier RL, Lown B. "Experimental studies of psychophysiological factors in sudden cardiac death." *Acta Med Scand Suppl.* 1982;660:57–68.

Verrier RL, Lown B. "Myocardial perfusion and neurally induced cardiac arrhythmias." *Ann NY Acad Sci.* 1984;427:171–86.

Verrier RL, Lown B. "Neural influences and sudden cardiac death." *Adv Cardiol.* 1978;25:155–68.

Virag R, Bouilly P, Frydman D, et al. "Is impotence an arterial disorder?" *Lancet.* 1985;1:181–84.

Williams RB. "The role of the brain in physical disease: folklore, normal science, or paradigm shift?" *JAMA.* 1990:263:1971–2.

Zimmerman FH, Gustafson GM, Kemp HG Jr. "Recurrent myocardial infarction associated with cocaine abuse in a young man with normal coronary arteries: evidence for coronary artery spasm culminating in thrombosis." *J Am Coll Cardiol.* 1987;9(4):964–68.

4. LIFESTYLE CHANGES OF THE RICH AND FAMOUS

Berkman LF, Syme SL. "Social networks, host resistance, and mortality: a nine year follow up study of Alameda County residents." *Am J Epidemiol.* 1979; 109(2):186–204.

Blazer DG. "Social support and mortality in an elderly community population." *Am J Epidemiol.* 1982;115(5):684–94.

Bloom JR, Spiegel D. "The relationship of two dimensions of social support to the psychological well-being and social functioning of women with advanced breast cancer." *Soc Sci Med.* 1984;19(8):831–37.

Blumenthal JA, Barefoot J, Burg MM, Williams RB Jr. "Psychological correlates of hostility among patients undergoing coronary angiography." *Br J Med Psychol.* 1987;60:349–55.

Cassel J. "The contribution of the social environment to host resistance: the Fourth Wade Hampton Frost Lecture." *Am J Epidemiol.* 1976;104(2):107–23.

Dembroski TM, MacDougall JM, Costa PT, et al. "Components of hostility as predictors of sudden death and myocardial infarction in the Multiple Risk Factor Intervention Trial." *Psychosom Med.* 1989;51:514–22.

Dimsdale JE, Ruberman W, Carleton RA. "Conference on behavioral medicine and cardiovascular disease: task force 1: sudden cardiac death: stress and cardiac arrhythmias." *Circulation.* Supplement 1. 1987;76(1):I198–I201.

Eliot, RS. "Conference on behavioral medicine and cardiovascular disease: coronary artery disease: biobehavioral factors: overview." *Circulation.* Supplement 1. 1987;76(1):I110–I111. American Heart Association Monograph 6.

Friedman M and Rosenman RH. *Type A Behavior and Your Heart.* New York: Fawcett, 1981.

Friedman M and Rosenman RH. *Treating Type A Behavior and Your Heart.* New York: Knopf, 1984.

Glaser R, Kiecolt-Glaser J. "Stress-associated depression in cellular immunity: implications for acquired immune deficiency syndrome (AIDS)." *Brain Behav Immun.* 1987;1(2):107–12.

Glaser R, Kiecolt-Glaser J. "Stress-associated immune suppression and acquired immune deficiency syndrome (AIDS)." *Adv Biochem Psychopharmacol.* 1988;44:203–15.

Goleman D. *Vital Lies, Simple Truths.* New York: Simon & Schuster, 1985.

Goodwin JS, Hunt WC, Key CR, Samet JM. "The effect of marital status on stage, treatment, and survival of cancer patients." *JAMA.* 1987;258(21):3125–30.

Graboys TB. "Stress and the aching heart." *N Engl J Med.* 1984;311:594–95.

Graham LE 2d., Scherwitz L, Brand R. "Self-reference and coronary heart disease incidence in the Western Collaborative Group Study." *Psychosom-Med.* 1989;51(2):137–44.

Henry JP. "The induction of acute and chronic cardiovascular disease in animals by psychosocial stimulation." *Int J Psychiatry Med.* 1975;6(1–2):147–58.

House JS, Landis KR, Umberson D. "Social relationships and health." *Science.* 1988;241(4865):540–45.

Iny LJ, Gianoulakis C, Palmour RM, Meaney MJ. "The beta-endorphin response to stress during postnatal development in the rat." *Brain Res.* 1987; 428(2):177–81.

Johnson JV, Hall EM. "Job strain, work place social support, and cardiovascular disease: a cross-sectional study of a random sample of the Swedish working population." *Am J Public Health.* 1988;78(10):1336–42.

Kaplan GA, Salonen JT, Cohen RD, Brand RJ, et al. "Social connections and mortality from all causes and from cardiovascular disease: prospective evidence from eastern Finland." *Am J Epidemiol.* 1988;128(2):370–80.

Kaplan GA. "Social contacts and ischaemic heart disease." *Ann Clin Res.* 1988;20(1–2),131–36.

Keefe DL, Schwartz J, Somberg J. "The substrate and the trigger: the role of myocardial vulnerability in sudden cardiac death." *American Heart Journal.* 1987; 113(1):218–25.

Kiecolt-Glaser J, Glaser R. "Major life changes, chronic stress, and immunity." *Adv Biochem Psychopharmacol.* 1988;44:217–24.

Krantz DS, DeQuattro V, Blackburn HW, et al. "Psychosocial factors in hypertension." *Circulation.* 1987;76(1 Pt 2):I84–88.

McAdams DP, Bryant FB. "Intimacy motivation and subjective mental health in a nationwide sample." *J Pers.* 1987;55(3):395–413.

Meaney MJ, Aitken DH, Bodnoff SR, et al. "Early postnatal handling alters glucocorticoid receptor concentrations in selected brain regions." *Behav Neurosci.* 1985;99(4):765–70.

Meaney MJ, Aitken DH, Bodnoff SR, et al. "The effects of postnatal handling on the development of the glucocorticoid receptor systems and stress recovery in the rat." *Prog Neuropsychopharmacol Biol Psychiatry.* 1985; 9(5–6). P 731–34.

Meaney MJ, Aitken DH, van Berkel C, et al. *Science.* 1988;239(4841 Pt 1):766–68.

Nerem RM, Levesque MJ, Cornhill JF. "Social environment as a factor in diet-induced atherosclerosis." *Science.* (1980;208(4451):1475–76.

Ornish DM. *Stress, Diet, & Your Heart.* New York: New American Library/ Signet Books, 1984.

Orth-Gomer K, Johnson JV. "Social network interaction and mortality. A six year follow-up study of a random sample of the Swedish population." *J Chronic Dis.* 1987;40(10):949–57.

Orth-Gomer K, Unden AL, Edwards ME. "Social isolation and mortality in ischemic heart disease. A 10-year follow-up study of 150 middle-aged men." *Acta Med Scand.* 1988;224(3):205–15.

Pennebaker JW, Kiecolt-Glaser JK, Glaser R. "Disclosure of traumas and immune function: health implications for psychotherapy." *J Consult Clin Psychol.* 1988;56(2):239–45.

Pennebaker JW, Susman JR. "Disclosure of traumas and psychosomatic processes." *Soc Sci Med.* 1988;26(3):327–32.

Reed D, McGee D, Yano K, Feinleib M. "Social networks and coronary heart disease among Japanese men in Hawaii." *Am J Epidemiol.* 1983;117(4):384–96.

Ruberman W, Weinblatt E, Goldberg J, et al. "Psychosocial influences on mortality after myocardial infarction." 1985 Year Book of Medicine. Article 29-14.

Ruberman W, Weinblatt E, Goldberg JD, Chaudhary BS. "Psychosocial influences on mortality after myocardial infarction." *N Engl J Med.* 1984;311(9):552–59.

Sacks FM, Ornish D, Rosner B, et al. "Plasma lipoprotein levels in vegetarians. The effect of ingestion of fats from dairy products." *JAMA.* 1985;254(10):1337–41.

Scherwitz L, Berton K, Leventhal H. "Type A behavior, self-involvement, and cardiovascular response." *Psychosom Med.* 1978;40(8):593–609.

Scherwitz L, Graham L E 2d, Grandits G, et al. "Self-involvement and coronary heart disease incidence in the multiple risk factor intervention trial." *Psychosom Med.* 1986;48(3–4):187–99.

Scherwitz L, Graham LE 2d, Grandits G, Billings J. "Speech characteristics and behavior-type assessment in the Multiple Risk Factor Intervention Trial (MRFIT) structured interviews." *J Behav Med.* 1987;10(2):173–95.

Scherwitz L, McKelvain R, Laman C, et al. "Type A behavior, self-involvement, and coronary atherosclerosis." *Psychosom Med.* 1983;45(1):47–57.

Seeman TE, Syme SL. "Social networks and coronary artery disease: a comparison of the structure and function of social relations as predictors of disease." *Psychosom Med.* 1987;49(4):341–54.

Sosa R, Kennell J, Klaus M, et al. "The effect of a supportive companion on perinatal problems, length of labor, and mother-infant interaction." *N Engl J Med.* 1980;303(11):597–600.

Spiegel D, et al. "Psychological support for cancer patients." *Lancet.* 1989;2(8677):1447.

Spiegel D, Bloom JR, Kraemer HC, Gottheil E. "Effect of psychosocial treatment on survival of patients with metastatic breast cancer." *Lancet.* 1989;2:8668, 888–90.

Spiegel D. "Modulation of gastric acid secretion by hypnosis." *Gastroenterology.* 1989;96(6), 1383–87.

Syme, SL. "Conference on behavioral medicine and cardiovascular disease: Coronary artery disease: a sociocultural perspective." *Circulation.* Supplement 1. 1987;76(1):I112–I116.

Syme SL. "Social determinants of disease." *Ann Clin Res.* 1987;19(2):44–52.

Thomas PD, Goodwin JM, Goodwin JS. "Effect of social support on stress-related changes in cholesterol level, uric acid level, and immune function in an elderly sample." *Am J Psychiatry.* 1985;142(6):735–37.

Waltz M. "Marital context and post-infarction quality of life: is it social support or something more?" *Soc Sci Med.* 1986;22(8):791–805.

West DA, Kellner R, Moore-West M. "The effects of loneliness: a review of the literature." *Compr Psychiatry.* 1986;27(4):351–63.

Wilber K. "Love story." *New Age Journal.* July/August 1989, p. 32.

Williams R. *The Trusting Heart.* New York: Times Books, 1989.

5. "THIS IS A WEED-OUT COURSE!"

Frankl VE. *Man's Search for Meaning.* New York: Washington Square Press, 1985.

Rodin J. "Aging and health: effects of the sense of control." *Science.* 1986; 233(4770):1271–6.

Rodin J, Timko C, Harris S. "The construct of control: biological and psychosocial correlates." *Ann Rev Gerontol Geriatr.* 1985;5:3–55.

Sharansky N. *Fear No Evil.* New York: Random House, 1989.

Simmons K. "Adolescent suicide: second leading death cause." *JAMA.* 1987; 257:3329–30.

Youth suicide: United States, 1970–80. *JAMA.* 1987;257:3333–34.

7. OPENING YOUR HEART TO YOUR FEELINGS AND TO INNER PEACE

Adelmann PK, Zajonc RB. "Facial efference and the experience of emotion." *Annu Rev Psychol.* 1989;40:249–80.

Assagioli R. *Psychosynthesis.* New York: Penguin, 1971.

Barbato J. *Mind-Body Fitness.* Mind Body Health Digest. 1989;3:1–6.

Benson H. *Beyond the Relaxation Response.* New York: Times Books, 1984.

Benson H. "Hypnosis and the relaxation response." *Gastroenterology.* 1989; 96(6):1609–11.

Benson H. "The relaxation response: history, physiological basis and clinical usefulness." *Acta Med Scand Suppl.* 1982;660:231–37.

Benson H. *Your Maximum Mind.* New York: Times Books, 1987.

Chesney MA, Agras WS, Benson H, et al. "Nonpharmacologic approaches to the treatment of hypertension." *Circulation.* 1987; 76(1 Pt 2): I104–109.

Ekman P, Levenson RW, Friesen WV. "Autonomic nervous system activity distinguishes among emotions." *Science.* 1983;221(4616):1208–10.

Falcone C, Sconocchia R, Guasti L, et al. "Dental pain threshold and angina pectoris in patients with coronary artery disease." *J Am Coll Cardiol.* 1988; 12(2):348–52.

Glaser R, Kiecolt-Glaser JK, Speicher CE, Holliday JE. "Stress, loneliness, and changes in herpesvirus latency." *J Behav Med.* 1985;8(3):249–60.

Glazier JJ, Chierchia S, Brown MJ, et al. "Importance of generalized defection perception of painful stimuli as a cause of silent myocardial ischemia in chronic stable angina pectoris." *Am J Cardiol.* 1986;58:667–72.

Jacob RG, Shapiro AP, Reeves RA, et al. "Relaxation therapy for hypertension." *Arch Intern Med.* 1986;146:2335–40.

Jacobson E. *You Must Relax!* New York: McGraw-Hill, 1976.

Jasnoski ML, Kugler J. "Relaxation, imagery, and neuroimmunomodulation." *Ann NY Acad Sci.* 1987;496:722–30.

Kiecolt-Glaser JK, Garner W, Speicher C, et al. "Psychosocial modifiers of immunocompetence in medical students." *Psychosom Med.* 1984;46(1):7–14.

Kiecolt-Glaser JK, Glaser R, Strain EC, et al. "Modulation of cellular immunity in medical students." *J Behav Med.* 1986;9(1):5–21.

Kutz I, Borysenko JZ, Benson H. "Meditation and psychotherapy: a rationale for the integration of dynamic psychotherapy, the relaxation response, and mindfulness meditation." *Am J Psychiatry.* 1985;142:1–7.

Langer EJ. *Mindfulness.* New York: Addison-Wesley Publishing Co., 1989.

Ornstein R and Sobel D. *The Healing Brain.* New York: Touchstone, 1987.

Oyle I. *The Healing Mind.* Berkeley: Celestial Arts, 1974.

Patel C, Marmot MG, Carruthers M, et al. "Trial of relaxation in reducing coronary risk: four year follow-up." *British Medical Journal.* 1985;290:1103–6.

Pelletier K. *Mind as Healer, Mind as Slayer.* New York: Dell, 1977.

Rama S, Ballentine R, Hymes A. *Science of Breath.* Honesdale, PA: The Himalayan Institute of Yoga Science and Philosophy, 1979.

Samuels M and Samuels N. *The Well Adult.* New York: Summit Books, 1988.

Satchidananda S. *Integral Yoga Hatha.* New York: Holt Rinehart & Winston, 1970.

Satchidananda S. *Integral Yoga: The Yoga Sutras of Patanjali.* Pomfret Center, CT: Integral Yoga Publications, 1978.

Welch R. *Raquel: The Raquel Welch Total Beauty and Fitness Program.* New York: Fawcett, 1986.

Zajonc RB. "Emotion and facial efference: a theory reclaimed." *Science.* 1985; 228(4695):15–21.

Zajonc RB, Murphy ST, Inglehart M. "Feeling and facial efference: implications of the vascular theory of emotion." *Psychol Rev.* 1989;96(3):395–416.

8. OPENING YOUR HEART TO OTHERS

Broyles W, Jr. *Brothers in Arms: A Journey from War to Peace.* New York: Avon Books, 1987.

Cumes-Rayner D, Price J. "Understanding hypertensive behaviour—I. Preference not to disclose." *J Psychosom Res.* 1989;33(1):63–74.

Harvard Medical School Mental Health Letter. 1989;5(7):1–4.

House JS, Robbins C, Metzner HL. "The association of social relationships and activities with mortality: prospective evidence from the Tecumseh Community Health Study." *Am J Epidemiol.* 1982;116(1):123–40.

Kabat-Zinn J. *Full Catastrophe Living: A Practical Guide to Mindfulness, Meditation, and Healing.* New York: Delacorte Press, 1990.

Keen S. *Faces of the Enemy: Reflections of the Hostile Imagination.* New York: Harper and Row, 1986.

Lynch JJ. *The Language of the Heart: The Body's Response to Human Dialogue.* New York: Basic Books, 1985.

Miller A. *For Your Own Good.* New York: Farrar, Straus, Giroux, 1983.

Miller A. *Prisoners of Childhood.* New York: Basic Books, 1981.

Miller A. *Thou Shalt Not Be Aware.* New York: Farrar, Straus, Giroux, 1984.

Percy W. *The Message in the Bottle.* New York: Farrar, Straus, Giroux, 1975.

Siegel B. *Peace, Love, and Healing.* New York: Harper & Row, 1989.

Tavris C. *Anger: The Misunderstood Emotion.* New York: Simon & Schuster, 1982.

Thomas L. *The Youngest Science.* New York: Bantam, 1984.

9. OPENING YOUR HEART TO A HIGHER SELF

Benson H, Lehmann JW, Malhotra MS, et al. "Body temperature changes during the practice of g Tum-mo yoga." *Nature.* 1982;295:234–36.

Borysenko J. *Goodbye to Guilt.* New York: Warner Books, 1990.

Borysenko J. *Minding the Body, Mending the Mind.* New York: Bantam Books, 1988.

Byrd RC. "Positive therapeutic effects of intercessory prayer in a coronary care unit population." *South Med J.* 1988;81(7):826–29.

Capra F. *The Tao of Physics.* Boston: Shambhala, 1983.

Chopra D. *Quantum Healing.* New York: Bantam Books, 1989.

Dossey L. *Beyond Illness: Discovering the Experience of Health.* Boston: Shambhala, 1985.

Dossey L. *Space, Time, and Medicine.* Boston: Shambhala, 1982.

Goleman D. *The Meditative Mind,* rev. ed. Los Angeles: Tarcher, 1988.

Hawking SM. *A Brief History of Time.* New York: Bantam, 1988.

Kuhn TS. *The Structure of Scientific Revolutions,* 2nd ed. Chicago: University of Chicago Press, 1970.

Locke S, et al. *Foundations of Psychoneuroimmunology.* Hawthorne, NY: Aldine de Gruyter, 1985.

Milton J. *Paradise Lost.* New York: New American Library, 1961.

Mitchell S. *Tao Te Ching: A New English Version.* New York: Harper and Row, 1989.

Needleman J. Interviewed by Stephen Bodian. *Yoga Journal.* Mar/Apr 1989, pp. 58–61.

Prabhavananda S and Isherwood C. *How to Know God: The Yoga Aphorisms of Patanjali.* Hollywood: Vedanta Society of Southern California, 1981.

Rossman ML. *Healing Yourself.* New York: Pocket Books, 1987.

Satchidananda S. *Beyond Words.* New York: Holt, Rinehart & Winston, 1977.

Satchidananda S. *The Golden Present.* Yogaville, VA: Integral Yoga Publications, 1987.

Satchidananda S. *To Know Your Self.* New York: Anchor Books/Doubleday, 1978.

Sivananda S. *Concentration and Meditation.* Himalayas: Divine Life Society, 1975.

Vivekananda S. *Jnana Yoga.* New York: Ramakrishna-Vivekananda Center, 1955.

Weil AT. *Natural Health, Natural Medicine.* Boston: Houghton Mifflin Company, 1990.

10. THE REVERSAL AND PREVENTION DIETS

Acheson K, Jequier E, Burger A, et al. "Thyroid hormones and thermogenesis: the metabolic cost of food and exercise." *Metabolism.* 1984;33(3):262–65.

Acheson KJ, Ravussin E, Schoeller DA, et al. "Two-week stimulation or blockade of the sympathetic nervous system in man: influence on body weight, body composition, and twenty-four-hour energy expenditure." *Metabolism.* 1988; 37(1):91–98.

American Dietetic Association. "Position of the American Dietetic Association: vegetarian diets—technical support paper." *ADA Reports.* 1988;88:352–55.

Anderson KM, Castelli WP, Levy D. "Cholesterol and mortality: 30 years of follow-up from the Framingham study." *JAMA.* 1987;257:2176–80.

Angier N. "Diet offers tantalizing clues to long life." *The New York Times,* April 17, 1990, page B5.

Blackburn GL, Wilson GT, Kanders BS, et al. "Weight cycling: the experience of human dieters." *Am J Clin Nutr.* 1989;49(5 Suppl):1105–9.

Breslau NA, Brinkley L, Hill KD, Pak CY. Relationship of animal protein–rich diet to kidney stone formation. *J Clin Endocrinal Metab.* 1988;66;140–46.

Brody J. "Huge study of diet indicts fat and meat." *The New York Times,*, May 8, 1990.

Brody J. *Jane Brody's Good Food Book.* New York: Bantam Books, 1987.

Brody J. *Jane Brody's Nutrition Book.* New York: Bantam Books, 1988.

Brownell KD. "Weight cycling." *Am J Clin Nutr.* 1989;49(5 Suppl):937.

Brownell KD, Greenwood MR, Stellar E, et al. "The effects of repeated cycles of weight loss and regain in rats." *Physiol Behav.* 1986;38(4):459–64.

Burr ML, Gilbert JF, Holliday RM, et al. "Effects of changes in fat, fish, and fibre intakes on death and myocardial infarction." *Lancet.* 1989;ii:757–61.

Burros M. *Twenty-Minute Menus.* New York: Simon & Schuster, 1989.

Chen J, Campbell TC, Li J, Peto R. *Diet, Lifestyle and Mortality in China: A Study of the Characteristics of 65 Chinese Countries.* Oxford: Oxford University Press (in press).

Chen J, Ohshima H, Yang H. "A correlation study on urinary excretion of N-nitroso compounds and cancer mortality in China: interim results." *IARC Sci Publ.* 1987;(84):503–6.

Connor SL and Connor WE. *The New American Diet.* New York: Fireside Books, 1986.

Dawber TR. *The Framingham Study: The Epidemiology of Atherosclerotic Disease.* Cambridge, Mass: Harvard University Press, 1980.

Department of Health and Human Services, Public Health Service. *The Surgeon General's Report on Nutrition and Health.* Washington, D.C.: Government Printing Office, 1988. (DHHS publication no. (PHS) 88-50210.)

Dreon DM, Frey-Hewitt B, Ellsworth N, et al. "Dietary fat:carbohydrate ratio and obesity in middle-aged men." *Am J Clin Nutr.* 1988;47(6):995–1000.

Dwyer JT. "Health aspects of vegetarian diets." *Am J Clin Nutr.* 1988;48(3 Suppl):712–38.

Fisher M, Leaf A. "n-3 fatty acids and cellular aspects of atherosclerosis." *Arch Intern Med.* 1989;149:1726–28.

Gear JS, Mann JI, Thorogood M, et al. "Biochemical and haematological variables in vegetarians." *Br Med J.* 1980;280(6229):1415.

Gill JS, Zezulka AZ, Shipley MJ, et al. "Stroke and alcohol consumption." *N Engl J Med.* 1986;315:1041–46.

Griffin GC and Castelli WP. *How to Lower Your Cholesterol and Beat the Odds of a Heart Attack.* Tucson: Fisher Books, 1989.

Haber GB, Heaton KW, Murphy D, Burroughs LF. "Depletion and disruption of dietary fibre. Effects on satiety, plasma-glucose, and serum-insulin." *Lancet.* 1977;2(8040):679–82.

Kinsella JE. "Effects of polyunsaturated fatty acids on factors related to cardiovascular disease." *Am J Cardiol.* 1987;60(12):23G–32G.

LaCroix AZ, Mead LA, Kung-Yee L, et al. "Coffee consumption and the incidence of coronary heart disease." *N Engl J Med.* 1986;315:977–82.

Leaf A, Weber PC. "Cardiovascular effects of n-3 fatty acids: an update." *N Engl J Med.* 1988;318:549–57.

Leaf A, Weber PC. "Cardiovascular effects of n-3 fatty acids: an update." *n-3 News.* 1988;3:1–4.

Marsh AG, Sanchez TV, Michelsen O, et al. Vegetarian lifestyle and bone mineral density. *Am J Clin Nutr.* 1988;48(3 Suppl):837–41.

Masoro EJ. "Biology of aging." *Arch Intern Med.* 1987;147:166–90.

Masoro EJ. "Overview of the effects of food restriction." *Prog Clin Biol.* 1989; 287:27–35.

Mueller BA, Talbert RL. "Biological mechanisms and cardiovascular effects of omega-3 fatty acids." *Clin Pharm.* 1988;7(11):795–807.

O'Connor TP, Roebuck BD, Peterson FJ, et al. "Effect of dietary omega-3 and omega-6 fatty acids on development of azaserine-induced preneoplastic lesions in rat pancreas." *J Natl Cancer Inst.* 1989;81(11):858–63.

Olney JW. "Dietary MSG and behavior [letter]." *Toxicol Appl Pharmacol.* 1980;53(1):177–78.

Peto R, Boreham J, Chen J, et al. "Plasma cholesterol, coronary heart disease, and cancer [letter]." *BMJ.* 1989;298(6682):1249.

Reif-Lehrer L. "A search for children with possible MSG Intolerance [letter]." *Pediatrics.* 1976;58(5):771–72.

Reif-Lehrer L. "Possible significance of adverse reactions to glutamate in humans." *Fed Proc.* 1976;35(11):2205–11.

Robbins J. *Diet for a New America.* Felton, CA: EarthSave, 1989.

Romieu I, Willett WC, Stampfer MJ, et al. "Energy intake and other determinants of relative weight." *Am J Clin Nutr.* 1988;47(3):406–12.

Sacks FM, Donner A, Castelli WP, et al. "Effect of ingestion of meat on plasma cholesterol of vegetarians." *JAMA.* 1981;246(6):640–44.

Sacks FM, Castelli WP, Donner A, Kass EH. "Plasma lipids and lipoproteins in vegetarians and controls." *N Engl J Med.* 1975;292(22):1148–51.

Sacks FM, Kass EH. "Low blood pressure in vegetarians: effects of specific foods and nutrients." *Am J Clin Nutr.* 1988;48(3 Suppl):795–800.

Schatzkin A, Jones DY, Hoover RN, et al. "Alcohol consumption and breast cancer in the epidemiologic follow-up study of the first national health and nutrition examination survey." *N Engl J Med.* 1987;316:1169–73.

Shekelle RB, Stamler J. "Dietary cholesterol and ischaemic heart disease." *Lancet.* 1989;1(8648):1177–79.

Stamler J, Wentworth D, Neaton JD. "Is relationship between serum cholesterol and risk of premature death from coronary heart disease continuous and graded? Findings in 356,222 primary screenees of the Multiple Risk Factor Intervention Trial (MRFIT)." *JAMA.* 1986;256(20):2823–28.

Stampfer MJ, Colditz GA, Willett WC, et al. "A prospective study of moderate alcohol consumption and the risk of coronary disease and stroke in women." *N Engl J Med.* 1988;319:267–73.

Steen SN, Oppliger RA, Brownell KD. "Metabolic effects of repeated weight loss and regain in adolescent wrestlers." *JAMA.* 1988;260(1):47–50.

Swain JF, Rouse IL, Curley CB, Sacks FM. "Comparison of the effects of oat bran and low fiber wheat on serum lipoprotein levels and blood pressure." *N Engl J Med.* 1990;322:147–52.

Thorogood M, Carter R, Benfield L, et al. "Plasma lipids and lipoprotein cholesterol concentrations in people with different diets in Britain." *Br Med J.* 1987;295(6594):351–53.

Tracy L. *The Gradual Vegetarian.* New York: M. Evans & Co., 1985.

Walford RL. "The extension of maximum life span." *Clin Geriatr Med.* 1985; 1:29–35.

Walford RL, Harris SB, Weindruch R. "Dietary restriction and aging." *J Nutrition.* 1987;117:1650–54.

Weiner MA. "Cholesterol in foods rich in omega-3 fatty acids." *N Engl J Med.* 1986;315:833.

Young E, Olney J, Akil H. "Increase in delta, but not mu, receptors in MSG-treated rats." *Life Sci.* 1982;31(12–13):1343–46.

Young E, Olney J, Akil H. "Selective alterations of opiate receptor subtypes in monosodium glutamate-treated rats." *J Neurochem.* 1983;40(6):1558–64.

11. HOW TO QUIT SMOKING

Benowitz NL. "Pharmacologic aspects of cigarette smoking and nicotine addiction." *N Engl J Med.* 1988;319:1318–30.

Colditz GA, Bonita R, Stampfer MJ, et al. "Cigarette smoking and risk of stroke in middle-aged women." *N Engl J Med.* 1988;318:937–41.

Elist J, Jarman WD, Edson M. "Evaluating medical treatment of impotence." *Urology.* 1984;23(4):374–5.

Ferguson T. *The No-Nag, No-Guilt, Do-It-Your-Own-Way Guide to Quitting Smoking.* New York: Ballantine Books, 1989.

Fielding J, Phenow KJ. "Health effects of involuntary smoking." *N Engl J Med.* 1988;319:1452–60.

Fielding JE. "Smoking: health effects and control." *N Engl J Med.* 1985;313: 491–96, 555–61.

Ornish SA. "Effects of transdermal clonidine treatment on withdrawal symptoms associated with smoking cessation." *Arch Intern Med.* 1988:148:2027–31.

Palmer JR, Rosenberg L, Shapiro S. " 'Low-yield' cigarettes and the risk of nonfatal myocardial infarction in women." *N Engl J Med.* 1989;320:1569–73.

Pomerleau OF, Pomerleau CS. "Neuroregulators and the reinforcement of smoking: towards a biobehavioral explanation." *Neurosci Biobehav Rev.* 1984;8(4):503–13.

Risner ME, Goldberg SR, Prada JA, et al. "Effects of nicotine, cocaine and some of their metabolites on schedule-controlled responding by beagle dogs and squirrel monkeys." *J Pharmacol Exp Ther.* 1985;234(1):113–19.

U.S. Dept. of Health and Human services. *Reducing the Health Consequences of Smoking: 25 Years of Progress. A Report of the Surgeon General.* U.S. Dept. of Health and Human Services, Public Health Service, Centers for Disease Control, Center for Chronic Disease Prevention and Health Promotion, Office on Smoking and Health. DHHS Publication # (CDC) 89-8411, 1989.

Willett WC, Green A, Stampfer MJ, et al. "Relative and absolute excess risks of coronary heart disease among women who smoke cigarettes." *N Engl J Med.* 1987;317:1303–9.

Wolf PA, D'Agostino RB, Kannel WB, et al. "Cigarette smoking as a risk factor for stroke." *JAMA.* 1988;259:1025–29.

12. HOW TO EXERCISE

American College of Sports Medicine. *Guidelines for Exercise Testing and Prescription.* Philadelphia: Lea & Febiger, 1986.

Blair SN, Kohl HW, Paffenbarger RS, et al. "Physical fitness and all-cause mortality." *JAMA.* 1989;262:2395–2401.

Borg GV. "The Borg Scale for rate of perceived exertion." *Med Sci Sports Exercise.* 1982 14:377–87.

Dupac Daily Dozen Plus the Basic Six. Carola Ekeluud, Duke University, Durham North Carolina, 1984.

Kramsch DM, Aspen AJ, Abramowitz BM, et al. "Reduction of coronary atherosclerosis by moderate conditioning exercise in monkeys on an atherogenic diet." *N Engl J Med.* 1981;305:1483–89.

Leon AS, Connett J, Jacobs DR, et al. "Leisure-time physical activity levels and risk of coronary heart disease and death. The multiple risk factor intervention trial." *JAMA.* 1987;258:2388–95.

Lupica M. "A brother's keeper." *Esquire.* March 1989, pp. 77–80.

Moderate exercise slows CAD. *Medical World News.* August 10, 1987, p. 26–7.

Paffenbarger RS, Hyde RT, Wing AL, et al. "Physical activity, all-cause mortality, and longevity of college alumni." *N Engl J Med.* 1986;314:605–13.

Rippe JM, Ward A, Porcari HP, and Freedson PS. "Walking for health and fitness." *JAMA.* 1988;259:2720–24.

Sadaniantz A, Thompson PD. "Sudden death during exercise." *Cardiov Rev and Reports.* 1985;6:1314–15.

Thompson PD. "The benefits and risks of exercise training in patients with chronic coronary artery disease." *JAMA.* 1988;259:1537–40.

Thompson PD, Funk EJ, Carleton RA, et al. "The incidence of death during jogging in Rhode Island joggers from 1975 through 1980." *JAMA.* 1982;247:2535–48.

U.S. Dept. of Health and Human Services. *Reducing the Health Consequences of Smoking: 25 Years of Progress. A Report of the Surgeon General.* U.S. Dept. of Health and Human Services, Public Health Service, Centers for Disease Control, Center for Chronic Disease Prevention and Health Promotion, Office on Smoking and Health. DHHS Publication # (CDC) 89-8411, 1989.

Permissions Acknowledgments

Subject Index

Recipe Index

ABOUT THE AUTHOR

DEAN ORNISH, M.D., is assistant clinical professor of medicine and an attending physician at the School of Medicine, University of California, San Francisco, and an attending physician at the Pacific Presbyterian Medical Center in San Francisco. He is president and director of the Preventive Medicine Research Institute in Sausalito. A graduate of Baylor College of Medicine, Dr. Ornish was a clinical fellow in medicine at Harvard Medical School and an intern and medical resident at Massachusetts General Hospital. He is the author of *Stress, Diet & Your Heart.*